WORLD HEALTH ORGANIZATION

INTERNATIONAL AGENCY FOR RESEARCH ON CANCER

IARC MONOGRAPHS

ON THE

EVALUATION OF THE CARCINOGENIC RISK OF CHEMICALS TO HUMANS

Some Chemicals Used in Plastics and Elastomers

VOLUME 39

This publication represents the views and expert opinions
of an IARC Working Group on the
Evaluation of the Carcinogenic Risk of Chemicals to Humans
which met in Lyon,

11-18 June, 1985

IARC MONOGRAPHS

In 1969, the International Agency for Research on Cancer (IARC) initiated a programme on the evaluation of the carcinogenic risk of chemicals to humans involving the production of critically evaluated monographs on individual chemicals. In 1980, the programme was expanded to include the evaluation of the carcinogenic risk associated with exposures to complex mixtures.

The objective of the programme is to elaborate and publish in the form of monographs critical reviews of data on carcinogenicity for chemicals and complex mixtures to which humans are known to be exposed, and on specific occupational exposures, to evaluate these data in terms of human risk with the help of international working groups of experts in chemical carcinogenesis and related fields, and to indicate where additional research efforts are needed.

This project was supported by PHS Grant No. 1 UO1 CA33193-03 awarded by the US National Cancer Institute, Department of Health and Human Services.

Distributed for the International Agency for Research on Cancer by the Secretariat of the World Health Organization

PRINTED IN SWITZERLAND

CONTENTS

NOTE TO THE READER

The term 'carcinogenic risk' in the *IARC Monographs* series is taken to mean the probability that exposure to the chemical will lead to cancer in humans.

Inclusion of a chemical in the *Monographs* does not imply that it is a carcinogen, only that the published data have been examined. Equally, the fact that a chemical has not yet been evaluated in a monograph does not mean that it is not carcinogenic.

Anyone who is aware of published data that may alter the evaluation of the carcinogenic risk of a chemical to humans is encouraged to make this information available to the Unit of Carcinogen Identification and Evaluation, Division of Environmental Carcinogenesis, International Agency for Research on Cancer, 150 cours Albert Thomas, 69372 Lyon Cedex 08, France, in order that the chemical may be considered for re-evaluation by a future Working Group.

Although every effort is made to prepare the monographs as accurately as possible, mistakes may occur. Readers are requested to communicate any errors to the Unit of Carcinogen Identification and Evaluation, so that corrections can be reported in future volumes.

IARC WORKING GROUP ON THE EVALUATION OF THE CARCINOGENIC RISK OF CHEMICALS TO HUMANS: SOME CHEMICALS USED IN PLASTICS AND ELASTOMERS

Lyon, 11-18 June 1985

Members

P.A. Bertazzi, Istituto di Medicina del Lavoro, Clinica del Lavoro 'Luigi Devoto', University of Milan, via S. Barnaba 8, 20122 Milan, Italy

M. Bignami, Istituto Superiore di Sanita, viale Regina Elena 299, 00161 Rome, Italy

H.M. Bolt, Institut für Arbeitsphysiologie an der Universität Dortmund, Ardeystrasse 67, 4600 Dortmund 1, Federal Republic of Germany

I.N. Chernozemsky, Head, Laboratory of Chemical Carcinogenesis and Testing, Institute of Oncology, Medical Academy, Sofia 1156, Bulgaria

J. Fajen, National Institute for Occupational Safety and Health, Robert A. Taft Laboratories, 4676 Columbia Parkway, Cincinnati, OH 45226, USA

E. Farber, Department of Pathology, Medical Sciences Building, Room 6217, 1 King's College Circle, University of Toronto, Toronto, Ontario M5S 1A8, Canada (*Chairman*)

R. Frentzel-Beyme, Institut für Dokumentation, Information und Statistik, Deutsches Krebsforschungszentrum, Im Neuenheimer Feld 280, 6900 Heidelberg 1, Federal Republic of Germany

B. Hardin, National Institute for Occupational Safety and Health, Robert A. Taft Laboratories, 4676 Columbia Parkway, Cincinnati, OH 45226, USA

P.Th. Henderson, Toxicology Department, Faculty of Medicine, University of Nijmegen, PO Box 9101, 6500 HB Nijmegen, The Netherlands

S. Hernberg, Scientific Director, Institute of Occupational Health, Haartmaninkatu 1, 00290 Helsinki 29, Finland

K. Hooper, Department of Health Services/Department of Industrial Relations, Hazard Evaluation System and Information Service (HESIS), 2151 Berkeley Way, Berkeley, CA 94704, USA

M.S. Legator, Department of Preventive Medicine and Community Health, Division of Environmental Toxicology, University of Texas Medical Branch, Galveston, TX 77550, USA

L.S. Levy, Institute of Occupational Health, The University of Birmingham, University Road West, PO Box 363, Birmingham B15 2TT, UK

T. Matsushima, Department of Molecular Oncology, Institute of Medical Science, University of Tokyo, 4-6-1 Shirokanedai, Minato-ku, Tokyo 108, Japan

E.E. McConnell, National Toxicology Program, National Institute of Environmental Health Sciences, PO Box 12233, Research Triangle Park, NC 27709, USA

J.M. Peters, Department of Preventive Medicine, Division of Occupational Health, University of Southern California School of Medicine, 2025 Zonal Avenue, Los Angeles, CA 90033, USA

M. Roberfroid, Unité de Biochimie toxicologique et cancérologique, Faculté de Médecine, Ecole de Pharmacie, Université Catholique de Louvain, UCL 7369, 73 avenue E. Mounier, 1200 Brussels, Belgium

B.W. Stewart, Principal Research Fellow, Children's Leukaemia and Cancer Research Unit, The Prince of Wales Children's Hospital, High Street, Randwick, NSW 2031, Australia

S. Venitt, Institute of Cancer Research, F Block, Clifton Avenue, Sutton, Surrey SM2 5PX, UK

M.D. Waters, Director, Genetic Toxicology Division (MD-68), Health Effects Research Laboratory, US Environmental Protection Agency, Research Triangle Park, NC 27711, USA

Representative of the National Cancer Institute

S.M. Sieber, Deputy Director, Division of Cancer Etiology, National Cancer Institute, Building 31, Room 11A03, Bethesda, MD 20205, USA

Representative of Tracor Jitco Inc.

S. Olin, Tracor Jitco, Inc., 1601 Research Boulevard, Rockville, MD 20850, USA

Observers

Representative of the Chemical Industry Ecology and Toxicology Centre

E. Longstaff, Central Toxicology Laboratory, ICI, Alderley Park, Macclesfield, Cheshire SK10 4TJ, UK

Representative of the Chemical Manufacturers' Association

J.M. Norris, The Dow Chemical Company, 1803 Building, Midland, MI 48640, USA

Representative of the International Programme on Chemical Safety

E. Smith, International Programme on Chemical Safety, World Health Organization, 1211 Geneva 27, Switzerland

Representative of the Organization for Economic Cooperation and Development

S. Furukawa, Chemicals Division, Environment Directorate, 2 rue André Pascal, 75775 Paris Cedex 16, France

Representative of Roussel UCLAF

P. Rajot, Directeur Environnement, Sécurité, Sûreté, Roussel UCLAF, Tour Roussel Nobel, 3 avenue du Général de Gaulle, 92800 Puteaux, France

Secretariat

H. Bartsch, Division of Environmental Carcinogenesis

J.R.P. Cabral, Division of Environmental Carcinogenesis

M. Friesen, Division of Environmental Carcinogenesis

L. Haroun, Division of Environmental Carcinogenesis (*Secretary*)

E. Heseltine, Editorial and Publications Services

J. Kaldor, Division of Epidemiology and Biostatistics

D. Mietton, Division of Environmental Carcinogenesis

I. O'Neill, Division of Environmental Carcinogenesis

C. Partensky, Division of Environmental Carcinogenesis

S. Poole, Birmingham, UK

R. Saracci, Division of Epidemiology and Biostatistics

L. Tomatis, Director

H. Vainio, Division of Environmental Carcinogenesis (*Head of the Programme*)

J. Wahrendorf, Division of Epidemiology and Biostatistics

J. Wilbourn, Division of Environmental Carcinogenesis

H. Yamasaki, Division of Environmental Carcinogenesis

Secretarial assistance

J. Cazeaux

M.-J. Ghess

M. Lézère

S. Reynaud

K. Zouhair

PREAMBLE

IARC MONOGRAPHS PROGRAMME ON THE EVALUATION OF THE CARCINOGENIC RISK OF CHEMICALS TO HUMANS[1]

PREAMBLE ·

1. BACKGROUND

In 1969, the International Agency for Research on Cancer (IARC) initiated a programme to evaluate the carcinogenic risk of chemicals to humans and to produce monographs on individual chemicals. Following the recommendations of an ad-hoc Working Group, which met in Lyon in 1979 to prepare criteria to select chemicals for *IARC Monographs*(1), the *Monographs* programme was expanded to include consideration of exposures to complex mixtures which may occur, for example, in many occupations or as a result of human habits.

The criteria established in 1971 to evaluate carcinogenic risk to humans were adopted by all the working groups whose deliberations resulted in the first 16 volumes of the *IARC Monographs* series. This preamble reflects subsequent re-evaluation of those criteria by working groups which met in 1977(2), 1978(3), 1982(4) and 1983(5).

2. OBJECTIVE AND SCOPE

The objective of the programme is to elaborate and publish in the form of monographs critical reviews of data on carcinogenicity for chemicals, groups of chemicals, industrial processes and other complex mixtures to which humans are known to be exposed, to evaluate the data in terms of human risk with the help of international working groups of experts, and to indicate where additional research efforts are needed. These evaluations are intended to assist national and international authorities in formulating decisions concerning preventive measures. No recommendation is given concerning legislation, since this depends on risk-benefit evaluations, which seem best made by individual governments and/or other international agencies.

---

[1]This project is supported by PHS Grant No. 1 U01 CA33193-03 awarded by the US National Cancer Institute, Department of Health and Human Services.

The *IARC Monographs* are recognized as an authoritative source of information on the carcinogenicity of environmental and other chemicals. A users' survey, made in 1984, indicated that the monographs are consulted by various agencies in 45 countries. As of April 1986, 39 volumes of the *Monographs* had been published or were in press. Five supplements have been published: two summaries of evaluations of chemicals associated with human cancer, an evaluation of screening assays for carcinogens, and two cross indexes of synonyms and trade names of chemicals evaluated in the series(6).

3. SELECTION OF CHEMICALS AND COMPLEX EXPOSURES FOR MONOGRAPHS

The chemicals (natural and synthetic including those which occur as mixtures and in manufacturing processes) and complex exposures are selected for evaluation on the basis of two main criteria: (a) there is evidence of human exposure, and (b) there is some experimental evidence of carcinogenicity and/or there is some evidence or suspicion of a risk to humans. In certain instances, chemical analogues are also considered. The scientific literature is surveyed for published data relevant to the *Monographs* programme; and the IARC *Survey of Chemicals Being Tested for Carcinogenicity*(7) often indicates those chemicals that may be scheduled for future meetings.

As new data on chemicals for which monographs have already been prepared become available, re-evaluations are made at subsequent meetings, and revised monographs are published.

4. WORKING PROCEDURES

Approximately one year in advance of a meeting of a working group, a list of the substances or complex exposures to be considered is prepared by IARC staff in consultation with other experts. Subsequently, all relevant biological data are collected by IARC; recognized sources of information on chemical carcinogenesis and on-line systems such as CANCERLINE, MEDLINE and TOXLINE are used in conjunction with US Public Health Service Publication No. 149(8). Bibliographical sources for data on mutagenicity and teratogenicity are the Environmental Mutagen Information Center and the Environmental Teratology Information Center, both located at the Oak Ridge National Laboratory, TN, USA.

The major collection of data and the preparation of first drafts for the sections on chemical and physical properties, on production and use, on occurrence, and on analysis are carried out by Tracor Jitco, Inc., and its subcontractor, Technical Resources, Inc., both in Rockville, MD, USA, under a separate contract with the US National Cancer Institute. Most of the data so obtained refer to the USA and Japan; IARC attempts to supplement this information with that from other sources in Europe. Representatives from industrial associations may assist in the preparation of sections describing industrial processes.

Six months before the meeting, articles containing relevant biological data are sent to an expert(s), or are used by IARC staff, to prepare first drafts of the sections on biological effects. The complete drafts are then compiled by IARC staff and sent, prior to the meeting, to all participants of the Working Group for their comments.

The Working Group meets in Lyon for seven to eight days to discuss and finalize the texts of the monographs and to formulate the evaluations. After the meeting, the master copy of each monograph is verified by consulting the original literature, edited by a professional editor and prepared for reproduction. The aim is to publish monographs within nine months of the Working Group meeting. Each volume of monographs is printed in 4000 copies for distribution to governments, regulatory agencies and interested scientists. The monographs are also available *via* the WHO Distribution and Sales Service.

These procedures are followed for the preparation of most volumes of monographs, which cover chemicals and groups of chemicals; however, they may vary when the subject matter is an industry or life-style factor.

5. DATA FOR EVALUATIONS

With regard to biological data, only reports that have been published or accepted for publication are reviewed by the working groups, although a few exceptions have been made: in certain instances, reports from government agencies that have undergone peer review and are widely available are considered. The monographs do not cite all of the literature on a particular chemical or complex exposure: only those data considered by the Working Group to be relevant to the evaluation of carcinogenic risk to humans are included.

Anyone who is aware of data that have been published or are in press which are relevant to the evaluations of the carcinogenic risk to humans of chemicals or complex exposures for which monographs have appeared is asked to make them available to the Unit of Carcinogen Identification and Evaluation, Division of Environmental Carcinogenesis, International Agency for Research on Cancer, Lyon, France.

6. THE WORKING GROUP

The tasks of the Working Group are five-fold: (a) to ascertain that all data have been collected; (b) to select the data relevant for evaluation; (c) to ensure that the summaries of the data enable the reader to follow the reasoning of the Working Group; (d) to judge the significance of the results of experimental and epidemiological studies; and (e) to make an evaluation of the carcinogenicity of the chemical or complex exposure.

Working Group participants who contributed to the consideration and evaluation of chemicals or complex exposures within a particular volume are listed, with their addresses, at the beginning of each publication. Each member serves as an individual scientist and not as a representative of any organization or government. In addition, observers are often invited from national and international agencies and industrial associations.

7. GENERAL PRINCIPLES APPLIED BY THE WORKING GROUP IN EVALUATING CARCINOGENIC RISK OF CHEMICALS OR COMPLEX MIXTURES

The widely accepted meaning of the term 'chemical carcinogenesis', and that used in these monographs, is the induction by chemicals (or complex mixtures of chemicals) of neoplasms that are not usually observed, the earlier induction of neoplasms that are commonly observed, and/or the induction of more neoplasms than are usually found —although fundamentally different mechanisms may be involved in these three situations. Etymologically, the term 'carcinogenesis' means the induction of cancer, that is, of malignant neoplasms; however, the commonly accepted meaning is the induction of various types of neoplasms or of a combination of malignant and benign tumours. In the monographs, the words 'tumour' and 'neoplasm' are used interchangeably. (In the scientific literature, the terms 'tumorigen', 'oncogen' and 'blastomogen' have all been used synonymously with 'carcinogen', although occasionally 'tumorigen' has been used specifically to denote a substance that induces benign tumours.)

(a) Experimental Evidence

(i) *Evidence for carcinogenicity in experimental animals*

The Working Group considers various aspects of the experimental evidence reported in the literature and formulates an evaluation of that evidence.

Qualitative aspects: Both the interpretation and evaluation of a particular study as well as the overall assessment of the carcinogenic activity of a chemical (or complex mixture) involve several considerations of qualitative importance, including: (a) the experimental parameters under which the chemical was tested, including route of administration and exposure, species, strain, sex, age, etc.; (b) the consistency with which the chemical has been shown to be carcinogenic, e.g., in how many species and at which target organ(s); (c) the spectrum of neoplastic response, from benign neoplasm to multiple malignant tumours; (d) the stage of tumour formation in which a chemical may be involved: some chemicals act as complete carcinogens and have initiating and promoting activity, while others may have promoting activity only; and (e) the possible role of modifying factors.

There are problems not only of differential survival but of differential toxicity, which may be manifested by unequal growth and weight gain in treated and control animals. These complexities are also considered in the interpretation of data.

Many chemicals induce both benign and malignant tumours. Among chemicals that have been studied extensively, there are few instances in which the only neoplasms induced are benign. Benign tumours may represent a stage in the evolution of a malignant neoplasm or they may be 'end-points' that do not readily undergo transition to malignancy. If a substance is found to induce only benign tumours in experimental animals, it should nevertheless be suspected of being a carcinogen, and it requires further investigation.

Hormonal carcinogenesis: Hormonal carcinogenesis presents certain distinctive features: the chemicals involved occur both endogenously and exogenously; in many instances, long exposure is required; and tumours occur in the target tissue in association with a stimulation of non-neoplastic growth, although in some cases hormones promote the proliferation of tumour cells in a target organ. For hormones that occur in excessive amounts, for hormone-mimetic agents and for agents that cause hyperactivity or imbalance in the endocrine system, evaluative methods comparable with those used to identify chemical carcinogens may be required; particular emphasis must be laid on quantitative aspects and duration of exposure. Some chemical carcinogens have significant side effects on the endocrine system, which may also result in hormonal carcinogenesis. Synthetic hormones and anti-hormones can be expected to possess other pharmacological and toxicological actions in addition to those on the endocrine system, and in this respect they must be treated like any other chemical with regard to intrinsic carcinogenic potential.

Complex mixtures: There is an increasing amount of data from long-term carcino-genicity studies on complex mixtures and on crude materials obtained by sampling in occupational environments. The representativity of such samples must be considered carefully.

Quantitative aspects: Dose-response studies are important in the evaluation of carcinogenesis: the confidence with which a carcinogenic effect can be established is strengthened by the observation of an increasing incidence of neoplasms with increasing exposure.

The assessment of carcinogenicity in animals is frequently complicated by recognized differences among the test animals (species, strain, sex, age) and route and schedule of administration; often, the target organs at which a cancer occurs and its histological type may vary with these parameters. Nevertheless, indices of carcinogenic potency in particular experimental systems (for instance, the dose-rate required under continuous exposure to halve the probability of the animals remaining tumourless[9]) have been formulated in the hope that, at least among categories of fairly similar agents, such indices may be of some predictive value in other species, including humans.

Chemical carcinogens share many common biological properties, which include metabolism to reactive (electrophilic[10-11]) intermediates capable of interacting with DNA. However, they may differ widely in the dose required to produce a given level of tumour induction. The reason for this variation in dose-response is not understood, but it may be due to differences in metabolic activation and detoxification processes, in different DNA repair capacities among various organs and species or to the operation of qualitatively distinct mechanisms.

Statistical analysis of animal studies: It is possible that an animal may die prematurely from unrelated causes, so that tumours that would have arisen had the animal lived longer may not be observed; this possibility must be allowed for. Various analytical techniques have been developed which use the assumption of independence of competing risks to allow for the effects of intercurrent mortality on the final numbers of tumour-bearing animals in particular treatment groups.

For externally visible tumours and for neoplasms that cause death, methods such as Kaplan-Meier (i.e., 'life-table', 'product-limit' or 'actuarial') estimates[9], with associated significance tests[12], have been recommended. For internal neoplasms that are discovered 'incidentally'[12] at autopsy but that did not cause the death of the host, different estimates[13] and significance tests[12] may be necessary for the unbiased study of the numbers of tumour-bearing animals.

The design and statistical analysis of long-term carcinogenicity experiments were reviewed in Supplement 2 to the *Monographs* series[14]. That review outlined the way in which the context of observation of a given tumour (fatal or incidental) could be included in an analysis yielding a single combined result. This method requires information on time to death for each animal and is therefore comparable to only a limited extent with analyses which include global proportions of tumour-bearing animals.

Evaluation of carcinogenicity studies in experimental animals: The evidence of carcinogenicity in experimental animals is assessed by the Working Group and judged to fall into one of four groups, defined as follows:

(1) *Sufficient evidence* of carcinogenicity is provided when there is an increased incidence of malignant tumours: (a) in multiple species or strains; or (b) in multiple experiments (preferably with different routes of administration or using different dose levels); or (c) to an unusual degree with regard to incidence, site or type of tumour, or age at onset. Additional evidence may be provided by data on dose-response effects.

(2) *Limited evidence* of carcinogenicity is available when the data suggest a carcinogenic effect but are limited because: (a) the studies involve a single species, strain or experiment; or (b) the experiments are restricted by inadequate dosage levels, inadequate duration of exposure to the agent, inadequate period of follow-up, poor survival, too few animals, or inadequate reporting; or (c) the neoplasms produced often occur spontaneously and, in the past, have been difficult to classify as malignant by histological criteria alone (e.g., lung adenomas and adenocarcinomas and liver tumours in certain strains of mice).

(3) *Inadequate evidence* of carcinogenicity is available when, because of major qualitative or quantitative limitations, the studies cannot be interpreted as showing either the presence or absence of a carcinogenic effect.

(4) *No evidence* of carcinogenicity applies when several adequate studies are available which show that, within the limits of the tests used, the chemical or complex mixture is not carcinogenic.

It should be noted that the categories *sufficient evidence* and *limited evidence* refer only to the strength of the experimental evidence that these chemicals or complex mixtures are carcinogenic and not to the extent of their carcinogenic activity nor to the mechanism involved. The classification of any chemical may change as new information becomes available.

(ii)   *Evidence for activity in short-term tests*[1]

Many short-term tests bearing on postulated mechanisms of carcinogenesis or on the properties of known carcinogens have been developed in recent years. The induction of cancer is thought to proceed by a series of steps, some of which have been distinguished experimentally (15-19). The first step — initiation — is thought to involve damage to DNA, resulting in heritable alterations in or rearrangements of genetic information. Most short-term tests in common use today are designed to evaluate the genetic activity of a substance.

[1]Based on the recommendations of a working group which met in 1983(5).

Data from these assays are useful for identifying potential carcinogenic hazards, in identifying active metabolites of known carcinogens in human or animal body fluids, and in helping to elucidate mechanisms of carcinogenesis. Short-term tests to detect agents with tumour-promoting activity are, at this time, insufficiently developed.

Because of the large number of short-term tests, it is difficult to establish rigid criteria for adequacy that would be applicable to all studies. General considerations relevant to all tests, however, include (a) that the test system be valid with respect to known animal carcinogens and noncarcinogens; (b) that the experimental parameters under which the chemical (or complex mixture) is tested include a sufficiently wide dose range and duration of exposure to the agent and an appropriate metabolic system; (c) that appropriate controls be used; and (d) that the purity of the compound or, in the case of complex mixtures, that the source and representativity of the sample being tested be specified. Confidence in positive results is increased if a dose-response relationship is demonstrated and if this effect has been reported in two or more independent studies.

Most established short-term tests employ as end-points well-defined genetic markers in prokaryotes and lower eukaryotes and in mammalian cell lines. The tests can be grouped according to the end-point detected:

Tests of *DNA damage*. These include tests for covalent binding to DNA, induction of DNA breakage or repair, induction of prophage in bacteria and differential survival of DNA repair-proficient/-deficient strains of bacteria.

Tests of *mutation* (measurement of heritable alterations in phenotype and/or genotype). These include tests for detection of the loss or alteration of a gene product, and change of function through forward or reverse mutation, recombination and gene conversion; they may involve the nuclear genome, the mitochondrial genome and resident viral or plasmid genomes.

Tests of *chromosomal effects*. These include tests for detection of changes in chromosome number (aneuploidy), structural chromosomal aberrations, sister chromatid exchanges, micronuclei and dominant-lethal events. This classification does not imply that some chromosomal effects are not mutational events.

Tests for *cell transformation*, which monitor the production of preneoplastic or neoplastic cells in culture, are also of importance because they attempt to simulate essential steps in cellular carcinogenesis. These assays are not grouped with those listed above since the mechanisms by which chemicals induce cell transformation may not necessarily be the result of genetic change.

The selection of specific tests and end-points for consideration remains flexible and should reflect the most advanced state of knowledge in this field.

The data from short-term tests are summarized by the Working Group and the test results tabulated according to the end-points detected and the biological complexities of the test systems. The format of the table used is shown below. In these tables, a '+' indicates that the compound was judged by the Working Group to be significantly positive in one or more assays for the specific end-point and level of biological complexity; '-' indicates that it was judged to be negative in one or more assays; and '?' indicates that there were contradictory results from different laboratories or in different biological systems, or that the result was judged to be equivocal. These judgements reflect the assessment by the Working Group of the quality of the data (including such factors as the purity of the test compound, problems of metabolic activation and appropriateness of the test system) and the relative significance of the component tests.

Overall assessment of data from short-term tests

	Genetic activity			Cell transformation
	DNA damage	Mutation	Chromosomal effects	
Prokaryotes				
Fungi/ Green plants				
Insects				
Mammalian cells (*in vitro*)				
Mammals (*in vivo*)				
Humans (*in vivo*)				

An overall assessment of the evidence for *genetic activity* is then made on the basis of the entries in the table, and the evidence is judged to fall into one of four categories, defined as follows:

(1) *Sufficient evidence* is provided by at least three positive entries, one of which must involve mammalian cells *in vitro* or *in vivo* and which must include at least two of three end-points — DNA damage, mutation and chromosomal effects.

(2) *Limited evidence* is provided by at least two positive entries.

(3) *Inadequate evidence* is available when there is only one positive entry or when there are too few data to permit an evaluation of an absence of genetic activity or when there are unexplained, inconsistent findings in different test systems.

(4) *No evidence* applies when there are only negative entries; these must include entries for at least two end-points and two levels of biological complexity, one of which must involve mammalian cells *in vitro* or *in vivo*.

It is emphasized that the above definitions are operational, and that the assignment of a chemical or complex mixture into one of these categories is thus arbitrary.

In general, emphasis is placed on positive results; however, in view of the limitations of current knowledge about mechanisms of carcinogenesis, certain cautions should be respected: (i) At present, short-term tests should not be used by themselves to conclude whether or not an agent is carcinogenic nor can they predict reliably the relative potencies of compounds as carcinogens in intact animals. (ii) Since the currently available tests do not detect all classes of agents that are active in the carcinogenic process (e.g., hormones), one must be cautious in utilizing these tests as the sole criterion for setting priorities in carcinogenesis research and in selecting compounds for animal bioassays. (iii) Negative results from short-term tests cannot be considered as evidence to rule out carcinogenicity, nor does lack of demonstrable genetic activity attribute an epigenetic or any other property to a substance (5).

(b) Evaluation of Carcinogenicity in Humans

Evidence of carcinogenicity can be derived from case reports, descriptive epidemiological studies and analytical epidemiological studies.

An analytical study that shows a positive association between an exposure and a cancer may be interpreted as implying causality to a greater or lesser extent, on the basis of the following criteria: (a) There is no identifiable positive bias. (By 'positive bias' is meant the operation of factors in study design or execution that lead erroneously to a more strongly positive association between an exposure and disease than in fact exists. Examples of positive bias include, in case-control studies, better documentation of the exposure for cases than for controls, and, in cohort studies, the use of better means of detecting cancer in exposed individuals than in individuals not exposed.) (b) The possibility of positive confounding has been considered. (By 'positive confounding' is meant a situation in which the relationship between an exposure and a disease is rendered more strongly positive than it truly is as a result of an association between that exposure and another exposure which either causes or prevents the disease. An example of positive confounding is the association between coffee consumption and lung cancer, which results from their joint association with cigarette smoking.) (c) The association is unlikely to be due to chance alone. (d) The association is strong. (e) There is a dose-response relationship.

In some instances, a single epidemiological study may be strongly indicative of a cause-effect relationship; however, the most convincing evidence of causality comes when several independent studies done under different circumstances result in 'positive' findings.

Analytical epidemiological studies that show no association between an exposure and a cancer ('negative' studies) should be interpreted according to criteria analogous to those listed above: (a) there is no identifiable negative bias; (b) the possibility of negative confounding has been considered; and (c) the possible effects of misclassification of exposure or outcome have been weighed. In addition, it must be recognized that the probability that a given study can detect a certain effect is limited by its size. This can be perceived from the confidence limits around the estimate of association or relative risk. In a study regarded as 'negative', the upper confidence limit may indicate a relative risk substantially greater than unity; in that case, the study excludes only relative risks that are above the upper limit. This usually means that a 'negative' study must be large to be convincing. Confidence in a 'negative' result is increased when several independent studies carried out under different circumstances are in agreement. Finally, a 'negative' study may be considered to be relevant only to dose levels within or below the range of those observed in the study and is pertinent only if sufficient time has elapsed since first human exposure to the agent. Experience with human cancers of known etiology suggests that the period from first exposure to a chemical carcinogen to development of clinically observed cancer is usually measured in decades and may be in excess of 30 years.

The evidence for carcinogenicity from studies in humans is assessed by the Working Group and judged to fall into one of four groups, defined as follows:

(1) *Sufficient evidence* of carcinogenicity indicates that there is a causal relationship between the exposure and human cancer.

(2) *Limited evidence* of carcinogenicity indicates that a causal interpretation is credible, but that alternative explanations, such as chance, bias or confounding, could not adequately be excluded.

(3) *Inadequate evidence* of carcinogenicity, which applies to both positive and negative evidence, indicates that one of two conditions prevailed: (a) there are few pertinent data; or (b) the available studies, while showing evidence of association, do not exclude chance, bias or confounding.

(4) *No evidence* of carcinogenicity applies when several adequate studies are available which do not show evidence of carcinogenicity.

(c) Relevance of Experimental Data to the Evaluation of Carcinogenic Risk to Humans

Information compiled from the first 38 volumes of the *IARC Monographs* shows that, of the chemicals or groups of chemicals now generally accepted to cause or probably to cause cancer in humans, all of those that have been tested appropriately produce cancer in at least one animal species. For several of the chemicals (e.g., aflatoxins, 4-aminobiphenyl, diethylstilboestrol, melphalan, mustard gas and vinyl chloride), evidence of carcinogenicity in experimental animals preceded evidence obtained from epidemiological studies or case reports.

For many of the chemicals (or complex mixtures) evaluated in the *IARC Monographs* for which there is *sufficient evidence* of carcinogenicity in animals, data relating to carcinogenicity for humans are either insufficient or nonexistent. **In the absence of adequate data on humans, it is reasonable, for practical purposes, to regard chemicals or exposures for which there is sufficient evidence of carcinogenicity in animals as if they presented a carcinogenic risk to humans.** The use of the expressions 'for practical purposes' and 'as if they presented a carcinogenic risk' indicates that, at the present time, a correlation between carcinogenicity in animals and possible human risk cannot be made on a purely scientific basis, but only pragmatically. Such a pragmatic correlation may be useful to regulatory agencies in making decisions related to the primary prevention of cancer.

In the present state of knowledge, it would be difficult to define a predictable relationship between the dose (mg/kg bw per day) of a particular chemical required to produce cancer in test animals and the dose that would produce a similar incidence of cancer in humans. Some data, however, suggest that such a relationship may exist(20,21), at least for certain classes of carcinogenic chemicals, although no acceptable method is currently available for quantifying the possible errors that may be involved in such an extrapolation procedure.

8. EXPLANATORY NOTES ON THE CONTENTS OF MONOGRAPHS ON CHEMICALS AND COMPLEX MIXTURES

These notes apply to the format of most monographs, except for those that address industries or life-style factors. Thus, sections 1 and 2, as described below, are applicable in monographs on chemicals or groups of chemicals; in other monographs, they may be replaced by sections on the history of an industry or habit, a description of a process and other relevant information.

(a) Chemical and Physical Data (Section 1)

The Chemical Abstracts Services Registry Number, the latest Chemical Abstracts Primary Name (Ninth Collective Index)(22) and the IUPAC Systematic Name(23) are recorded in section 1. Other synonyms and trade names are given, but the list is not necessarily comprehensive. Some of the trade names may be those of mixtures in which the compound being evaluated is only one of the ingredients.

The structural and molecular formulae, molecular weight and chemical and physical properties are given. The properties listed refer to the pure substance, unless otherwise specified, and include, in particular, data that might be relevant to identification, environmental fate and human exposure, and biological effects, including carcinogenicity.

A separate description of the composition of technical products includes available information on impurities and formulated products.

(b) Production, Use, Occurrence and Analysis (Section 2)

The purpose of section 2 is to provide indications of the extent of past and present human exposure to the chemical.

Monographs on occupational exposures to complex mixtures or exposures to complex mixtures resulting from human habits include sections on: historical perspectives; description of the industry or habit; manufacturing processes and use patterns; exposures in the workplace; chemistry of the complex mixture.

(i)   Synthesis

Since cancer is a delayed toxic effect, the dates of first synthesis and of first commercial production of the chemical are provided. This information allows a reasonable estimate to be made of the date before which no human exposure could have occurred. In addition, methods of synthesis used in past and present commercial production are described.

(ii)   Production

Since Europe, Japan and the USA are reasonably representative industrialized areas of the world, most data on production, foreign trade and uses are obtained from those regions. It should not, however, be inferred that those areas or nations are the sole or even necessarily the major sources or users of any individual chemical.

Production and foreign trade data are obtained from both governmental and trade publications. In some cases, separate production data on organic chemicals manufactured in the USA are not available because their publication could disclose confidential information. In such cases, an indication of the minimum quantity produced can be inferred from the number of companies reporting commercial production. Each company is required to report on individual chemicals if the annual sales value or production volume exceeds a specified minimum level. These levels vary for chemicals classified for different uses, e.g., medicinals and plastics; in fact, the minimal reportable level for annual sales value ranges from $1000-$50 000, and the minimal reportable level for annual production volume ranges from 450-22 700 kg for different classes of use. Data on production are also obtained by means of general questionnaires sent to companies thought to produce the compounds being evaluated. Information from the completed questionnaires is compiled, by country, and the resulting estimates of production are included in the individual monographs.

(iii)   Use

Information on uses is usually obtained from published sources but is often complemented by direct contact with manufacturers. Some uses identified may not be current or major applications, and the coverage is not necessarily comprehensive. In the case of drugs, mention of their therapeutic uses does not necessarily represent current practice nor does it imply judgement as to their clinical efficacy.

Statements concerning regulations and standards (e.g., pesticide registrations, maximum levels permitted in foods, occupational standards and allowable limits) in specific countries may not reflect the most recent situation, since such standards are continuously reviewed and modified. The absence of information on regulatory status for a country should not be taken to imply that that country does not have regulations with regard to the chemical.

(iv)   Occurrence

Information on the occurrence of a chemical in the environment is obtained from published data, including that derived from the monitoring and surveillance of levels of the chemical in occupational environments, air, water, soil, foods and tissues of animals and humans. When no published data are available to the Working Group, unpublished reports, deemed appropriate, may be considered. When available, data on the generation, persistence and bioaccumulation of a chemical are also included.

(v) *Analysis*

The purpose of the section on analysis is to give the reader an overview, rather than a complete list, of current methods cited in the literature. No critical evaluation or recommendation of any of the methods is meant or implied.

(c) Biological Data Relevant to the Evaluation of Carcinogenic Risk to Humans (Section 3)

In general, the data recorded in section 3 are summarized as given by the author; however, comments made by the Working Group on certain shortcomings of reporting, of statistical analysis or of experimental design are given in square brackets. The nature and extent of impurities/contaminants in the chemicals being tested are given when available.

(i) *Carcinogenicity studies in animals*

The monographs are not intended to cover all reported studies. A few studies are purposely omitted because they are inadequate (e.g., too short a duration, too few animals, poor survival) or because they are judged irrelevant for the purpose of the evaluation. In certain cases, however, such studies are mentioned briefly, particularly when the information is considered to be a useful supplement to other reports or when it is the only data available. Their inclusion does not, however, imply acceptance of the adequacy of their experimental design or of the analysis and interpretation of their results.

Mention is made of all routes of administration by which the test material has been adequately tested and of all species in which relevant tests have been done(24). In most cases, animal strains are given. Quantitative data are given to indicate the order of magnitude of the effective carcinogenic doses. In general, the doses and schedules are indicated as they appear in the original report; sometimes units have been converted for easier comparison. Experiments in which the compound was administered in conjunction with known carcinogens and experiments on factors that modify the carcinogenic effect are also reported. Experiments on the carcinogenicity of known metabolites and derivatives are also included.

(ii) *Other relevant biological data*

LD_{50} data are given when available, and other data on toxicity are included when considered relevant.

Data on effects on reproduction, on teratogenicity and embryo- and fetotoxicity and on placental transfer, from studies in experimental animals and from observations in humans, are included when considered relevant.

Information is given on absorption, distribution and excretion. Data on metabolism are usually restricted to studies that show the metabolic fate of the chemical in experimental animals and humans, and comparisons of data from animals and humans are made when possible.

Data from short-term tests are also included. In addition to the tests for genetic activity and cell transformation described previously (see pages 18-19), data from studies of related effects, but for which the relevance to the carcinogenic process is less well established, may also be mentioned.

The criteria used for considering short-term tests and for evaluating their results have been described (see pages 19-21). In general, the authors' results are given as reported. An assessment of the data by the Working Group which differs from that of the authors, and comments concerning aspects of the study that might affect its interpretation are given in square brackets. Reports of studies in which few or no experimental details are given, or in which the data on which a reported positive or negative result is based are not available for examination, are cited, but are identified as 'abstract' or 'details not given' and are not considered in the summary tables or in making the overall assessment of genetic activity.

For several recent reviews on short-term tests, see IARC(24), Montesano *et al.*(25), de Serres and Ashby(26), Sugimura *et al.*(27), Bartsch *et al.*(28) and Hollstein *et al.*(29).

(iii) *Case reports and epidemiological studies of carcinogenicity to humans*

Observations in humans are summarized in this section. These include case reports, descriptive epidemiological studies (which correlate cancer incidence in space or time to an exposure) and analytical epidemiological studies of the case-control or cohort type. In principle, a comprehensive coverage is made of observations in humans; however, reports are excluded when judged to be clearly not pertinent. This applies in particular to case reports, in which either the clinico-pathological description of the tumours or the exposure history, or both, are poorly described; and to published routine statistics, for example, of cancer mortality by occupational category, when the categories are so broadly defined as to contribute virtually no specific information on the possible relation between cancer occurrence and a given exposure. Results of studies are assessed on the basis of the data and analyses that are presented in the published papers. Some additional analyses of the published data may be performed by the Working Group to gain better insight into the relation between cancer occurrence and the exposure under consideration. The Working Group may use these analyses in its assessment of the evidence or may actually include them in the text to summarize a study; in such cases, the results of the supplementary analyses are given in square brackets. Any comments by the Working Group are also reported in square brackets; however, these are kept to a minimum, being restricted to those instances in which it is felt that an important aspect of a study, directly impinging on its interpretation, should be brought to the attention of the reader.

(d) Summary of Data Reported and Evaluation (Section 4)

Section 4 summarizes the relevant data from animals and humans and gives the critical views of the Working Group on those data.

(i) *Exposures*

Human exposure to the chemical or complex mixture is summarized on the basis of data on production, use and occurrence.

(ii) *Experimental data*

Data relevant to the evaluation of the carcinogenicity of the test material in animals are summarized in this section. The animal species mentioned are those in which the carcinogenicity of the substance was clearly demonstrated. Tumour sites are also indicated. If the substance has produced tumours after prenatal exposure or in single-dose experiments, this is indicated. Dose-response data are given when available.

Significant findings on effects on reproduction and prenatal toxicity, and results from short-term tests for genetic activity and cell transformation assays are summarized, and the latter are presented in tables. An overall assessment is made of the degree of evidence for genetic activity in short-term tests.

(iii) *Human data*

Case reports and epidemiological studies that are considered to be pertinent to an assessment of human carcinogenicity are described. Other biological data that are considered to be relevant are also mentioned.

(iv) *Evaluation*

This section comprises evaluations by the Working Group of the degrees of evidence for carcinogenicity of the exposure to experimental animals and to humans. An overall evaluation is then made of the carcinogenic risk of the chemical or complex mixture to humans. This section should be read in conjunction with pages 18 and 22 of this Preamble for definitions of degrees of evidence.

When no data are available from epidemiological studies but there is *sufficient evidence* that the exposure is carcinogenic to animals, a footnote is included, reading: 'In the absence of adequate data on humans, it is reasonable, for practical purposes, to regard chemicals or exposures for which there is *sufficient evidence* of carcinogenicity in animals as if they presented a carcinogenic risk to humans' (pp. 22-23).

References

1. IARC (1979) Criteria to select chemicals for *IARC Monographs. IARC intern. tech. Rep. No. 79/003*

2. IARC (1977) IARC Monographs Programme on the Evaluation of the Carcinogenic Risk of Chemicals to Humans. Preamble. *IARC intern. tech. Rep. No. 77/002*

3. IARC (1978) Chemicals with *sufficient evidence* of carcinogenicity in experimental animals — *IARC Monographs* volumes 1-17. *IARC intern. tech. Rep. No. 78/003*

4. IARC (1982) *IARC Monographs on the Evaluation of the Carcinogenic Risk of Chemicals to Humans*, Supplement 4, *Chemicals, Industrial Processes and Industries Associated with Cancer in Humans* (IARC Monographs Volumes 1 to 29)

5.   IARC (1983) Approaches to classifying chemical carcinogens according to mechanism of action. *IARC intern. tech. Rep. No. 83/001*

6.   IARC (1972-1986) *IARC Monographs on the Evaluation of the Carcinogenic Risk of Chemicals to Humans*, Volumes 1-38, Lyon, France

Volume 1 (1972) Some Inorganic Substances, Chlorinated Hydrocarbons, Aromatic Amines, *N*-Nitroso Compounds and Natural Products (19 monographs), 184 pages

Volume 2 (1973) Some Inorganic and Organometallic Compounds (7 monographs), 181 pages

Volume 3 (1973) Certain Polycyclic Aromatic Hydrocarbons and Heterocyclic Compounds (17 monographs), 271 pages

Volume 4 (1974) Some Aromatic Amines, Hydrazine and Related Substances, *N*-Nitroso Compounds and Miscellaneous Alkylating Agents (28 monographs), 286 pages

Volume 5 (1974) Some Organochlorine Pesticides (12 monographs), 241 pages

Volume 6 (1974) Sex Hormones (15 monographs), 243 pages

Volume 7 (1974) Some Anti-thyroid and Related Substances, Nitrofurans and Industrial Chemicals (23 monographs), 326 pages

Volume 8 (1975) Some Aromatic Azo Compounds (32 monographs), 357 pages

Volume 9 (1975) Some Aziridines, *N*-, *S*- and *O*-Mustards and Selenium (24 monographs), 268 pages

Volume 10 (1976) Some Naturally Occurring Substances (22 monographs), 353 pages

Volume 11 (1976) Cadmium, Nickel, Some Epoxides, Miscellaneous Industrial Chemicals and General Considerations on Volatile Anaesthetics (24 monographs), 306 pages

Volume 12 (1976) Some Carbamates, Thiocarbamates and Carbazides (24 monographs), 282 pages

Volume 13 (1977) Some Miscellaneous Pharmaceutical Substances (17 monographs), 255 pages

Volume 14 (1977) Asbestos (1 monograph), 106 pages

Volume 15 (1977) Some Fumigants, the Herbicides, 2,4-D and 2,4,5-T, Chlorinated Dibenzodioxins and Miscellaneous Industrial Chemicals (18 monographs), 354 pages

Volume 16 (1978) Some Aromatic Amines and Related Nitro Compounds — Hair Dyes, Colouring Agents, and Miscellaneous Industrial Chemicals (32 monographs), 400 pages

Volume 17 (1978) Some *N*-Nitroso Compounds (17 monographs), 365 pages

Volume 18 (1978) Polychlorinated Biphenyls and Polybrominated Biphenyls (2 monographs), 140 pages

Volume 19 (1979) Some Monomers, Plastics and Synthetic Elastomers, and Acrolein (17 monographs), 513 pages

Volume 20 (1979) Some Halogenated Hydrocarbons (25 monographs), 609 pages

Volume 21 (1979) Sex Hormones (II) (22 monographs), 583 pages

Volume 22 (1980) Some Non-nutritive Sweetening Agents (2 monographs), 208 pages

Volume 23 (1980) Some Metals and Metallic Compounds (4 monographs), 438 pages

Volume 24 (1980) Some Pharmaceutical Drugs (16 monographs), 337 pages

Volume 25 (1981) Wood, Leather and Some Associated Industries (7 monographs), 412 pages

Volume 26 (1981) Some Antineoplastic and Immunosuppressive Agents (18 monographs), 411 pages

Volume 27 (1981) Some Aromatic Amines, Anthraquinones and Nitroso Compounds, and Inorganic Fluorides Used in Drinking-Water and Dental Preparations (18 monographs), 344 pages

Volume 28 (1982) The Rubber Industry (1 monograph), 486 pages

Volume 29 (1982) Some Industrial Chemicals and Dyestuffs (18 monographs), 416 pages

Volume 30 (1982) Miscellaneous Pesticides (18 monographs), 424 pages

Volume 31 (1983) Some Food Additives, Feed Additives and Naturally Occurring Substances (21 monographs), 314 pages

Volume 32 (1983) Polynuclear Aromatic Compounds, Part 1, Chemical, Environmental and Experimental Data (42 monographs), 477 pages

Volume 33 (1984) Polynuclear Aromatic Compounds, Part 2, Carbon Blacks, Mineral Oils and Some Nitroarenes (8 monographs), 245 pages

Volume 34 (1984) Polynuclear Aromatic Compounds, Part 3, Industrial Exposures in Aluminium Production, Coal Gasification, Coke Production, and Iron and Steel Founding (4 monographs), 219 pages

Volume 35 (1984) Polynuclear Aromatic Compounds, Part 4, Bitumens, Coal-Tars and Derived Products, Shale-Oils and Soots (4 monographs), 271 pages

Volume 36 (1985) Allyl Compounds, Aldehydes, Epoxides and Peroxides (15 monographs), 369 pages

Volume 37 (1985) Tobacco Habits other than Smoking; Betel-quid and Areca-nut Chewing; and Some Nitroso Compounds (8 monographs), 291 pages

Volume 38 (1986) Tobacco Smoking (1 monograph), 421 pages

Volume 39 (1986) Some Chemicals Used in Plastics and Elastomers (19 monographs), 403 pages

Supplement No. 1 (1979) Chemicals and Industrial Processes Associated with Cancer in Humans (IARC Monographs, Volumes 1 to 20), 71 pages

Supplement No. 2 (1980) Long-term and Short-term Screening Assays for Carcinogens: A Critical Appraisal, 426 pages

Supplement No. 3 (1982) Cross Index of Synonyms and Trade Names in Volumes 1 to 26, 199 pages

Supplement No. 4 (1982) Chemicals, Industrial Processes and Industries Associated with Cancer in Humans (IARC Monographs, Volumes 1 to 29), 292 pages

Supplement No. 5 (1985) Cross Index of Synonyms and Trade Names in Volumes 1 to 36, 259 pages

7.   IARC (1973-1984) *Information Bulletin on the Survey of Chemicals Being Tested for Carcinogenicity*, Numbers 1-11, Lyon, France

Number 1 (1973) 52 pages
Number 2 (1973) 77 pages
Number 3 (1974) 67 pages
Number 4 (1974) 97 pages
Number 5 (1975) 88 pages
Number 6 (1976) 360 pages
Number 7 (1978) 460 pages
Number 8 (1979) 604 pages
Number 9 (1981) 294 pages
Number 10 (1983) 326 pages
Number 11 (1984) 370 pages

8.   PHS 149 (1951-1983) Public Health Service Publication No. 149, *Survey of Compounds which have been Tested for Carcinogenic Activity*, Washington DC, US Government Printing Office

1951 Hartwell, J.L., 2nd ed., Literature up to 1947 on 1329 compounds, 583 pages

1957 Shubik, P. & Hartwell, J.L., Supplement 1, Literature for the years 1948-1953 on 981 compounds, 388 pages

1969 Shubik, P. & Hartwell, J.L., edited by Peters, J.A., Supplement 2, Literature for the years 1954-1960 on 1048 compounds, 655 pages

1971 National Cancer Institute, Literature for the years 1968-1969 on 882 compounds, 653 pages

1973 National Cancer Institute, Literature for the years 1961-1967 on 1632 compounds, 2343 pages

1974 National Cancer Institute, Literature for the years 1970-1971 on 750 compounds, 1667 pages

1976 National Cancer Institute, Literature for the years 1972-1973 on 966 compounds, 1638 pages

1980 National Cancer Institute, Literature for the year 1978 on 664 compounds, 1331 pages

1983 National Cancer Institute, Literature for years 1974-1975 on 575 compounds, 1043 pages

9. Pike, M.C. & Roe, F.J.C. (1963) An actuarial method of analysis of an experiment in two-stage carcinogenesis. *Br. J. Cancer, 17*, 605-610

10. Miller, E.C. (1978) Some current perspectives on chemical carcinogenesis in humans and experimental animals: Presidential address. *Cancer Res., 38*, 1479-1496

11. Miller, E.C. & Miller, J.A. (1981) Searches for ultimate chemical carcinogens and their reactions with cellular macromolecules. *Cancer, 47*, 2327-2345

12. Peto, R. (1974) Guidelines on the analysis of tumour rates and death rates in experimental animals. *Br. J. Cancer, 29*, 101-105

13. Hoel, D.G. & Walburg, H.E., Jr (1972) Statistical analysis of survival experiments. *J. natl Cancer Inst., 49*, 361-372

14. Peto, R., Pike, M.C., Day, N.E., Gray, R.G., Lee, P.N., Parish, S., Peto, J., Richards, S. & Wahrendorf, J. (1980) *Guidelines for simple sensitive significance tests for carcinogenic effects in long-term animal experiments.* In: *IARC Monographs on the Evaluation of the Carcinogenic Risk of Chemicals to Humans, Supplement 2, Long-term and Short-term Screening Assays for Carcinogens: A Critical Appraisal,* Lyon, pp. 311-426

15. Berenblum, I. (1975) *Sequential aspects of chemical carcinogenesis: Skin.* In: Becker, F.F., ed., *Cancer. A Comprehensive Treatise,* Vol. 1, New York, Plenum Press, pp. 323-344

16. Foulds, L. (1969) *Neoplastic Development,* Vol. 2, London, Academic Press

17. Farber, E. & Cameron, R. (1980) The sequential analysis of cancer development. *Adv. Cancer Res., 31*, 125-126

18. Weinstein, I.B. (1981) The scientific basis for carcinogen detection and primary cancer prevention. *Cancer, 47*, 1133-1141

19. Slaga, T.J., Sivak, A. & Boutwell, R.K., eds (1978) *Mechanisms of Tumor Promotion and Cocarcinogenesis,* Vol. 2, New York, Raven Press

20. Rall, D.P. (1977) *Species differences in carcinogenesis testing.* In: Hiatt, H.H., Watson, J.D. & Winsten, J.A., eds, *Origins of Human Cancer,* Book C, Cold Spring Harbor, NY, Cold Spring Harbor Laboratory, pp. 1383-1390

21. National Academy of Sciences (NAS) (1975) *Contemporary Pest Control Practices and Prospects: The Report of the Executive Committee*, Washington DC

22. Chemical Abstracts Services (1978) *Chemical Abstracts Ninth Collective Index (9CI), 1972-1976*, Vols 76-85, Columbus, OH

23. International Union of Pure & Applied Chemistry (1965) *Nomenclature of Organic Chemistry*, Section C, London, Butterworths

24. IARC (1980) *IARC Monographs on the Evaluation of the Carcinogenic Risk of Chemicals to Humans*, Supplement 2, *Long-term and Short-term Screening Assays for Carcinogens: A Critical Appraisal*, Lyon

25. Montesano, R., Bartsch, H. & Tomatis, L., eds (1980) *Molecular and Cellular Aspects of Carcinogen Screening Tests (IARC Scientific Publications No. 27)*, Lyon

26. de Serres, F.J. & Ashby, J., eds (1981) *Evaluation of Short-Term Tests for Carcinogens. Report of the International Collaborative Program*, Amsterdam, Elsevier/North-Holland Biomedical Press

27. Sugimura, T., Sato, S., Nagao, M., Yahagi, T., Matsushima, T., Seino, Y., Takeuchi, M. & Kawachi, T. (1976) *Overlapping of carcinogens and mutagens*. In: Magee, P.N., Takayama, S., Sugimura, T. & Matsushima, T., eds, *Fundamentals in Cancer Prevention*, Tokyo/Baltimore, University of Tokyo/University Park Press, pp. 191-215

28. Bartsch, H., Tomatis, L. & Malaveille, C. (1982) *Qualitative and quantitative comparison between mutagenic and carcinogenic activities of chemicals*. In: Heddle, J.A., ed., *Mutagenicity: New Horizons in Genetic Toxicology*, New York, Academic Press, pp. 35-72

29. Hollstein, M., McCann, J., Angelosanto, F.A. & Nichols, W.W. (1979) Short-term tests for carcinogens and mutagens. *Mutat. Res.*, *65*, 133-226

GENERAL REMARKS ON THE SUBSTANCES CONSIDERED

Background

Chemicals used in the manufacture of plastics and elastomers were the subject of a previous volume of *IARC Monographs* (IARC, 1979). A second volume of *Monographs* on this class of chemicals was undertaken because of developments in the two areas that provide the basis for selection of substances for evaluation: evidence of exposure, and evidence or suspicion of carcinogenicity. This thirty-ninth volume of *IARC Monographs* comprises considerations of a number of industrial chemicals used in the production of plastics and elastomers; some of the compounds are also used in paints and adhesives. Two compounds — dichloroacetylene and 4-vinylcyclohexene — can occur as by-products in the production or use of some of these chemicals. New data were available on some of the chemicals evaluated previously: methyl acrylate, ethyl acrylate, caprolactam, 4,4'-methylene-dianiline, toluene diisocyanate, vinyl acetate, vinyl bromide and vinylidene chloride, and these have been summarized and taken into consideration in the re-evaluations. 4,4'-Methylenediphenyl diisocyanate [evaluated in Volume 19 of the *Monographs* (IARC, 1979)], a monomer produced from 4,4'-methylenedianiline (MDA) [evaluated in Volume 4 of the *Monographs* (IARC, 1974)], can hydrolyse to MDA when in contact with moisture; however, 4,4'-methylenediphenyl diisocyanate was not re-evaluated in the present volume because no new data on carcinogenicity have become available.

Amounts produced

Plastics and elastomers are petroleum-based materials that are produced in large quantities in many parts of the world and which have a wide range of applications in both industrial and consumer products. Of the 19 compounds considered, three are monomers that are produced annually in amounts of more than one million tonnes (1,3-butadiene, caprolactam, vinyl acetate), and seven are chemicals produced in amounts in excess of 100 000 tonnes (acrylamide, ethyl acrylate, *n*-butyl acrylate, toluene diisocyanate, 4,4'-methylenedianiline, melamine and vinylidene chloride).

Uses

Since the 1950s, synthetic plastics and elastomers have been used in textiles, coatings, adhesives, packaging, building, transportation and machinery products. Their importance is illustrated by the ubiquity of the compounds and of their polymeric derivatives in consumer goods. For example, latex paints for interior decoration are made of acrylic, 1,3-butadiene or vinyl acetate copolymers. Flexible polyurethane foams for furnishings are manufactured by copolymerization of polyols with toluene diisocyanate. Melamine plastics are common in durable table tops and dinnerware. Vinyl acetate and isocyanate adhesives are used for chloride polymers. Caprolactam is used in the production of fibres for nylon carpets. Nylon 11, derived from 11-aminoundecanoic acid, finds use in a variety of industrial materials. Textiles may be treated with resins from vinyl bromide for flame retardation or finished with resins derived from melamine. Electrical wires and weather-resistant exterior panels can be coated with polymerized vinyl or vinylidene fluoride. Modern car paints, primers and topcoat finishes are often based on polyurethanes. Tyres made of polybutadiene and styrene-butadiene rubber constitute the largest use of 1,3-butadiene.

Exposures

Human exposure to the chemicals used in plastics and elastomers occurs during synthesis and polymerization of volatile monomers; in addition, the general population may be exposed by direct contact with manufactured products or through air, water and food. Although the residual amounts of unreacted monomers in finished products are generally very small, fresh paints and glues may contain low levels to which people may be exposed occupationally or in houses.

The production, use and disposal of polymers may result in mixed exposures to monomers, catalysts, activators, stabilizers, antioxidants, plasticizers, fillers and other processing chemicals. Consequently, it is difficult to study the health effects of any specific compound in such complex mixtures.

Reactivity

The acrylates, 1,3-butadiene, halogenated vinyl and vinylidene compounds can polymerize spontaneously and are highly inflammable or react explosively with air. The diisocyanates react readily with water and are hydrolysed to the corresponding amines.

The reactivity of the compounds must be taken into account in the design and evaluation of biological studies. Technical grades may contain degradation products and stabilizers, which, although normally present in very small quantities, may be important. Caprolactam can be nitrosated. 1,3-Butadiene, 4-vinylcyclohexene and the vinylic and acrylic compounds may react with nucleophiles and serve as substrates for enzymatic epoxidation. Diisocyanates and vinyl acetate can be hydrolysed to give the corresponding carcinogenic aromatic amines and acetaldehyde as breakdown products. Due to its low solubility in water, melamine can precipitate in urine to form inflammatory crystals or stones.

Health effects

Humans are exposed to plastics and elastomers, and to precursors and by-products associated with their production. This fact was recognized by the Working Group that made the initial IARC evaluations of plastics and related compounds and is reflected in the 'General Remarks' to the corresponding volume. New evidence is now available of human exposure to several of the substances considered in the present volume, and more data are being generated on the environmental levels of certain of the substances in particular contexts. In previous volumes, no data were available on reproductive effects or developmental toxicity of these chemicals in humans; in the present volume, such reports were available only for caprolactam. Studies in which reproductive toxicity in experimental animals was evaluated were available previously only for vinylidene chloride and caprolactam; in the present volume, such reports are given for acrylamide, n-butyl acrylate, ethyl acrylate, 1,3-butadiene, vinylidene chloride, caprolactam, melamine and 4,4′-methylenedianiline. There is a lack of information on the absorption, distribution and, most importantly, the metabolism of many of these compounds, with the exception of most olefins (acrylic and vinylic derivatives).

The Working Group noted that, except for a few compounds, the available data were inadequate to evaluate mutagenicity. In particular, the scarcity of information on effects *in vivo* makes it difficult to evaluate genetic effects adequately.

New information is now available on the carcinogenic activity of several of the chemicals considered previously. Completion and publication of a number of bioassays, many of which have formed part of the US National Toxicology Program, have been the major reason for making the present evaluations and re-evaluations.

For several of the monomers considered in this volume, there is evidence of carcinogenicity in experimental animals (1,3-butadiene, toluene diisocyanate, vinyl bromide); for others, the data are inadequate, and more testing is needed. Surprisingly, for several substances (methyl and butyl acrylate and melamine), long-term studies have been completed but are, as yet, unpublished and consequently could not be used in these evaluations. Publication of these studies is a clear priority, especially for 1,3-butadiene and toluene diisocyanate.

In their 'General Remarks on the Substances Considered', the previous Working Group noted the need for both chronic animal studies and epidemiological investigations. To supplement the bioassay data now available, further experimental studies might address a wide range of secondary questions, including the effect of lower doses, effects of modifying factors, interactions between related compounds and mechanisms of carcinogenesis. However, while the perceived need for animal bioassays might be deemed to have been met, at least in part, there is no comparable body of epidemiological investigations on these compounds.

The dearth of epidemiological data on the effects on humans of exposure to elastomers, plastics and related compounds is a cause for concern. There is no indication that such studies are in progress (Muir & Wagner, 1984). In drawing attention to the need for such studies, the present Working Group was aware that the mixed exposures of many occupationally exposed groups tend to limit severely the possibility of making associations between exposure to single chemicals and increased risk of cancer. A range of studies designed specifically to evaluate occupational exposure to particular plastics and elastomers during their production and use may be required. In the absence of comprehensive epidemiological information, the extrapolation from experimental animal data implicit in the evaluation *'sufficient evidence* of carcinogenicity' (see Preamble, pp. 22-23) mandates action.

References

IARC (1974) *IARC Monographs on the Evaluation of Carcinogenic Risk of Chemicals to Man*, Vol. 4, *Some Aromatic Amines, Hydrazine and Related Substances,* N-*Nitroso Compounds and Miscellaneous Alkylating Agents,* Lyon, pp. 79-85

IARC (1979) *IARC Monographs on the Evaluation of the Carcinogenic Risk of Chemicals to Humans*, Vol. 19, *Some Monomers, Plastics and Synthetic Elastomers, and Acrolein,* Lyon

Muir, C.S. & Wagner, G., eds (1984) *Directory of On-Going Research in Cancer Epidemiology 1984 (IARC Scientific Publications No. 62)*, Lyon, International Agency for Research on Cancer

THE MONOGRAPHS

VINYL COMPOUNDS

ACRYLAMIDE

1. Chemical and Physical Data

1.1 Synonyms and trade names

Chem. Abstr. Services Reg. No.: 79-06-1

Chem. Abstr. Name: 2-Propenamide

IUPAC Systematic Name: Acrylamide

Synonyms: Acrylamide monomer; acrylic acid amide; acrylic amide; ethylene-carboxamide; propenamide; propeneamide; propenoic acid amide

1.2 Structural and molecular formulae and molecular weight

$$CH_2 = CH - \overset{\overset{\textstyle O}{\|}}{C} - NH_2$$

C_3H_5NO Mol. wt: 71.08

1.3 Chemical and physical properties of the pure substance

(a) *Description*: Colourless-to-white, odourless crystalline solid (Hawley, 1981; Sax, 1984); leaf or flake-like crystals from benzene (Windholz, 1983; Weast, 1984)

(b) *Boiling-point*: 125°C at 25 mm Hg (Hawley, 1981; Windholz, 1983; Sax, 1984)

(c) *Melting-point*: 84-85°C (Grasselli & Ritchey, 1975; Verschueren, 1983; Weast, 1984)

(d) *Density*: d_4^{30} 1.122 (Hawley, 1981; Windholz, 1983; Sax, 1984)

(e) *Spectroscopy data*: Ultraviolet (Sadtler Research Laboratories, 1980; [3515[a]]), infrared (Sadtler Research Laboratories, 1980; prism [2998,13447], grating [8284]), nuclear magnetic resonance (Sadtler Research Laboratories, 1980; proton [3166], C-13 [6618]) and mass spectral data (NIH/EPA Chemical Information System, 1983) have been reported.

(f) *Solubility*: Very soluble in water (215.5 g/100 ml at 30°C); soluble in chloroform (2.7 g/100 ml at 30°C), ethanol (86.2 g/100 ml at 30°C), acetone (63.1 g/100 ml at 30°C) and diethyl ether; insoluble in heptane (Grasselli & Ritchey, 1975; MacWilliams, 1978; Hawley, 1981; Windholz, 1983)

(g) *Volatility*: Vapour pressure, 0.007 mm Hg at 25°C (MacWilliams, 1978); relative vapour density (air = 1), 2.45 (Sax, 1984)

(h) *Stability*: The solid is stable at room temperature but polymerizes on melting or exposure to ultraviolet light (Hawley, 1981; Buckingham, 1982; Windholz, 1983)

(i) *Conversion factor*: mg/m³ = 2.91 × ppm[b]

1.4 Technical products and impurities

Acrylamide is available in crystalline form (solid) and in aqueous solution. The crystalline acrylamide is a white, free flowing crystal and has the following typical properties: assay, 98% min; water, 0.8% max; iron, 15 mg/kg max; water insolubles, 0.2% max; butanol insolubles, 1.5% max. The 50% aqueous acrylamide solution has the following properties: assay, 48-52%; pH, 5.0-6.5; polymer, 0.05% max; Cu^{++}, inhibitor with oxygen, 25-30 mg/kg (MacWilliams, 1978). Other possible polymerization inhibitors include hydroquinone, *tert*-butyl pyrocatechol (Windholz, 1983), ferrous salts and *N*-phenyl-2-naphthylamine (Bikales, 1970). Possible contaminants include sodium sulphate, acrylic acid, sulphuric acid and water, depending on the mode of synthesis (MacWilliams, 1978).

The commercial product has been reported to contain residual levels of 1-100 mg/kg acrylonitrile (US Environmental Protection Agency, 1980).

---

[a]Spectrum number in Sadtler compilation

[b]Calculated from: mg/m³ = (molecular weight/24.45) × ppm, assuming standard temperature (25°C) and pressure (760 mm Hg)

2. Production, Use, Occurrence and Analysis

2.1 Production and use

(a) Production

Acrylamide was first produced in 1893 by Moureu in Germany. A US firm made research quantities from 1952 and began commercial production in 1954 (Bikales, 1970).

All industrial methods for the production of acrylamide involve the hydration of acrylonitrile. Before 1970, such hydration was carried out with sulphuric acid; acrylamide was extracted from the resulting sulphate solution by neutralization with ammonia and subsequent cooling to isolate the crystalline monomer. This process can produce unwanted side-reaction products, such as polyacrylamide and acrylic acid. These side reactions, often initiated by increased reaction temperatures (the reaction of acrylonitrile with sulphuric acid and water is highly exothermic), can be suppressed by inhibitors such as copper salts (MacWilliams, 1978).

Methods previously used for preparing acrylamide from acrylamide sulphate, using a lime process or ion exchange, have been described (MacWilliams, 1978).

Currently, acrylamide is manufactured by direct catalytic conversion of acrylonitrile, thereby eliminating the sulphate by-product (Mannsville Chemical Products Corp., 1982). In a technique developed in 1971, an aqueous solution of acrylonitrile is passed over a fixed bed of copper or copper-metal admixtures at 25-200°C, resulting in direct hydration of the acrylonitrile. Unreacted aqueous acrylonitrile can be recycled into the reactor. The catalyst can be recovered by subsequent oxidation/reduction (MacWilliams, 1978).

While manganese dioxide, rhodium complexes and cobalt oxides have also been described as catalysts for use in this process, in most commercial acrylamide plants copper-based or Raney copper catalysts are used. With the catalytic technique, solid acrylamide monomer can be isolated, but a 50% aqueous acrylamide solution is produced most widely because of its lower cost and ease of handling. The aqueous form can be used for most applications (MacWilliams, 1978).

A Japanese firm has started using microorganisms as biocatalysts in the conversion of acrylonitrile to acrylamide and expected to reach an annual production of 4 million kg acrylamide by April 1985 (Anon., 1984).

The production of acrylamide in the USA in 1983 was reported to be 39.1 million kg (US International Trade Commission, 1984), as compared to 10 million kg in 1972 (Mannsville Chemical Products, Corp., 1982). Three US companies have the combined capacity to produce 102.2 million kg acrylamide annually. All of the acrylamide produced by one firm is used internally to make polyacrylamide (Anon., 1985).

Two major Japanese manufacturers had a combined annual capacity of 55 million kg as of January 1984. Of the 41 million kg acrylamide manufactured in 1982, 36 million kg were used domestically and 5 million kg were exported; 1 million kg were imported.

Total acrylamide production capacity in western Europe in 1984 was 42.5 million kg. Two plants in the Federal Republic of Germany had a combined capacity of 8 million kg; one plant in the UK had a capacity of 7.5 million kg, and production capacity in The Netherlands was 27 million kg.

(b)   Use

Acrylamide monomer is used primarily for the production of polyacrylamides. These high-molecular-weight polymers can be modified to develop nonionic, anionic or cationic properties for specific uses. Polymerization (homopolymerization and copolymerization) is brought about through a free-radical mechanism in aqueous solution. The solubility and polyelectrolyte characteristics of these polymers are imparted by residual carboxyl groups or hydrolysed amide groups. Water-soluble cationic polymers can be produced by copolymerization with unsaturated quaternary ammonium compounds, such as diallyl-dimethyl ammonium chloride and vinylbenzyltrimethyl ammonium chloride. Anionic polyacrylamides are formed by copolymerization with carboxylic or sulphonic acids (Mannsville Chemical Products Corp., 1982).

Water and wastewater treatment

The largest use for polyacrylamides is in treating municipal drinking-water and wastewater. They act as a flocculants or coagulants to condition sludge, to clarify raw water and to treat effluent streams from sewage plants. Polyacrylamide can also be used to remove suspended solids in industrial waste-water prior to discharge, reuse or disposal (Mannsville Chemical Products Corp., 1982).

These high-molecular-weight polymers bind with colloidal particles to form heavy aggregates (American Cyanamid Co., 1969); the polymer-particle flocs quickly settle out from solution to leave a clear supernatant. When polyacrylamides are used as sludge conditioning/dewatering agents, they produce a more concentrated sludge than inorganic coagulants (Mannsville Chemical Products Corp., 1982).

Crude-oil production processes

Polyacrylamides are used to increase water viscosity in oil recovery processes, and 10-30% of the total annual production volume is used in this way (Mannsville Chemical Products Corp., 1982).

Partially hydrolysed polyacrylamides and acrylamide-acrylic acid copolymers can be used to control fluid loss in oil-well drilling muds (American Cyanamid Co., 1969).

Paper and pulp processing

Polyacrylamides are used in the pulp and paper production industry as binders and as retention aids for fibres (Mannsville Chemical Products Corp., 1982); they are also used as drainage aids/flocculants. Cationic polyacrylamides increase pigment retention on paper fibre (American Cyanamid Co., 1969).

Approximately 20% of the acrylamide used in the USA (Anon., 1985) and western Europe in 1984 was in the paper industry; however, this is the primary use (55%) of polyacrylamides in Japan.

Mineral processing

Polyacrylamides are used for the clarification of waste water, the recovery of tailings and the flocculation of ores in mineral processing (Mannsville Chemical Products Corp., 1982). They are used to thicken mineral concentrates and to permit reuse of water in the extraction process.

Concrete processing

The curing of cement often involves premature dehydration of the cement slurry; the loss of water results in decreased structural strength. Addition of polyacrylamides to the cement mixture to control loss of water prevents such weakening and limits the formation of scale on the concrete. A waterproof concrete with high compression strength can be produced by the addition of methylolated polymer and subsequent curing by radiation (American Cyanamid Co., 1982).

Cosmetic additives

Polyacrylamides have been used in soap and cosmetic preparations as thickeners and in pre-shave lotions, hair grooming preparations and denture fixtures (American Cyanamid Co., 1969).

Soil and sand treatment

Acrylamide resins can be used to stabilize soil, as the polymers bind loose grains when injected under the surface (American Cyanamid Co., 1969). Polyacrylamides can be used to allow foundry sand to flow freely into moulds (American Cyanamid Co., 1982).

Coating applications

Polyacrylamides are used as dispersants and binders in coatings. Water-based paints containing 0.1-0.5% polyacrylamides have better pigment suspension and flow (American Cyanamid Co., 1982). Since 1952, numerous patents have been awarded which describe the use of acrylamide resins in surface coatings and thermosetting acrylics. These resins are used as coatings in home appliances, building materials and automotive parts (American Cyanamid Co., 1969).

Textile processing

Polyacrylamides are used as sizing agents for cotton and as shrink-proofing agents for wool; they are also used to bind textile fibres and as water repellants (American Cyanamid Co., 1969).

Miscellaneous uses

A small percentage of acrylamide is used as grout (a thin fluid for filling interstices), thickeners for latex, emulsion stabilizers for printing inks, gelling agents for explosives, electrophoretic gels and retardants for crystal growth in the production of diazo compounds. Adhesives and adhesive tapes may contain acrylamide polymers as binders (American Cyanamid Co., 1969, 1982). Polyacrylamides are also used to clarify solutions in chemical and food manufacturing (Mannsville Chemical Products Corp., 1982). Electrophoresis in acrylamide gels is a widely used procedure in hospital laboratories.

Some polyacrylamides can be used as dispersants, anti-precipitants and deflocculants in aqueous systems (American Cyanamid Co., 1982). These properties are used for fluidizing pigment presscakes and reducing the viscosity of latexes. When added to herbicidal gels, polyacrylamides allow them to sink before breaking up, thereby limiting treatment to the bottom of a lake or reservoir (American Cyanamid Co., 1982).

(c) Regulatory status and guidelines

Occupational exposure limits for acrylamide have been set by regulation or recommended guideline in 13 countries (Table 1).

Table 1. National occupational exposure limits for acrylamide[a]

Country	Year	Concentration (mg/m^3)	Interpretation[b]
Australia	1978	0.3[c]	TWA
Belgium	1978	0.3[c]	TWA
Finland	1981	0.3[c]	TWA
France	1984	0.3[c]	TWA
Germany, Federal Republic of	1984	0.3[c]	TWA
Italy	1978	0.3[c]	TWA
Japan	1984	0.3	-
The Netherlands	1978	0.3[c]	TWA
Sweden	1984	0.3[c]	TWA
Switzerland	1978	0.3[c]	TWA
UK	1985	0.3[c]	TWA
		0.6[c]	STEL
USA			
ACGIH	1984	0.3[c]	TWA
		0.6[c]	STEL
NIOSH	1976	0.3[c]	TWA
OSHA	1983	0.3[c]	TWA
Yugoslavia	1971	0.3[c]	Ceiling

[a]From National Institute for Occupational Safety and Health (NIOSH) (1976); International Labour Office (1980); Työsuojeluhallitus (1981); NIOSH (1982); US Occupational Safety and Health Administration (OSHA) (1983); American Conference of Governmental Industrial Hygienists (ACGIH) (1984); Arbetarskyddsstyrelsens Författningssamling (1984); Deutsches Forschungsgemeinschaft (1984); Institut National de Recherche et de Sécurité (1984); Japan Ministry of Labour (1984); Health and Safety Executive (1985); NIOSH (1985)

[b]TWA, time-weighted average; STEL, short-term exposure limit

[c]Skin notation (absorption is possible)

The US Food and Drug Administration (1984) has established regulations for the use of acrylamide:

- Polyacrylamide can be used in washing or to assist in the peeling of fruits and vegetables using lye, if the concentration does not exceed 10 mg/l in the wash water and if no more than 0.2% of the acrylamide monomer is present.

- Acrylamide-sodium acrylate resins can be used as boiler water additives in the preparation of steam that will be in contact with food, if the water contains not more than 0.05% by weight of the acrylamide monomer.

- Polyacrylamide can be used as a film former in the imprinting of soft-shell gelatin capsules, if not more than 0.2% of the monomer is present.

- Homopolymers and copolymers of acrylamide may be safely used as food packaging adhesives, providing the amount used does not exceed that 'reasonably required to accomplish the intended effect'.

- Acrylamide-acrylic acid resins may be safely used as components in the production of paper or paperboard used for packing food, providing the resin contains less than 0.2% residual monomer and that the resin does not exceed 2% by weight of the paper or paperboard.

The US Environmental Protection Agency (1984) has designated acrylamide as a hazardous waste under the Resource Conservation and Recovery Act of 1976, because of its toxicity.

The recommended maximum concentration of acrylamide in potable waters was set at an average of 0.25 μg/l by the Ministry of Housing and Local Government in the UK in 1969.

2.2 Occurrence

(a) Natural occurrence

It is not known whether acrylamide occurs as a natural product.

(b) Occupational exposure

The National Institute for Occupational Safety and Health (1976) estimated that approximately 20 000 workers were potentially exposed to acrylamide in the USA. Primary exposure occurs during the handling of the monomer, but 500 mg/kg acrylamide have been detected in polymerized material (Mallevialle et al., 1984).

Personal sampling conducted at two US acrylamide manufacturing plants showed breathing-zone concentrations of 0.1-3.6 mg/m³. On the basis of monitoring of stationary air, concentrations to which workers at another plant were exposed were estimated not to have exceeded 0.3 mg/m³ in the control room, bagging room and processing area during normal operations (National Institute for Occupational Safety and Health, 1976). More recent data on occupational exposures in four manufacturing plants and during a grouting operation are shown in Table 2.

Acrylamide was not detected in personal and area air samples taken at a plant where specialty chemicals and flocculants were manufactured for paper and water treatment plants (National Institute for Occupational Safety and Health, 1982).

Table 2. Occupational exposure to acrylamide[a]

Job title	No. of samples	8-hour TWA (mg/m^3)	
		Range	Mean
Monomer operators	19	0.001-0.227	0.084
Polymer operators	27	0.001-0.181	0.045
Monomer material handlers	4	0.17-0.26	0.116
Polymer material handlers	4	0.018-0.035	0.024
Maintenance	14	0.001-0.132	0.024
Utility operators	4	0.004-0.392	0.176
Grouting operators	2	0.002-0.007	0.005

[a]Compiled by the Working Group from Hills *et al.* (1985)

(c)   Water

Commercial polyelectrolytes used as coagulants during the preparation of potable water contained less than 0.05% monomeric acrylamide. Polymers used for effluent treatment, however, contained up to 5% acrylamide (Brown *et al.*, 1982).

Acrylamide was detected at levels of <5 μg/l in both river-water and tap-water in an area where polyacrylamides were used in the treatment of potable water (Brown & Rhead, 1979). It was also detected in sewage effluent from a treatment facility at which polyacrylamides were not used and in a number of other industrial sites (Table 3).

2.3 Analysis

Selected methods for the analysis of acrylamide in various matrices are listed in Table 4.

Differential pulse polarography (DPP) can also be used to analyse for acrylamide in surface-wipe samples (McLean *et al.*, 1978) or in methanol-water extracts of polyacrylamide (Betso & McLean, 1976). In preparing samples for DPP analysis, treatment with the mixed ion-exchange resin removes interfering impurities such as acrylic acid, acrylonitrile, and sodium and potassium ions. Other substances that are reducible at or near the same polarographic potential, such as substituted acrylamides and acrylate esters, will interfere if present (Betso & McLean, 1976).

The gas chromatography/electron capture detection method for determining low levels of acrylamide in water requires conversion of acrylamide to 2,3-dibromopropionamide, preferably by an ionic reaction with acidic aqueous bromine. When interferences (of unspecified nature) were noted, the crude 2,3-dibromopropionamide was chromatographed to clean up the sample prior to analysis. Quantitative recoveries of acrylamide from spiked samples (4 μg/l) of river-water, sewage effluent and sea-water were reported (Hashimoto,

Table 3. Acrylamide concentrations in water samples

Location	Source of sample	Concentration ($\mu g/l$)	Reference
Municipal water treatment (UK)	River-water Tap-water	3.4 4.5	Brown & Rhead (1979)
Sewage works (UK)	Effluent	2.3-17.4	Brown & Rhad (1979)
Clay pit (UK)	Effluent Stream-water	16 1.2	Croll et al. (1974)
Acrylamide manufacture (UK)	Wastewater effluent Treated effluent	1100 280	Croll et al. (1974)
Pulp mill (UK)	Effluent	0.47-1.2	Croll et al. (1974)
Coal mine (UK)	Coal-washing effluent Tailings lagoon	1.8 39-42	Croll et al. (1974)
Reservoir (USA)	During polyacrylamide waterproofing	4	Jewett et al. (1978)

1976). A similar method was reported for the analysis of acrylamide (1.5-100 ng/g) in a variety of vegetable crops (Arikawa & Shiga, 1980).

A high-performance liquid chromatography/ultraviolet absorbance detection (HPLC/UV) procedure has been reported for the analysis of acrylamide in water after conversion to 2,3-dibromopropionamide. Extraction of a water sample with ethyl acetate and hexane before bromination is reported to reduce interference (Brown & Rhead, 1979). The direct HPLC/UV method for separation/analysis of residual acrylamide in polymers (Skelly & Husser, 1978) has also been used on air samples collected in impingers (water) and on surface-wipe samples.

3. Biological Data Relevant to the Evaluation of Carcinogenic Risk to Humans

3.1 Carcinogenicity studies in animals

(a) Oral administration

Mouse: In a study designed to test the activity of acrylamide as an initiator on skin, groups of 40 female Sencar mice, six to eight weeks of age, received six doses of 12.5, 25.0 or

Table 4. Methods for the analysis of acrylamide[a]

Sample matrix	Sample preparation	Assay procedure[a]	Limit of detection	Reference
Air	Collect (impinger with water); dilute (methanol); stir with ion-exchange resin to remove impurities	DPP	0.03 mg/m^3[b]	National Institute for Occupational Safety and Health (1976); McLean et al. (1978)
Water	Convert to dibromide (bromine/ potassium bromide/hydrobromic acid); decompose excess bromine (sodium thiosulphate); add sodium sulphate; extract (ethyl acetate); dry extract (sodium sulphate)	GC/EC	0.03 μg/l[c]	Hashimoto (1976)
	Convert to dibromide (bromine/ potassium bromide/hydrobromic acid); decompose excess bromine (sodium thiosulphate); add sodium sulphate; extract (ethyl acetate); dry extract (sodium sulphate)	HPLC/UV	0.2 μg/l	Brown & Rhead (1979)
Polymer	Extract (solvent and conditions determined by matrix); separate from polymer (centrifuge, decant)	HPLC/UV	0.1 mg/kg in polyacrylamide or aqueous polymer dispersions;	Husser et al. (1977)
			10 mg/kg in nonaqueous polymer dispersions;	Skelly & Husser (1978)
			4.5 mg/kg in aqueous polymer dispersions	Frind & Hensel (1984)

[a]Abbreviations: DPP, differential pulse polarography; GC/EC, gas chromatography/electron capture detection; HPLC/UV, high-performance liquid chromatography/ultraviolet absorbance detection

[b]0.5 μg/ml of impinger solvent (water)

[c]Calculated, for aqueous standard solution

50.0 mg/kg bw acrylamide (purity, >99%, determined by linked gas chromatography-mass spectrometry) dissolved in 0.2 ml distilled water by gastric intubation over a period of two weeks (total dose, 75, 150 or 300 mg/kg bw). Two weeks later, animals received thrice-weekly skin applications of 1 μg 12-O-tetradecanoylphorbol 13-acetate (TPA) in 0.2 ml acetone on the back skin for 20 weeks. Vehicle-control groups received distilled water and acetone by the same schedule. As a positive control, groups of 25 mice received a single intragastric application of 30, 100 or 300 mg/kg bw ethyl carbamate (purity, 98%) in 10% polyoxygenated vegetable oil followed by treatment with TPA as described above. Nearly all animals survived until 52 weeks (33-38 per group), at which time they were sacrificed, and all gross lesions of the skin were examined histopathologically. A significant ($p < 0.01$, Cox regression model) dose-response relationship was observed for the time of appearance of the first tumour and for the combined incidence of squamous-cell papillomas and carcinomas of the skin. Treatment-related increases in the incidence of squamous-cell carcinoma were observed: TPA alone, 0/34; acrylamide alone, 0/17; 12.5 mg/kg acrylamide/TPA, 2/35; 25 mg/kg acrylamide/TPA, 7/33; and 50 mg/kg acrylamide/TPA, 6/38 (see Table 5). The incidence of squamous-cell carcinomas in positive controls receiving 300 mg/kg bw ethyl carbamate was reported as 3/16 (Bull *et al.*, 1984).

In a lung adenoma bioassay, groups of 40 female and 40 male A/J mice, eight weeks of age, received oral doses of 6.25, 12.5 or 25.0 mg/kg bw acrylamide (purity, >99%, determined by linked gas chromatography-mass spectrometry) in 0.2 ml distilled water three times per week for eight weeks. Similar groups of mice received either oral doses of 10.5, 21.0 or 42.0 mg/kg bw ethyl carbamate (purity, 98%) in distilled water and served as positive controls or distilled water only and served as vehicle controls. Animals were sacrificed seven months after the beginning of treatment; lungs were fixed in formalin and surface adenomas were counted. Although no value was given for lung adenoma frequency, the authors reported a significant ($p < 0.01$) dose-response relationship (Bull *et al.*, 1984) (see Table 5). [The Working Group noted that survival data were not presented and that only lungs were examined.]

Rat: Groups of 90 male and 90 female Fischer 344 rats, five to six weeks of age, were administered 0, 0.01, 0.1, 0.5 or 2 mg/kg bw per day acrylamide in drinking-water for two years. The solutions were prepared twice a week from recrystallized acrylamide that was 96-99% pure with a water content of 0.4-3.8%. Groups of 10 males and 10 females were killed at six, 12 and 18 months, such that 60 animals of each sex were available for the full study. At the end of the study, 20-25% of males in each group were dead, except in the highest-dose group, in which 40% were dead; among females, 15-30% of each group were dead, except those receiving the highest dose, of which 55% died. Increased incidences of adrenal pheochromocytomas, mesotheliomas of the tunica of the testes and follicular adenomas of the thyroid were observed in males. In animals receiving 0, 0.01, 0.1, 0.5 and 2 mg/kg bw, the numbers with pheochromocytomas were: 3, 7, 7, 5 and 10 ($p < 0.05$); those with mesotheliomas of the tunica of the testes: 3, 0, 7, 11 ($p < 0.05$) and 10 ($p < 0.05$); and those with adenomas of the thyroid: 1, 0, 2, 1 and 7 ($p < 0.05$). Central nervous system tumours of glial origin, or glial proliferation suggestive of early tumours, were found in 5, 2, 0, 3 and 8 rats (not significant). In female rats, increased incidences of pituitary adenomas,

Table 5.

(A) Skin tumours initiated in Sencar mice by administration of acrylamide by various routes[a]

Total dose (mg/kg bw)	Route	TPA	Squamous-cell carcinomas/ number of animals
0	oral	+	0/34
75	oral	+	2/35
150	oral	+	7/33
300	oral	+	6/38
300	oral	−	0/17
0	intraperitoneal	+	0/35
75	intraperitoneal	+	2/38
150	intraperitoneal	+	4/36
300	intraperitoneal	+	4/35
300	intraperitoneal	−	0/17
0	topical	+	0/36
75	topical	+	1/38
150	topical	+	2/35
300	topical	+	3/34
300	topical	−	0/20

(B) Lung tumours in A/J mice after oral or intraperitoneal administration of acrylamide[a]

Total dose (mg/kg bw)	Route	Number of tumours/animal	
		Male	Female
0	oral	0.2^b	0.3^b
6.25	oral	0.5^b	0.3^b
12.5	oral	0.75^b	0.7^b
25.0	oral	1.4^b	1.3^b
0 - untreated	−	0.31	0.50
0 - vehicle	intraperitoneal	0.06	0.13
1	intraperitoneal	0.75	0.35
3	intraperitoneal	0.69	0.88
10	intraperitoneal	0.88	1.57
30	intraperitoneal	1.87	2.53

[a]From Bull *et al.* (1984)

[b]Estimated from Chart 5 in Bull *et al.* (1984)

thyroid follicular tumours, mammary adenomas and adenocarcinomas, oral-cavity papillomas, uterine adenocarcinomas and clitoral-gland adenomas were observed. In animals receiving 0, 0.01, 0.1, 0.5 and 2 mg/kg bw, the numbers with pituitary adenomas were: 25, 30, 32, 27 and 32 ($p < 0.05$); with thyroid follicular tumours: 1, 0, 1, 1 and 5 ($p < 0.05$); with mammary fibroadenomas: 10, 11, 9, 19 and 23 ($p < 0.05$); with mammary adenocarcinomas: 2, 1, 1, 2 and 6 ($p < 0.05$ by a trend test); with oral cavity papillomas: 0, 3, 2, 1 and 7 ($p < 0.05$); with adenocarcinomas of the uterus: 1, 2, 1, 0 and 5 ($p < 0.05$); and with clitoral-gland adenomas: 0, 1, 3, 4 and 5 ($p < 0.05$). The numbers of female rats with a tumour of the central nervous system of glial origin or glial proliferation suggestive of an early tumour were also increased: 1, 2, 1, 1 and 9 rats, respectively (Johnson *et al.*, 1986)

(b) Skin application

Mouse: A group of 40 female Sencar mice, six to eight weeks of age, received six topical applications of 12.5, 25.0 or 50.0 mg/kg bw acrylamide (purity, >99%, determined by linked gas chromatography-mass spectrometry) dissolved in 0.2 ml ethanol on the back skin over a period of two weeks (total dose, 75, 150 or 300 mg/kg bw), followed two weeks later by thrice-weekly applications of 1 μg TPA in 0.2 ml acetone for 20 weeks. Vehicle-control mice were treated with ethanol and acetone alone. Positive-control groups of 25 mice received a single application of 30, 100 or 300 mg/kg bw ethyl carbamate (purity, 98%) dissolved in acetone on the back skin, followed two weeks later by treatment with TPA as described above. Nearly all animals survived until 52 weeks (34-38 per group), at which time they were sacrificed, and all gross lesions of the skin were examined histopathologically. A significant ($p < 0.01$, Cox regression model) dose-response relationship was seen for the time of appearance of the first tumour and for the combined incidence of squamous-cell papillomas and carcinomas of the skin. The incidences of squamous-cell carcinomas were: TPA alone, 0/36; low-dose, 1/38; mid-dose, 2/35; and high-dose, 3/34. No skin tumour was seen in the absence of TPA promotion (see Table 5) (Bull *et al.*, 1984). [The Working Group noted that the incidence of tumours produced in the positive controls was not given.]

(c) Intraperitoneal administration

Mouse: Groups of 40 female Sencar mice, six to eight weeks of age, were given six intraperitoneal injections of 12.5, 25.0 or 50.0 mg/kg bw acrylamide (purity, >99%, determined by linked gas chromatography-mass spectrometry) dissolved in 0.2 ml distilled water over a period of two weeks (total dose, 75, 150 or 300 mg/kg bw), followed two weeks later by thrice-weekly topical applications 1 μg TPA in 0.2 ml acetone to the back skin for 20 weeks. A vehicle-control group received distilled water and acetone by the same schedule. Positive-control groups of 25 mice were injected intraperitoneally with single doses of 30, 100 or 300 mg/kg bw ethyl carbamate (purity, 98%), followed by treatment with TPA as described above. Nearly all animals survived until 52 weeks (35-38 per group), at which time they were sacrificed, and all gross lesions of the skin were examined histopathologically. A significant ($p < 0.01$, Cox regression model) dose-response relationship was observed for the time of appearance of the first tumour and for the combined incidence of squamous-cell papillomas and carcinomas of the skin. The incidences of squamous-cell carcinomas were:

TPA alone, 0/35; low-dose, 2/38; mid-dose, 4/36; and high-dose, 4/35. No skin tumour was seen in the absence of TPA promotion (see Table 5) (Bull *et al.*, 1984). [The Working Group noted that the incidence of tumours produced in the positive control group was not reported.]

In a lung adenoma bioassay, groups of 16 female and 16 male A/J mice, eight weeks of age, received thrice-weekly intraperitoneal injections of 1, 3, 10, 30 or 60 mg/kg bw acrylamide (purity, >99%, determined by linked gas chromatography-mass spectrometry) dissolved in distilled water for eight weeks. Control groups were either untreated, injected with distilled water (vehicle controls) or received a single intraperitoneal injection of 500 or 1000 mg/kg bw ethyl carbamate (purity, 98%) (positive controls). The group treated with 60 mg/kg bw acrylamide was abandoned due to the appearance of peripheral neuropathy and poor survival. Animals in all other groups survived until six months after the beginning of treatment, at which time they were sacrificed, their lungs were fixed and the surface adenomas were counted. The incidences of lung adenomas were: males — untreated controls, 5/16; vehicle controls, 2/16; 1 mg, 8/16; 3 mg, 6/16; 10 mg, 10/17; and 30 mg, 14/15; females — untreated controls, 7/14; vehicle controls, 1/15; 1 mg, 6/17; 3 mg, 9/17; 10 mg, 11/14; and 30 mg, 14/15. In comparison, all 56 of the male and female positive controls treated with ethyl carbamate developed lung adenomas. The average number of lung adenomas/mouse in the untreated controls, vehicle controls, 1-mg, 3-mg, 10-mg and 30-mg groups was: (males) 0.31, 0.06, 0.75, 0.69, 0.88 and 1.87; (females) 0.5, 0.13, 0.35, 0.88, 1.57 and 2.53, respectively. Acrylamide treatment increased the yield of lung adenomas in animals of each sex. Significant dose-response relationships ($p < 0.01$) were found when either animals with tumours or multiplicity of tumours were tested in the model analysis of Cox (see Table 5) (Bull *et al.*, 1984).

3.2   Other relevant biological data

A review on the toxicity of acrylamide was published recently (WHO, 1985).

(a)   Experimental systems

Toxic effects

Oral LD_{50} values for acrylamide have been reported to range from 100-170 mg/kg bw in various strains of mice and from 120-250 mg/kg bw in various strains of rats; the subcutaneous LD_{50} in guinea-pigs was 170 mg/kg bw (Ghiringhelli, 1956; Hamblin, 1956; Fullerton & Barnes, 1966; Paulet & Vidal, 1975; Tilson & Cabe, 1979; Hashimoto *et al.*, 1981). Intraperitoneal LD_{50} values in various strains of rat ranged from 90-220 mg/kg bw (Druckrey *et al.*, 1953; Paulet & Vidal, 1975; Pryor *et al.*, 1983). The dermal LD_{50} in rats was 400 mg/kg bw (Novikova, 1979).

A monkey [strain unspecified] given two intraperitoneal injections of 100 mg/kg bw acrylamide died after three days. Gross examination revealed congested lungs and kidneys and necrosis of the liver. Microscopic examination of the liver revealed congestion of the sinusoids with fatty degeneration and necrosis. The kidneys showed degeneration of the convoluted tubular epithelium and glomerular degeneration (McCollister *et al.*, 1964).

Acrylamide is well established as a cumulative neurotoxin, and reviews on its neurotoxicity have been published (Spencer & Schaumburg, 1974; National Institute for Occupational Safety and Health, 1976; Hashimoto, 1980). Acrylamide causes predominantly peripheral neuropathy in most experimental animals, including non-human primates. This effect is produced in most animal species with repeated doses of 10-50 mg/kg bw per day, irrespective of the route of administration, including dermal application. In some instances, when acrylamide administration is discontinued, the animals recover completely and nerve conduction parameters return to normal (Hamblin, 1956; Kuperman, 1958; McCollister *et al.*, 1964; Fullerton & Barnes, 1966; Leswing & Ribelin, 1969; Hopkins, 1970; Kaplan & Murphy, 1972; Spencer & Schaumburg, 1974; Guirguis, 1983).

The visual system was also found to be a target of acrylamide. Impairments of visual function (measured using behavioural and electrophysiological techniques) were observed in female Macaque monkeys treated with 10 mg/kg bw per day for five days a week for six to ten weeks; dosing was continued until each animal was markedly ataxic (Merigan *et al.*, 1982).

Male ddY mice receiving oral doses of 35 mg/kg (0.5 mmol/kg) bw acrylamide twice weekly for eight weeks developed testicular atrophy and degeneration of the germinal epithelium. Sertoli and interstitial cells did not appear to be affected by acrylamide treatment. Neurotoxic signs were observed in treated mice; when mice were treated by concurrent intraperitoneal injection of phenobarbital as a metabolic initiator, the neurotoxic signs were significantly reduced and testicular toxicity was prevented, probably due to accelerated detoxification (Hashimoto *et al.*, 1981). Testicular atrophy was also observed in rats (Burek *et al.*, 1980).

Other subchronic effects of acrylamide, probably secondary to nerve degeneration, include atrophy of skeletal muscles and distension of the urinary bladder in male and female Fischer 344 rats after administration of 20 mg/kg bw per day for three months in the drinking-water (Burek *et al.*, 1980).

Effects on reproduction and prenatal toxicity

When fertilized chicken eggs were injected with 0.03-0.6 mg acrylamide on day 5, 6 or 7 of incubation, increased embryonic mortality and leg deformities were observed in hatched chicks (Parker *et al.*, 1978). In contrast, mortality was elevated but no malformation occurred when eggs were injected on day 3 of incubation with 0.007, 0.07 or 0.7 mg (0.1, 1.0 or 10.0 μmol) (Kankaanpää *et al.*, 1979).

Reduced content of striatal dopamine receptors was seen in 14- but not in 21-day-old neonates after oral administration of 20 mg/kg bw acrylamide per day to pregnant Fischer 344 rats on days 7-16 of gestation (Agrawal & Squibb, 1981). Previously, these investigators had observed an increased content of dopamine receptors in the corpus striatum of acrylamide-treated adult rats (Agrawal *et al.*, 1981).

Ikeda *et al.* (1983) injected near-term pregnant Osborne-Mendel rats, New Zealand rabbits, beagle dogs and pigs intravenously with 5 or 10 mg/kg bw ^{14}C-acrylamide and demonstrated that the radioactivity crossed the placenta in all four species within 1-2 h. Edwards (1976) injected pregnant Porton rats intravenously with acrylamide on day 9 of gestation and detected the compound in foetal tissue 1 h later. He also conducted a limited teratology study (six rats received 400 mg/kg in the diet on days 1-21 of gestation) and found no evidence of embryotoxicity or teratogenicity. Foetal toxicity was suggested by reduced foetal body weight, but frank maternal toxicity was also demonstrated by ataxia and reduced food consumption. Another group of eight rats received 200 mg/kg acrylamide in the diet from day 1 of gestation through parturition, and their offspring were observed up to six weeks of age. Although the mothers exhibited slightly abnormal gaits, their offspring had normal postnatal weight gain and had no gait abnormalities. After intravenous injection of four rats with 100 mg/kg bw on day 9 of gestation, their offspring developed normal righting reflexes and, at six weeks of age, showed no gross or microscopic abnormalities in the brain, spinal cord or sciatic nerve. [The Working Group noted that, while these results suggest that maternally neurotoxic doses of acrylamide are not necessarily neurotoxic to the foetus, group sizes in this series of studies were inadequate to evaluate the teratogenicity of acrylamide.]

Absorption, distribution, excretion and metabolism

When applied to rabbits as an aqueous solution (10-30%), acrylamide penetrated the skin rapidly and appeared in the blood both as the free compound and bound to proteins (Hashimoto & Ando, 1975).

Radioautographic investigation of the distribution of acrylamide in mice showed accumulation in the blood, spleen, liver, kidney, gut epithelium and salivary glands. The distal part of the sciatic nerve appeared to have accumulated acrylamide selectively (Ando, 1979).

A dose of 10 mg/kg bw [2,3-^{14}C]-acrylamide administered orally to Fischer 344 rats was rapidly distributed (as total radioactivity) throughout the body. The concentration of radioactivity in neural tissue did not differ significantly from that in non-neural tissues and the authors concluded that the relative distribution of the compound does not account for its neurotoxic activity. Radioactivity was associated with erythrocytes, and the whole-blood concentration reached a plateau after 1 h and remained constant for several days, although the quantity of radioactivity in plasma declined steadily. Total tissue radioactivity decreased following biphasic kinetics: the first component had a half-life of less than 5 h and the second one of approximately eight days. Within 24 h, 62% of the dose was excreted in urine (acrylamide and/or its metabolites) and 71% within seven days; approximately 15% of the dose appeared in the bile (as total radioactivity) within 6 h; however, after seven days only 6% had been excreted in the faeces. It was concluded that acrylamide must undergo enterohepatic circulation. No radioactivity was recovered in expired CO_2. The elimination of unchanged acrylamide from whole blood in rats was found to be monophasic, with an elimination half-life of 1.7 h (Miller *et al.*, 1982). In Porton strain rats that received an intravenous injection of 100 mg/kg bw, an elimination half-life of 1.9 h was reported (Edwards, 1975).

When Porton strain albino rats were injected intravenously with 100 mg/kg bw [1-^{14}C]-acrylamide, urinary excretion of radioactivity was very rapid: 40% of the dose was excreted over the first day and 65% by day 4. Within the first 8 h, 6% of the radioactivity was exhaled as CO_2, and this increased only slightly over 24 h, indicating that a minor pathway of acrylamide metabolism exists. It was also shown that acrylamide binds covalently to haemoglobin *in vitro* (Hashimoto & Aldridge, 1970).

Acrylamide reacts with glutathione both enzymatically and nonenzymatically and inhibits glutathione-S-transferase in rat liver and brain (Dixit *et al.*, 1981) and in mouse liver and skin (Mukhtar *et al.*, 1981). It may therefore counteract its own detoxification (Dixit *et al.*, 1981). It also inhibits aryl hydrocarbon hydroxylase in mouse skin and liver (Mukhtar *et al.*, 1981). Administration of acrylamide to rats resulted in biliary excretion of glutathione conjugates, accompanied by significant depletion of hepatic glutathione (Edwards, 1975). Prior depletion of glutathione led to earlier onset of acrylamide neurotoxicity (Dixit *et al.*, 1980). The enzymatic conjugation of acrylamide with glutathione increased after induction with phenobarbital or *trans*-stilbene oxide (Dixit *et al.*, 1981), which is consistent with the finding that liver enzyme inducers reduced the neurotoxic effects of acrylamide in rats (Kaplan *et al.*, 1973) and testicular atrophy in mice (Hashimoto *et al.*, 1981).

The presence of a reactive vinyl group in acrylamide enables it to react as a strong electrophile with nucleophilic groups. The proposed metabolic pathways are as follows: acrylamide reacts with glutathione to form S-β-propionamide glutathione conjugate which is excreted in the urine as cysteine or N-acetylcysteine derivatives. The major urinary metabolite (accounting for 48% of the excreted dose) is N-acetylcysteine-S-β-propionamide (Langvardt *et al.*, 1979; Dixit *et al.*, 1982; Miller *et al.*, 1982). Unidentified metabolites, not containing sulphur atoms, were also excreted in urine (Miller *et al.*, 1982).

Acrylamide was not metabolized *in vitro* by mouse-liver microsomes (Tanii & Hashimoto, 1981).

Mutagenicity and other short-term tests

In standard plate and liquid preincubation assays, acrylamide (tested at up to 3000 μg/plate) was not mutagenic to *Salmonella typhimurium* TA1535, TA1537, TA1538, TA98 or TA100 in the presence or absence of a metabolic system (S9) from Aroclor-induced rats or hamsters (Lijinsky & Andrews, 1980; Bull *et al.*, 1984).

A diet containing 500 mg/kg acrylamide fed to male ddY mice for three weeks increased the frequency of chromatid exchanges and chromosome breaks in spermatogonia and induced polyploidy and aneuploidy in both bone-marrow and spermatogonial cells. There was no increase in the number of sister chromatid exchanges in bone-marrow or spermatogonial cells or of chromosomal aberrations in bone-marrow cells following intraperitoneal administration of 100, 150 or 200 mg/kg bw, but these doses caused severe reduction in mitotic spermatogonia. Dietary and parenteral administration of acrylamide induced chain-quadrivalents, ring-quadrivalents, fragments and univalents in primary spermatocytes (Shiraishi, 1978).

(b) Humans

Toxic effects

Monomeric acrylamide is a primary skin and respiratory irritant and neurotoxin with an affinity for the peripheral ends of the spinal nerves in the extremities (Table 6). Acrylamide

Table 6. Reports on toxic effects of acrylamide

Reference	No. of cases	Toxicity (acute, chronic)
Auld & Bedwell (1967)	1	Neurotoxic effects; reversible
Garland & Patterson (1967)	6	Peripheral neuropathy; two cases reversible
Morviller (1969)	4	'Light intoxications', dermal desquamation, hyperhidrosis, weight loss, signs of polyneuritis and ataxia, ocular 'irritation'; reversible
Graveleau et al. (1970)	1	Desquamations (hands), hyperhidrosis (hands and feet), paraesthesias, ataxia
Takahashi et al. (1971)	15	Absence of deep reflexes, decreased sensory functions, ataxia and gastrointestinal symptoms (subjective)
Cavigneaux & Cabasson (1972)	1	Paraesthesias, sensomotor defects, polyneuritis
Igisu et al. (1975)	5	Encephaloneuropathy (including mental disturbances), coughing, rhinorrhoea, ataxia, reduced sensory conduction velocity; reversible
Davenport et al. (1976)	1	Peripheral neuropathy, ataxia, hyperhidrosis (hands and feet); reversible
Kesson et al. (1977)	6	Hyperhidrosis, desquamation, sensorial disturbances; residual neurological problems persisted in the two eldest persons
Mapp et al. (1977)	5	Dermal erythema and desquamations, peripheral neuropathy, encephaloneuropathy, dyspnoea, impotence

intoxication in the workplace is due mainly to repetitive, daily, local dermal contact (Garland & Patterson, 1967; Spencer & Schaumburg, 1975). It induces axonal neuropathy characterized by dying-back degeneration (Spencer & Schaumburg, 1975; Spencer et al., 1978).

The clinical signs of intoxication with acrylamide have been summarized by Spencer and Schaumburg (1975) and Hashimoto (1980). They include generalized fatigue, foot weakness, sensory changes, including numbness of the limbs and tingling of the fingers, as well as impairment of fine motor activities and, later, motor paralysis. In addition to signs of peripheral neuropathy, some affected individuals develop signs of central nervous system damage such as tremor, an ataxic gait or mild organic mental syndrome (Garland & Patterson, 1967; Morviller, 1969; Igisu et al., 1975; Spencer & Schaumburg, 1975). If exposure is interrupted, the neuropathy is often reversible, but recovery is slow.

The doses toxic to humans have not been well defined.

Effects on reproduction and prenatal toxicity

No data were available to the Working Group.

Absorption, distribution, excretion and metabolism

No data were available to the Working Group.

Mutagenicity and chromosomal effects

No data were available to the Working Group.

3.3 Case reports and epidemiological studies of carcinogenicity to humans

No data were available to the Working Group.

4. Summary of Data Reported and Evaluation

4.1 Exposure data

Acrylamide has been available commercially since 1954. Its major use is in the production of polyacrylamides for water treatment. Occupational exposure to acrylamide occurs in the manufacture of the monomer and polymers. Acrylamide has been detected in drinking-water samples.

4.2 Experimental data

Acrylamide showed initiating activity to the skin in female mice after oral, topical or intraperitoneal administration followed by chronic topical treatment with 12-*O*-tetra-decanoylphorbol 13-acetate. Acrylamide increased both the incidence and multiplicity of lung adenomas in mice of both sexes following intragastric or intraperitoneal administration.

Acrylamide was tested in rats by administration in the drinking-water. It increased the incidences of benign or malignant neoplasms at several sites including thyroid gland, mammary gland, scrotum, oral cavity and adrenal gland.

Acrylamide has not been adequately tested for reproductive effects or prenatal toxicity in experimental animals.

Acrylamide was not mutagenic to *Salmonella typhimurium* in the presence or absence of an exogenous metabolic system. It induced chromatid exchanges and chromosomal breaks in germ cells and aneuploidy and polyploidy in spermatogonial and bone-marrow cells following its oral administration to male mice.

Overall assessment of data from short-term tests: Acrylamide[a]

	Genetic activity			Cell transformation
	DNA damage	Mutation	Chromosomal effects	
Prokaryotes		−		
Fungi/ Green plants				
Insects				
Mammalian cells (*in vitro*)				
Mammals (*in vivo*)			+	
Humans (*in vivo*)				
Degree of evidence in short-term tests for genetic activity: **Inadequate**				Cell transformation: No data

[a]The groups into which the table is divided and the symbols '+', '−' and '?' are defined on pp. 19-20 of the Preamble; the degrees of evidence are defined on pp. 20-21.

4.3 Human data

Acrylamide is a potent neurotoxin. No data were available to evaluate the reproductive effects or prenatal toxicity of acrylamide to humans.

No case report or epidemiological study was available to evaluate the carcinogenicity of acrylamide to humans.

4.4 Evaluation[1]

There is *sufficient evidence*[2] for the carcinogenicity of acrylamide to experimental animals.

No data on humans were available.

---

[1]For definition of the italicized term, see Preamble, p. 18.

[2]In the absence of adequate data in humans, it is reasonable, for practical purposes, to regard chemicals for which there is sufficient evidence of carcinogenicity in animals as if they represented a carcinogenic risk to humans.

5. References

Agrawal, A.K. & Squibb, R.E. (1981) Effects of acrylamide given during gestation on dopamine receptor binding in rat pups. *Toxicol. Lett.*, *7*, 233-238

Agrawal, A.K., Squibb, R.E. & Bondy, S.C. (1981) The effects of acrylamide treatment upon the dopamine receptor. *Toxicol. appl. Pharmacol.*, *58*, 89-99

American Conference of Governmental Industrial Hygienists (1984) *Threshold Limit Values for Chemical Substances and Physical Agents in the Work Environment and Biological Exposure Indices with Intended Changes for 1984-1985*, Cincinnati, OH, p. 9

American Conference of Governmental Industrial Hygienists (1985) *Threshold Limit Values for Chemical Substances and Physical Agents in the Work Environment and Biological Exposure Indices with Intended Changes for 1985-1986*, Cincinnati, OH, p. 9

American Cyanamid Co. (1969) *Chemistry of Acrylamide*, Wayne, NJ

American Cyanamid Co. (1982) *Cyanamer® acrylamides, for the Processing Industries*, Wayne, NJ

Ando, K. (1979) Distribution of acrylamide in mouse after repeated doses. *Arch. Hig. Rada. Toksikol.*, *30*, 417-425

Anon. (1984) Biocatalysts for acrylamide. *Chem. Week*, *134*, 30

Anon. (1985) Chemical profile: Acrylamide. *Chem. Mark. Rep.*, *227*, 62

Arbetarskyddsstyrelsens Författningssamling (National Swedish Board of Occupational Safety and Health) (1984) *Hygiene Limit Values (AFS 1984:5)* (Swed.), Stockholm, p. 10

Arikawa, A. & Shiga, M. (1980) Determination of trace acrylamide in crops by gas chromatography (Jpn.). *Bunseki Kagaku*, *29*, T33-T39

Auld, R.B. & Bedwell, S.F. (1967) Peripheral neuropathy with sympathetic overactivity from industrial contact with acrylamide. *Can. med. Assoc. J.*, *96*, 652-654

Betso, S.R. & McLean, J.D. (1976) Determination of acrylamide monomer by differential pulse polarography. *Anal. Chem.*, *48*, 766-770

Bikales, N.M. (1970) *Acrylamide and related amides*. In: Leonard, E.C., ed., *Vinyl and Diene Monomers*, Part 1, New York, Wiley Interscience, pp. 81-104

Brown, L. & Rhead, M. (1979) Liquid chromatographic determination of acrylamide monomer in natural and polluted aqueous environments. *Analyst*, *104*, 391-399

Brown, L., Rhead, M.H. & Bancroft, K.C.C. (1982) Rapid screening technique utilizing high-performance liquid chromatography for assessing acrylamide contamination in effluents. *Analyst*, *107*, 749-754

Buckingham, J., ed. (1982) *Dictionary of Organic Compounds*, 5th ed., Vol. 5, New York, Chapman and Hall, pp. 4784-4785

Bull, R.J., Robinson, M., Laurie, R.D., Stoner, G.D., Greisiger, E., Meier, J.R. & Stober, J. (1984) Carcinogenic effects of acrylamide in SENCAR and A/J mice. *Cancer Res.*, *44*, 107-111

Burek, J.D., Albee, R.R., Beyer, J.E., Bell, T.J., Carreon, R.M., Morden, D.C., Wade, C.E., Hermann, E.A. & Gorzinski, S.J. (1980) Subchronic toxicity of acrylamide administered to rats in the drinking water followed by up to 144 days of recovery. *J. environ. Pathol. Toxicol.*, *4*, 157-182

Cavigneaux, A. & Cabasson, G.B. (1972) Acrylamide poisoning (Fr.). *Arch. Mal. prof. Méd. Trav. Séc. soc.*, *33*, 115-116

Croll, B.T., Arkell, G.M. & Hodge, R.P.J. (1974) Residues of acrylamide in water. *Water Res.*, *8*, 989-993

Davenport, J.G., Farrell, D.F. & Sumi, S.M. (1976) 'Giant axonal neuropathy' caused by industrial chemicals: Neurofilamentous axonal masses in man. *Neurology*, *26*, 919-923

Deutsches Forschungsgemeinschaft (1984) *Maximal Concentrations in the Workplace and Biological Occupational Limit Values* (Ger.), Part XX, Weinheim, Verlag Chemie GmbH, p. 15

Dixit, R., Husain, R., Seth, P.K. & Mukhtar, H. (1980) Effects of diethyl maleate an acrylamide induced neuropathy in rats. *Toxicol. Lett.*, *6*, 417-421

Dixit, R., Mukhtar, H., Seth, P.K. & Murti, C.R.K. (1981) Conjugation of acrylamide with glutathione catalysed by glutathione-*S*-transferases of rat liver and brain. *Biochem. Pharmacol.*, *30*, 1739-1744

Dixit, R., Seth, P.K. & Mukhtar, H. (1982) Metabolism of acrylamide into urinary mercapturic acid and cysteine conjugates in rats. *Drug Metab. Disposition*, *10*, 196-197

Druckrey, H., Cronsbruch, U. & Schmähl, D. (1953) Reactions of monomeric acrylamide on proteins (Ger.). *Z. Naturforsch.*, *8b*, 145-150

Edwards, P.M. (1975) The distribution and metabolism of acrylamide and its neurotoxic analogues in rats. *Biochem. Pharmacol.*, *24*, 1277-1282

Edwards, P.M. (1976) The insensitivity of the developing rat foetus to the toxic effects of acrylamide. *Chem.-biol. Interactions*, *12*, 13-18

Frind, H. & Hensel, R. (1984) Determination of monomeric acrylamide in water soluble polymers (Ger.). *Fresenius Z. anal. Chem.*, *318*, 335-338

Fullerton, P.M. & Barnes, J.M. (1966) Peripheral neuropathy in rats produced by acrylamide. *Br. J. ind. Med.*, *23*, 210-221

Garland, T.O. & Patterson, M.W. (1967) Six cases of acrylamide poisoning. *Br. med. J.*, *iv*, 134-138

Ghiringhelli, L. (1956) Comparative studies on the toxicity of some nitriles and amides (Ital.). *Med. Lav.*, *47*, 192-199

Grasselli, J.G. & Ritchey, W.M., eds (1975) *CRC Atlas of Spectral Data and Physical Constants for Organic Compounds*, Vol. 4, Cleveland, OH, CRC Press, p. 309

Graveleau, J., Loirat, P. & Nusinovici, V. (1970) Acrylamide polyneuritis (Fr.). *Rev. Neurol.*, *123*, 62-65

Guirguis, S. (1983) *Acrylamide and acrylonitrile*. In: Rom, W.N., ed., *Environmental and Occupational Medicine*, Boston, MA, Little, Brown and Co., pp. 603-607

Hamblin, D.O. (1956) *The Toxicity of Acrylamide. A Preliminary Report*, Paris, Société d'Etudes pour le Développement économique et social, pp. 195-199

Hashimoto, A. (1976) Improved method for the determination of acrylamide monomer in water by means of gas-liquid chromatography with an electron-capture detector. *Analyst*, *101*, 932-938

Hashimoto, K. (1980) The toxicity of acrylamide (Jpn.). *Jpn. J. ind. Health*, *22*, 233-248

Hashimoto, K. & Aldridge, W.N. (1970) Biochemical studies on acrylamide, a neurotoxic agent. *Biochem. Pharmacol.*, *19*, 2591-2604

Hashimoto, K. & Ando, K. (1975) *Studies on the percutaneous absorbtion of acrylamide* (Abstract). In: McCallum, R.I., ed., *Proceedings of XVIII International Congress on Occupational Health, Brighton, UK*, London, Permanent Commission and International Association on Occupational Health, p. 453

Hashimoto, K., Sakamoto, J. & Tanii, H. (1981) Neurotoxicity of acrylamide and related compounds and their effects on male gonads in mice. *Arch. Toxicol.*, *47*, 179-189

Hawley, G.G., ed. (1981) *The Condensed Chemical Dictionary*, 10th ed., New York, Van Nostrand Reinhold Co., p. 16

Health and Safety Executive (1985) *Occupational Exposure Limits 1985 (Guidance Note EH 40/85)*, London, Her Majesty's Stationery Office, p. 7

Hills, B., Greife, A., Fajen, J., Wennberg, P. & Reeve, G. (1985) *Industrial Hygiene Report In-Depth Study*, Cincinnati, OH, National Institute for Occupational Safety and Health

Hopkins, A. (1970) The effect of acrylamide on the peripheral nervous system of the baboon. *J. Neurol. Neurosurg. Psychiatr.*, *33*, 805-816

Husser, E.R., Stehl, R.H., Price, D.R. & DeLap, R.A. (1977) Liquid chromatographic determination of residual acrylamide monomer in aqueous and nonaqueous dispersed phase polymeric systems. *Anal. Chem.*, *49*, 154-158

Igisu, H., Goto, I., Kawamaura, Y., Kato, M., Izumi, K. & Kuroiwa, Y. (1975) Acrylamide encephaloneuropathy due to well water pollution. *J. Neurol. Neurosurg. Psychiatr.*, *38*, 581-584

Ikeda, G.J., Miller, E., Sapienza, P.P., Michel, T.C., King, M.T., Turner, V.A., Blumenthal, H., Jackson, W.E., III & Levin, S. (1983) Distribution of ^{14}C-labelled acrylamide and betaine in foetuses of rats, rabbits, beagle dogs, and miniature pigs. *Food chem. Toxicol.*, *21*, 49-58

Institut National de Recherche et de Sécurité (1984) *Limit Values for Concentrations of Toxic Substances in Air at Working Places (Cahiers de Notes Documentaires No. 114)* (Fr.), Paris, p. 66

International Labour Office (1980) *Occupational Exposure Limits for Airborne Toxic Substances, a Tabular Compilation of Values from Selected Countries*, 2nd (rev.) ed. (*Occupational Safety and Health Series No. 37*), Geneva, pp. 36-37

Japan Ministry of Labour (1984) Guideline for establishing adequate supervision of work environment in the workplace of airborne toxic substances. *Kihatsuno, 69*

Jewett, G.L., Bell, D.R. & Beafore, F.J. (1978) *Determination of acrylamide in a potable water reservoir during a clay/polymer soil-sealing treatment.* In: *Proceedings of 175th American Chemical Society National Meeting, Anaheim, CA, March 12-17, 1978* (Abstract No. 82), Baltimore, MD, Port City Press

Johnson, K.A., Gorzinski, S.J., Bodner, K.M., Campbell, R.A., Wolf, C.H., Friedman, M.A. & Mast, R.W. (1986) Chronic toxicity and oncogenicity study on acrylamide incorporated in the drinking water of Fischer 344 rats. *Toxicol. appl. Pharmacol.* (in press)

Kankaanpää, J., Elovaara, E., Hemminki, K. & Vainio, H. (1979) Embryotoxicity of acrolein, acrylonitrile and acrylamide in developing chick embryos. *Toxicol. Lett., 4*, 93-96

Kaplan, M.L. & Murphy, S.D. (1972) Effects of acrylamid on rotarod performance and sciatic nerve β-glucuronidase activity of rats. *Toxicol. appl. Pharmacol., 22*, 259-268

Kaplan, M.L., Murphy, S.D. & Gilles, F.H. (1973) Modification of acrylamide neuropathy in rats by selected factors. *Toxicol. appl. Pharmacol., 24*, 564-579

Kesson, C.M., Baird, A.W. & Lawson, D.H. (1977) Acrylamide poisoning. *Postgrad. med. J., 53*, 16-17

Kuperman, A.S. (1958) Effects of acrylamide on the central nervous system of the cat. *J. Pharmacol. exp. Ther., 123*, 180-192

Langvardt, P.W., Putzig, C.L., Young, J.D. & Braun, W.H. (1979) Isolation and identification of urinary metabolites of vinyl-type compounds: Application to metabolites of acrylonitrile and acrylamide (Abstract No. 323). *Toxicol. appl. Pharmacol., 48*, A161

Leswing, R.J. & Ribelin, W.E. (1969) Physiologic and pathologic changes in acrylamide neuropathy. *Arch. environ. Health, 18*, 22-29

Lijinsky, W. & Andrews, A.W. (1980) Mutagenicity of vinyl compounds in *Salmonella typhimurium. Teratog. Carcinog. Mutagenesis, 1*, 259-267

MacWilliams, D.C. (1978) *Acrylamide.* In: Mark, H.F., Othmer, D.F., Overberger, C.G. & Seaborg, G.T., eds, *Kirk-Othmer Encyclopedia of Chemical Technology*, 3rd ed., Vol. 1, New York, John Wiley & Sons, pp. 298-311

Mallevialle, J., Bruchet, A. & Fiessinger, F. (1984) How safe are organic polymers in water treatment? *J. Am. Water Works Assoc., 76*, 87-93

Mannsville Chemical Products Corp. (1982) *Acrylamide* (*Chemical Products Synopsis*), Cortland, NY

Mapp, C., Mazzotta, M., Bartolucci, G.B. & Fabbri, L. (1977) Neuropathy with acrylamide: First observations in Italy (Ital.). *Med. Lav., 68*, 1-12

McCollister, D.D., Oyen, F. & Rowe, V.K. (1964) Toxicology of acrylamide. *Toxicol. appl. Pharmacol, 6*, 172-181

McLean, J.D., Mann, J.R. & Jacoby, J.A. (1978) A monitoring method for the determination of acrylamide in an industrial environment. *Am. ind. Hyg. Assoc. J., 39*, 247-250

Merigan, W.H., Barkdoll, E. & Maurissen, J.P.J. (1982) Acrylamide-induced visual impairment in primates. *Toxicol. appl. Pharmacol., 62*, 342-345

Miller, M.J., Carter, D.E. & Sipes, I.G. (1982) Pharmacokinetics of acrylamide in Fisher-344 rats. *Toxicol. appl. Pharmacol., 63*, 36-44

Ministry of Housing and Local Government (1969) New chemicals for water treatment. *Water Treat. Exam., 18*, 90-91

Morviller, P. (1969) On a little-known industrial toxin in France: Acrylamide (Fr.). *Arch. Mal. prof. Méd. Trav. Séc. soc., 30*, 527-530

Mukhtar, H., Dixit, R. & Seth, P.K. (1981) Reduction in cutaneous and hepatic glutathione contents, glutathione *S*-transferase and aryl hydrocarbon hydroxylase activities following topical application of acrylamide to mouse. *Toxicol. Lett., 9*, 153-156

National Institute for Occupational Safety and Health (1976) *Criteria for a Recommended Standard for Occupational Exposure to Acrylamide* (*DHEW (NIOSH) Pub. No. 77-112*), Washington DC, US Department of Health, Education, and Welfare

National Institute for Occupational Safety and Health (1982) *Health Hazard Evaluation Report. American Cyanamid Company, Kalamazoo, MI* (*NIOSH Report No. HETA-80-190-1135*), Washington DC, US Department of Health, Education, and Welfare

NIH/EPA Chemical Information System (1983) *Carbon-13 NMR Spectral Search System, Mass Spectral Search System,* and *Infrared Spectral Search System*, Arlington, VA, Information Consultants

Novikova, E.E. (1979) Toxic effect of acrylamide entering through skin surfaces (Russ.). *Gig. Sanit., 10*, 73-74

Parker, R.D.R., Sharma, R.P. & Obersteiner, E.J. (1978) Acrylamide toxicity in developing chick embryo (Abstract No. 522). *Pharmacologist, 20*, 249

Paulet, G. & Vidal (1975) On the toxicity of some acrylic and methacrylic esters, acrylamide and polyacrylamides (Fr.). *Arch. Mal. prof. Méd. Trav. Séc. soc., 36*, 58-60

Pryor, G.T., Uyeno, E.T., Tilson, H.A. & Mitchell, C.L. (1983) Assessment of chemicals using a battery of neurobehavioral tests: A comparative study. *Neurobehav. Toxicol. Teratol., 5*, 91-117

Sadtler Research Laboratories (1980) *The Sadtler Standard Spectra Collection, Cumulative Index*, Philadelphia, PA

Sax, N.I. (1984) *Dangerous Properties of Industrial Materials*, 6th ed., New York, Van Nostrand Reinhold Co., pp. 128-129

Shiraishi, Y. (1978) Chromosome aberrations induced by monomeric acrylamide in bone marrow and germ cells of mice. *Mutat. Res., 57*, 313-324

Skelly, N.E. & Husser, E.R. (1978) Determination of acrylamide monomer in poly-acrylamide and in environmental samples by high performance liquid chromatography. *Anal. Chem., 50*, 1959-1962

Spencer, P.S. & Schaumburg, H.H. (1974) A review of acrylamide neurotoxicity. Part II. Experimental animal neurotoxicity and pathologic mechanisms. *Can. J. neurol. Sci., 1*, 152-169

Spencer, P.S. & Schaumburg, H.H. (1975) Nervous system degeneration produced by acrylamide monomer. *Environ. Health Perspect., 11*, 129-133

Spencer, P.S., Sabri, M.I., Schaumburg, H.H. & Morre, C.L. (1978) Does a defect of energy metabolism in the nerve fiber underlie axonal degeneration in polyneuropathies? *Ann. Neurol., 5*, 501-507

Takahashi, M., Ohara, T. & Hashimoto, K. (1971) Electrophysiological study of nerve injuries in workers handling acrylamide. *Int. Arch. Arbeitsmed., 28*, 1-11

Tanii, H. & Hashimoto, K. (1981) Studies on in vitro metabolism of acrylamide and related compounds. *Arch. Toxicol., 48*, 157-166

Tilson, H.A. & Cabe, P.A. (1979) The effects of acrylamide given acutely or in repeated doses on fore- and hindlimb function of rats. *Toxicol. appl. Pharm., 47*, 253-260

Työsuojeluhallitus (National Finnish Board of Occupational Safety and Health) (1981) *Airborne Contaminants in the Workplace (Safety Bull. 3)* (Finn.), Tampere, p. 7

US Environmental Protection Agency (1980) *TSCA Chemical Assessment Series. Assessment of Testing Needs — Acrylamide (EPA Report No. 560/11-80-016)*, Washington DC, Office of Pesticides and Toxic Substances

US Environmental Protection Agency (1984) Protection of environment. *US Code Fed. Regul., Title 40*, Part 261.33, p. 361

US Food and Drug Administration (1984) Food and drugs. *US Code Fed. Regul., Title 21*, Parts 172.255, 173.310, 173.315, 175.105, 176.110, pp. 35-36, 115-117, 132, 163

US International Trade Commission (1984) *Synthetic Organic Chemicals, US Production and Sales, 1983 (USITC Publication 1588)*, Washington DC, US Government Printing Office, p. 255

US Occupational Safety and Health Administration (1983) *General Industry. OSHA Safety and Health Standards (29 CFR 1910) (OSHA 2206)* (rev.), Washington DC, US Government Printing Office, part 1910.100, p. 599

Verschueren, K. (1983) *Handbook of Environmental Data on Organic Chemicals*, 2nd ed., New York, Van Nostrand Reinhold, pp. 160-161

Weast, R.C., ed. (1984) *CRC Handbook of Chemistry and Physics*, 65th ed., Boca Raton, FL, CRC Press, p. C-80

WHO (1985) *Acrylamide (Environmental Health Criteria 49)*, Geneva, International Programme on Chemical Safety

Windholz, M., ed. (1983) *The Merck Index*, 10th ed., Rahway, NJ, Merck & Co., p. 19

n-BUTYL ACRYLATE

1. Chemical and Physical Data

1.1 Synonyms and trade names

Chem. Abstr. Services Reg. No.: 141-32-2

Chem. Abstr. Name: 2-Propenoic acid, butyl ester

IUPAC Systematic Name: Butyl acrylate

Synonyms: Acrylic acid, *n*-butyl ester; butyl acrylate (*n*-); butyl 2-propenoate; *n*-butyl propenoate

1.2 Structural and molecular formulae and molecular weight

$$CH_2 = CH - \overset{\overset{\textstyle O}{\|}}{C} - O - CH_2 - CH_2 - CH_2 - CH_3$$

$C_7H_{12}O_2$ Mol. wt: 128.17

1.3 Chemical and physical properties of the pure substance

(a) *Description*: Colourless liquid monomer (Sax, 1975; National Fire Protection Association, 1984) with an odour threshold of 0.1 ppb (0.5 μg/m³) (Badische Corp. *et al.*, 1984)

(b) *Boiling-point*: 146-148°C (Weast, 1984)

(c) *Melting-point*: -64.6°C (Weast, 1984)

(d) *Density*: d_4^{20} 0.8898 (Weast, 1984)

(e) *Spectroscopy data*: Ultraviolet (Sadtler Research Laboratories, 1980; [1294[a]]), infrared (Sadtler Research Laboratories, 1980; prism [4694], grating [10779]), nuclear magnetic resonance (Sadtler Research Laboratories, 1980; proton [5141], C-13 [633]) and mass spectral data (NIH/EPA Chemical Information System, 1983) have been reported.

(f) *Solubility*: Very slightly soluble in water (0.14 g/100 ml at 20°C) (Windholz, 1983); soluble in ethanol, diethyl ether and acetone (Grasselli & Ritchey, 1975)

(g) *Volatility*: Vapour pressure, 4 mm Hg at 20°C; relative vapour density (air = 1), 4.42 (Sax, 1975; Nemec & Bauer, 1978; Verschueren, 1983)

(h) *Stability*: Flash-point, 49°C (open-cup) (Hawley, 1981); vapour forms inflammable mixtures with air; combustible, polymerizes readily on heating; can react with oxidizing materials (Sax, 1975; National Fire Protection Association, 1984)

(i) *Conversion factor:* mg/m^3 = 5.24 × ppm[b]

1.4 Technical products and impurities

Commercial *n*-butyl acrylate has the following specifications: *n*-butyl acrylate, 99.5 wt % min; water, 0.10 wt % max; acrylic acid, 0.009 wt % max; hydroquinone monomethyl ether (MEHQ) 15-20 mg/kg (also available with 50 or 100 mg/kg MEHQ or 100 mg/kg hydroquinone (HQ)); and substantially free of suspended matter. The assay value for butyl acrylate includes *iso* and secondary butyl acrylate (up to 0.4 wt % combined), which are equivalent to normal butyl acrylate in reactivity (Celanese Chemical Co., 1984).

n-Butyl acrylate can undergo spontaneous polymerization. To prevent premature polymerization, inhibitors such as HQ (see IARC, 1977) and MEHQ, are added and kept active under atmospheres containing 5-20% oxygen concentration in the vapour space. Polymerization is also inhibited by the exclusion of water and by keeping temperature below 25°C. When these precautions are taken, *n*-butyl acrylate can be stored in tanks made of stainless-steel, aluminium or glass for up to six months. HQ and MEHQ can be removed from the *n*-butyl acrylate prior to use in polymerization or neutralized by the addition of polymerization catalyst (Badische Corp. *et al.*, 1984).

---

[a]Spectrum number in Sadtler compilation

[b]Calculated from: mg/m^3 = (molecular weight/24.45) × ppm, assuming standard temperature (25°C) and pressure (760 mm Hg)

2. Production, Use, Occurrence and Analysis

2.1 Production and use

(a) Production

In the USA, a propylene oxidation process is used almost exclusively for the production of acrylic compounds. This technique, developed commercially in 1970, involves the oxidation of propylene to acrolein and the subsequent oxidation of acrolein to acrylic acid. The reactions occur in the vapour phase in shell-and-tube exchangers at near atmospheric pressure. Bismuth/cobalt oxides on silica or alumina carrier are used as catalysts for the first oxidation reaction, and a molybdenum/vanadium system for the second. The acrylic acid leaving the second reactor is absorbed with water, extracted with an organic solvent and purified by vacuum distillation (Mannsville Chemical Products Corp., 1984). The butyl ester is formed by reacting acrylic acid with butanol.

A technique used in the past is the modified Reppe process, in which *n*-butyl acrylate is produced by the reaction of acetylene with nickel carbonyl (see IARC, 1976) and butanol in the presence of an acid. In a variation of this process, acetylene, carbon monoxide and water are combined in the presence of a nickel halide to form acrylic acid. Butanol is used to produce the butyl ester.

Two techniques have been developed recently for the production of acrylate esters. One involves use of organic carbonates as esterifying agents, and the other yields acrylate esters from 2-halo-1-alkenes isolated from hydrocarbon feedstocks (Haggin, 1985).

There were four major producers of *n*-butyl acrylate in the USA in 1984. The US International Trade Commission (1984) reported production of 182 million kg in 1983. During the 1970s, *n*-butyl acrylate production grew by about 15% per year due to the use of vinyl acetate-butyl acrylate emulsions in place of other emulsion polymers in architectural coatings, especially interior house paints. Butyl acrylate production has exceeded that of ethyl acrylate since 1980 (Mannsville Chemical Products Corp., 1984).

In Japan, about 30 million kg *n*-butyl acrylate were used in 1982, and 5.4 million kg were exported (Anon., 1983). There are currently four major producers of *n*-butyl acrylate in Japan.

One company in France has been identified as the primary producer of *n*-butyl acrylate in western Europe, with production in 1984 of 25 million kg.

(b) Use

Acrylic esters undergo polymerization with water to form emulsion polymers, and these are the primary form in which acrylic monomers are used. When the emulsion, or substance containing an emulsion polymer, such as paint or adhesives, is applied to a surface, the water evaporates, leaving a tough film. Acrylic emulsion polymers are used in coatings, textiles, paper, adhesives, leather (Mannsville Chemical Products Corp., 1984), polishes and sealants.

Coatings

Acrylic polymers in latex paint form a coating that is resistant to water, sunlight and weather but remains flexible at low temperatures (Union Carbide Corp., 1982). Acrylic emulsion polymers are also used as industrial finishes and in can and coil coatings.

n-Butyl acrylate-vinyl acetate emulsion polymers are used to an increasing extent in architectural coatings such as interior house paints, and they are replacing styrene-butadiene, methacrylate and maleate modified emulsions for coating applications (Mannsville Chemical Products Corp., 1984).

Textiles

Acrylic resin emulsion polymers are used in textile finishing to impart texture to fabric. They can be used to improve the abrasion and dirt resistance of fabric as well as for bonding, laminating and back coating. They have also been used as binders in pigments and nonwoven fabric.

Paper

Paper coated with a suspension of acrylic emulsion polymers and finely ground solids is receptive to ink and water resistant (Mannsville Chemical Products Corp., 1984). Such coatings are used most often for book and magazine stock, but also for business machine paper, folding boxboard and frozen-food packaging. These emulsions can be added to paper pulp to impart resistance to grease and oil.

Adhesives

Acrylic emulsions are used as resins in adhesives on envelopes, labels and decals (Mannsville Chemical Products Corp., 1984). Emulsion-based sealants are also used for bathtub caulk, baseboard seams and glazing; sealants with acrylic solvents are found in skylight joints, concrete roofing and exterior panel joints.

Leather

Emulsion polymers bind topcoatings to leather and prevent their migration; they are used in automotive upholstery, furniture, clothing and shoes.

(c) Regulatory status and guidelines

Occupational exposure limits for *n*-butyl acrylate have been set by seven countries by regulation or recommended guideline (Table 1).

n-Butyl acrylate polymers or copolymers are permitted by the US Food and Drug Administration (1984) as components of adhesives, resinous and polymeric coatings, paper and paperboard in contact with dry, aqueous or fatty foods, and semirigid and rigid acrylic and modified acrylic plastics. Homopolymers and acrylic copolymers of *n*-butyl acrylate may be used as modifiers in semirigid and rigid vinyl chloride plastics.

2.2 Occurrence

(a) Natural occurrence

It is not known whether *n*-butyl acrylate occurs as a natural product.

Table 1. National occupational exposure limits for *n*-butyl acrylate[a]

Country	Year	Concentration (mg/m^3)	Interpretation[b]
Belgium	1978	55	TWA
Finland	1981	55	TWA
Sweden	1984	50	TWA
UK	1985	55	TWA
USSR	1977	10	Ceiling
USA (ACGIH)	1984	55	TWA
Yugoslavia	1971	10	Ceiling

[a]From International Labour Office (1980); Työsuojeluhallitus (1981); American Conference of Governmental Industrial Hygienists (ACGIH) (1984); Arbetarskyddsstyrelsens Författningssamling (1984); Health and Safety Executive (1985)

[b]TWA, time-weighted average

(*b*)   *Occupational exposure*

The monomer has been detected at levels of <0.5-2 mg/m^3 (<0.1-0.4 ppm) in the breathing zone of workers in a batch process polymer manufacturing plant (Boxer & Reed, 1983). It was not detected in 15 air samples taken near the reactor vessels in a resin department where *n*-butyl acrylate was used as part of the monomer mix in a paint manufacturing process; at the same plant, however, *n*-butyl acrylate monomer was found at a concentration of 4.8 mg/m^3 (0.92 ppm) in a laboratory air sample (Belanger & Coye, 1981).

Time-weighted average (TWA) concentrations of *n*-butyl acrylate monomer in air collected in charcoal tubes from areas near chemical reactors in a polystyrene production plant were: not detected-1.4 mg/m^3 (not detected-270 ppb; mean, 0.22 mg/m^3 [41 ppb]) for personal breathing-zone samples and not detected-2.8 mg/m^3 (not detected-525 ppb; mean, 0.22 mg/m^3 [42 ppb]) for workplace samples. At an outdoor unloading site for lorries and containers, the TWA concentration of *n*-butyl acrylate in breathing-zone samples was a mean of 0.4 mg/m^3 (77 ppb) and a maximum of 1.8 mg/m^3 (350 ppb) (Samimi & Falbo, 1982).

n-Butyl acrylate was detected at concentrations of up to 50 mg/m^3 in the atmosphere of a pilot plant producing and processing acrylate monomer (Kuzelová *et al.*, 1981).

2.3 Analysis

n-Butyl acrylate has been detected in the gases released from building materials after adsorption onto graphitized thermal carbon black, thermal desorption and gas chromatography-mass spectrometry (Kiselev *et al.*, 1983). The presence of *n*-butyl acrylate as residual monomer (10-150 ppm [mg/kg]) in polymers used in coatings was analysed using capillary columns with flame ionization detection (Rygle, 1980). Personal dosimeters (adsorption on charcoal and desorption with carbon disulphide) can be used to analyse for *n*-butyl acrylate at 50 mg/m^3 (the only level tested) (Samimi & Falbo, 1983); charcoal tubes have been used for personal sampling of lower concentrations (Samimi & Falbo, 1982).

3. Biological Data Relevant to the Evaluation of Carcinogenic Risk to Humans

3.1 Carcinogenicity studies in animals

(a) Skin application

Mouse: A group of 40 male C3H/HeJ mice, 74-79 days of age, received thrice-weekly topical applications of 25 μl of a 1% solution (approximately 0.2 mg per mouse per application; 6.6 mg/kg bw; 'maximum tolerated concentration') of *n*-butyl acrylate (purity, 99.5-99.8%) in spectrophotometric-grade acetone on the back skin for life. Control groups received applications of acetone alone (vehicle controls) or of 0.1% 3-methylcholanthrene in acetone (positive controls). The mean survival time for *n*-butyl acrylate-treated animals was 503 days, compared with 484 days for vehicle controls; early deaths due to tumour development were seen only in 3-methylcholanthrene-treated animals. Complete necropsies were performed, and the dorsal skin and all gross lesions were examined histologically. No treatment-related tumour was observed in *n*-butyl acrylate-treated animals; skin tumours (mainly squamous-cell carcinomas) were observed in 39/40 mice treated with 3-methyl-cholanthrene (DePass *et al.*, 1984). [The Working Group noted that no mention was made of control for possible losses of the parent compound by volatilization or polymerization.]

(b) Inhalation exposure

Rat: In a study reported as an abstract, groups of 86 male and 86 female Sprague-Dawley rats [age unspecified] were exposed to 0, 15, 45 or 135 ppm (0, 79, 236 or 707 mg/m^3) *n*-butyl acrylate [purity unspecified] in air for 6 h per day on five days per week for two years. Interim kills [no figures provided] were performed 12, 18 and 24 months after the start of the experiment, which was terminated after 30 months. No data on survival or the mode of post-mortem examination were given. The authors stated that no effect was established on either the overall tumour incidence or any of a variety of observed tumour types [numbers and types of tumours not given] (Klimisch & Reininghaus, 1984). [The Working Group noted the incomplete reporting of this study.]

3.2 Other relevant biological data

(a) Experimental systems

The toxic effects of acrylic monomers, including *n*-butyl acrylate, have been reviewed (Autian, 1975).

Toxic effects

Oral LD_{50} values for *n*-butyl acrylate have been reported in the range of 3.7-8.1 g/kg bw in rats (Smyth *et al.*, 1951; Carpenter *et al.*, 1974; Chernikova *et al.*, 1979), 5.4 g/kg bw in mice of unspecified sex or strain (Chernikova *et al.*, 1979) and 7.5 g/kg bw in male ddY mice (Tanii & Hashimoto, 1982). Intraperitoneal LD_{50}s of 550 mg/kg bw have been reported in Wistar rats (Paulet & Vidal, 1975) and 1.6 g/kg bw in rats of unspecified sex or strain (Chernikova *et al.*, 1979); values in mice were 853 mg/kg bw (Lawrence *et al.*, 1972) and 1.6 g/kg bw (Chernikova *et al.*, 1979). In rabbits, dermal LD_{50} values of 1.8 (Carpenter *et al.*, 1974) and 3 g/kg bw (Smyth *et al.*, 1951) have been reported. The LC_{50} of *n*-butyl acrylate in rats [duration of exposure unspecified] was found to be 138.5 mg/m³ (26 ppm) (Chernikova *et al.*, 1979).

In the guinea-pig 'maximization test' [intradermal injections of acrylate in peanut oil, acrylate in Freund's complete adjuvant (FCA) and FCA alone] and the FCA test (see Klecak *et al.*, 1977), *n*-butyl acrylate was shown to be a sensitizing agent (van der Walle *et al.*, 1982). Guinea-pigs sensitized to *n*-butyl acrylate showed cross reactions to other monoacrylates (van der Walle & Bensink, 1982).

In contrast with methyl acrylate and ethyl acrylate, *n*-butyl acrylate did not produce gastric oedema in male F344 rats when administered at 520 mg/kg bw by gavage in corn oil, but did when given in water (Ghanayem *et al.*, 1985).

Effects on reproduction and prenatal toxicity

Merkle and Klimisch (1983) exposed pregnant Sprague-Dawley rats by inhalation to *n*-butyl acrylate at 0, 130, 700 or 1310 mg/m³ (0, 25, 135 or 250 ppm) for 6 h per day on gestation days 7 to 16. Maternal body-weight gain was reduced at 700 and 1310 mg/m³, and both groups showed signs of irritation during exposure. There was a concentration-related reduction in the number of live foetuses per litter, but these differences were not statistically significant. Postimplantation deaths were significantly increased at the two higher concentrations. No evidence of a teratogenic response was detected during gross external, visceral or skeletal examinations.

Absorption, distribution, excretion and metabolism

Wistar rats that received an intraperitoneal injection of 90 mg/kg bw (0.7 mmol/kg bw) *n*-butyl acrylate excreted 6% of the dose as mercapturic acids in the urine within 24 h; this amount was increased to 38% when animals were pretreated with tri-*ortho*-tolyl phosphate, an inhibitor of esterases (Delbressine, 1981).

n-Butyl acrylate disappeared rapidly from rat blood *in vitro* and from rat-liver homogenates through hydrolysis, presumably *via* nonspecific esterases. Binding to erythrocytes may also account for the disappearance from the blood (Miller *et al.*, 1981).

In vitro, *n*-butyl acrylate decreased glutathione concentration in rat-liver homogenates (Delbressine, 1981).

Mutagenicity and other short-term tests

n-Butyl acrylate (30-2000 ug/plate) was not mutagenic to *Salmonella typhimurium* TA1535, TA1537, TA1538, TA98 or TA100 in the presence or absence of a metabolic system (S9) from the liver of Aroclor- or phenobarbital-induced rats when plates were incubated in closed jars. Negative results were also obtained in a preincubation assay (using stoppered tubes) with strain TA100, in the presence and absence of Aroclor-induced rat-liver S9 (Waegemaekers & Bensink, 1984).

In Chinese hamsters and Sprague-Dawley rats exposed to 4300 mg/m³ (820 ppm) *n*-butyl acrylate by inhalation for 5-6 h per day for four days, no chromosomal damage was observed in single bone-marrow samples taken 5 h after cessation of exposure (Engelhardt & Klimisch, 1983). [The Working Group noted that single samples were tested and the short period between cessation of exposure and sampling.]

(*b*) *Humans*

Toxic effects

Fourteen of 33 workers exposed over an average period of five years to 50 mg/m³ *n*-butyl acrylate (and 4-58 mg/m³ ethyl acrylate) complained of autonomic and neurotic symptoms, but electroencephalographic examination showed no organic dysfunction (Kuželová *et al.*, 1981).

Effects on reproduction and prenatal toxicity

No data were available to the Working Group.

Absorption, distribution, excretion and metabolism

No data were available to the Working Group.

Mutagenicity and chromosomal effects

No data were available to the Working Group.

3.3 Case reports and epidemiological studies of carcinogenicity to humans

No data were available to the Working Group.

4. Summary of Data Reported and Evaluation

4.1 Exposure data

Production of *n*-butyl acrylate has increased significantly since the 1970s due to its use in emulsion polymers for architectural coatings, including interior house paints. Occupational exposure occurs in the manufacture of *n*-butyl acrylate and in the manufacture and use of its emulsion polymers.

4.2 Experimental data

n-Butyl acrylate was tested for carcinogenicity by repeated skin applications in one experiment in male mice; no treatment-related tumour was observed. In a study reported as an abstract, in which male and female rats were exposed to *n*-butyl acrylate by inhalation for two years, no neoplastic effect was observed.

In one experiment in rats, inhalation of maternally toxic concentrations of *n*-butyl acrylate produced signs of embryotoxicity; there was no sign of foetotoxicity or teratogenicity.

n-Butyl acrylate was not mutagenic to *Salmonella typhimurium* in the presence or absence of an exogenous metabolic system.

Overall assessment of data from short-term tests: *n*-Butyl acrylate[a]

	Genetic activity			Cell transformation
	DNA damage	Mutation	Chromosomal effects	
Prokaryotes		−		
Fungi/ Green plants				
Insects				
Mammalian cells (*in vitro*)				
Mammals (*in vivo*)				
Humans (*in vivo*)				
Degree of evidence in short-term tests for genetic activity: **Inadequate**				Cell transformation: No data

[a]The groups into which the table is divided and the symbols '+', '−' and '?' are defined on pp. 19-20 of the Preamble; the degrees of evidence are defined on pp. 20-21.

4.3 Human data

No data were available to evaluate the reproductive effects or prenatal toxicity of *n*-butyl acrylate to humans.

No case report or epidemiological study was available to evaluate the carcinogenicity of *n*-butyl acrylate to humans.

4.4 Evaluation[1]

There is *inadequate evidence* for the carcinogenicity of *n*-butyl acrylate to experimental animals.

No data on humans were available.

In the absence of epidemiological data, no evaluation of the carcinogenicity of *n*-butyl acrylate to humans could be made.

5. References

American Conference of Governmental Industrial Hygienists (1984) *Threshold Limit Values for Chemical Substances and Physical Agents in the Work Environment and Biological Exposure Indices with Intended Changes for 1984-85*, Cincinnati, OH, p. 11

Anon. (1983) Acrylate ester promising. *Plastics Ind. News*, *27*, 97-98

Arbetarskyddsstyrelsens Författningssamling (National Swedish Board of Occupational Safety and Health) (1984) *Hygienic Limit Values (AFS 1984:5)* (Swed.), Stockholm, p. 12

Autian, J. (1975) Structure-toxicity relationships of acrylic monomers. *Environ. Health Perspect.*, *11*, 141-152

Badische Corp., Celanese Chemical Co., Inc., Rohm & Haas Co. & Union Carbide Corp. (1984) *Acrylate Esters, A Guide to Safety and Handling*, Williamsburg, VA, Dallas, TX, Philadelphia, PA, Danbury, CT

Belanger, P.L. & Coye, M.J. (1981) *Health Hazard Evaluation Report No. HHE-80-68-871 (US NTIS PB82-214396)*, Washington, DC, US Department of Health and Human Services, Public Health Service, Centers for Disease Control, National Institute for Occupational Safety and Health

Boxer, P.A. & Reed, L.D. (1983) *Health Hazard Evaluation Report No. HETA-82-051-1269 (US NTIS PB84-209923)*, Washington DC, US Department of Health and Human Services, Public Health Service, Centers for Disease Control, National Institute for Occupational Safety and Health

Carpenter, C.P., Weil, C.S. & Smyth, H.F., Jr (1974) Range-finding toxicity data: List VIII. *Toxicol. appl. Pharmacol.*, *28*, 313-319

[1]For definition of the italicized term, see Preamble, p. 18.

Celanese Chemical Co. (1984) *Butyl Acrylate Sales Specification* (*Technical Bulletin No. CCC-93*), Dallas, TX

Chernikova, V.V., Astapova, S.A., Gizatullina, N.S., Efremenko, A.A., Kustova, Z.R., Lobanova, I.Y., Ostroumova, N.A., Savchenko, N.A., Stepanov, S.V. & Tiunova, L.V. (1979) Experimental studies of acute and chronic effect of butyl acrylate (Russ.). *Khim. Prom-st. Ser. Toksikol. Sanit. Khim. Plastmass*, *2*, 22-24

Delbressine, L.P.C. (1981) *Metabolic Detoxification of Olefinic Compounds*, PhD Thesis, Nijmegen, University of Nijmegen, The Netherlands, p. 99

DePass, L.R., Fowler, E.H., Meckley, D.R. & Weil, C.S. (1984) Dermal oncogenicity bioassays of acrylic acid, ethyl acrylate, and butyl acrylate. *J. Toxicol. environ. Health*, *14*, 115-120

Engelhardt, G. & Klimisch, H.-J. (1983) *n*-Butyl acrylate: Cytogenetic investigations in the bone marrow of Chinese hamsters and rats after 4-day inhalation. *Fundam. appl. Toxicol.*, *3*, 640-641

Ghanayem, B.I., Maronpot, R.R. & Matthews, H.B. (1985) Ethyl acrylate-induced gastric toxicity. II. Structure-toxicity relationships and mechanism. *Toxicol. appl. Pharmacol. 80*, 336-344

Grasselli, J.G. & Ritchey, W.M., eds (1975) *CRC Atlas of Spectral Data and Physical Constants for Organic Compounds*, Vol. 4, Cleveland, OH, CRC Press, p. 313

Haggin, J. (1985) New Dow acrylate ester processes derive from C_1 efforts. *Chem. Eng. News*, *63*, 25-26

Hawley, G.G., ed. (1981) *The Condensed Chemical Dictionary*, 10th ed., New York, Van Nostrand Reinhold, p. 160

Health and Safety Executive (1985) *Occupational Exposure Limits 1985* (*Guidance Note EH 40/85*), London, Her Majesty's Stationery Office, p. 9

IARC (1976) *IARC Monographs on the Evaluation of Carcinogenic Risk of Chemicals to Man*, Vol. 11, *Cadmium, Nickel, Some Epoxides, Miscellaneous Industrial Chemicals and General Considerations on Volatile Anaesthetics*, Lyon, pp. 75-112

IARC (1977) *IARC Monographs on the Evaluation of the Carcinogenic Risk of Chemicals to Man*, Vol. 15, *Some Fumigants, the Herbicides 2,4-D and 2,4,5-T, Chlorinated Dibenzodioxins and Miscellaneous Industrial Chemicals*, Lyon, pp. 155-175

International Labour Office (1980) *Occupational Exposure Limits for Airborne Toxic Substances, A Tabular Compilation of Values from Selected Countries*, 2nd (rev.) ed. (*Occupational Safety and Health Series No. 37*), Geneva, pp. 56-57

Kiselev, A.V., Maltsev, V.V., Saada, B. & Valovoy, V.A. (1983) Gas chromatography-mass spectrometry of volatiles released from plastics used as building materials. *Chromatographia*, *17*, 539-544

Klecak, G., Geleick, H. & Frey, J.R. (1977) Screening of fragrance materials for allergenicity in the guinea pig. I. Comparison of four testing methods. *J. Soc. cosmet. Chem.*, *28*, 53-64

Klimisch, H.-J. & Reininghaus, W. (1984) Carcinogenicity of acrylates: Long-term inhalation studies on methyl acrylate (MA) and *n*-butyl acrylate (BA) in rats (Abstract). *Toxicologist, 4,* 53

Kuželová, M.J., Kovařik, D., Fiedlerová, A. & Popler (1981) Acrylic compounds and general health of the exposed persons (Czech.). *Pracov. Lék., 33,* 95-99

Lawrence, W.H., Bass, G.E., Purcell, W.P. & Autian, J. (1972) Use of mathematical models in the study of structure-toxicity relationships of dental compounds: I. Esters of acrylic and methacrylic acids. *J. dent. Res., 51,* 526-535

Mannsville Chemical Products Corp. (1984) *Acrylates and Acrylic Acid (Chemical Products Synopsis)*, Cortland, NY

Merkle, J. & Klimisch, H.-J. (1983) *n*-Butyl acrylate: Prenatal inhalation toxicity in the rat. *Fundam. appl. Toxicol., 3,* 443-447

Miller, R.R., Ayres, J.A., Rampy, L.W. & McKenna, M.J. (1981) Metabolism of acrylate esters in rat tissue homogenates. *Fundam. appl. Toxicol., 1,* 410-414

National Fire Protection Association (1984) *Fire Protection Guide on Hazardous Materials*, 8th ed., Quincy, MA, pp. 325M-20, 49-23

Nemec, J.W. & Bauer, W., Jr (1978) *Acrylic acid and derivatives.* In: Mark, H.F., Othmer, D.F., Overberger, C.G. & Seaborg, G.T., eds, *Kirk-Othmer Encyclopedia of Chemical Technology*, 3rd ed., Vol. 1, New York, John Wiley & Sons, pp. 330-334

NIH/EPA Chemical Information System (1983) *Carbon-13 NMR Spectral Search System, Mass Spectral Search System,* and *Infrared Spectral Search System*, Arlington, VA, Information Consultants

Paulet, G. & Vidal (1975) On the toxicity of some acrylic and methacrylic esters of acrylamide and polyacrylamides (Fr.). *Arch. Mal. prof., 36,* 58-60

Rygle, K.J. (1980) Trace residual monomer analysis by capillary gas chromatography. *J. Coatings Technol., 52,* 47-52

Sadtler Research Laboratories (1980) *The Sadtler Standard Spectra Collection, Cumulative Index*, Philadelphia, PA

Samimi, B. & Falbo, L. (1982) Monitoring of workers exposed to low levels of airborne monomers in a polystyrene production plant. *Am. ind. Hyg. Assoc. J., 43,* 858-862

Samimi, B. & Falbo, L. (1983) Validation of Abcor (NMS) organic vapor dosimeter under various concentrations and air velocity conditions. *Am. ind. Hyg. Assoc. J., 44,* 402-408

Sax, N.I. (1975) *Dangerous Properties of Industrial Materials*, 4th ed., New York, Van Nostrand Reinhold, p. 484

Smyth, H.F., Jr, Carpenter, C.P. & Weil, C.S. (1951) Range-finding toxicity data: List IV. *Arch. ind. Hyg. occup. Med., 4,* 119-122

Tanii, H. & Hashimoto, K. (1982) Structure-toxicity relationships of acrylates and methacrylates. *Toxicol. Lett., 11,* 125-129

Työsuojeluhallitus (National Finnish Board of Occupational Safety and Health) (1981) *Airborne Contaminants in the Workplace (Safety Bull. 3)* (Finn.), Tampere, p. 9

Union Carbide Corp. (1982) *Product Information: Ethyl, Butyl and 2-Ethylhexyl Acrylates* (*Tech. Bull. No. F-40242C*), Danbury, CT

US Food and Drug Administration (1984) Food and drugs. *US Code Fed. Regul., Title 21*, Parts 175.105, 175.300. 176.170, 176.180, 177.1010, 178.3790, pp. 132, 145, 176, 188, 198, 342

US International Trade Commission (1984) *Synthetic Organic Chemicals, US Production and Sales, 1983* (*USITC Publication 1588*), Washington DC, US Government Printing Office, pp. 258, 283

Verschueren, K. (1983) *Handbook of Environmental Data on Organic Chemicals*, 2nd ed., New York, Van Nostrand Reinhold, p. 307

Waegemaekers, T.H.J.M. & Bensink, M.P.M. (1984) Non-mutagenicity of 27 aliphatic acrylate esters in the *Salmonella*-microsome test. *Mutat. Res., 137*, 95-102

van der Walle, H.B. & Bensink, T. (1982) Cross reaction pattern of 26 acrylic monomers on guinea pig skin. *Contact Dermatol., 8*, 376-382

van der Walle, H.B., Klecak, G., Geleick, H. & Bensink, T. (1982) Sensitizing potential of 14 mono(meth)acrylates in the guinea pig. *Contact Dermatol., 8*, 223-235

Weast, R.C., ed. (1984) *CRC Handbook of Chemistry and Physics*, 65th ed., Boca Raton, FL, CRC Press, p. C-80

Windholz, M., ed. (1983) *The Merck Index*, 10th ed., Rahway, NJ, Merck & Co., p. 214

ETHYL ACRYLATE

This substance was considered by a previous Working Group, in February 1978 (IARC, 1979). Since that time, new data have become available, and these have been incorporated into the monograph and taken into consideration in the present evaluation.

1. Chemical and Physical Data

1.1 Synonyms and trade names

Chem. Abstr. Services Reg. No.: 140-88-5
Chem. Abstr. Name: 2-Propenoic acid, ethyl ester
IUPAC Systematic Name: Ethyl acrylate
Synonyms: Acrylic acid, ethyl ester; European Council no. CE 245; ethoxy-carbonylethylene; ethyl propenoate; ethyl 2-propenoate
Trade Names: Carboset 511; Latol 28-tall oil fatty acid

1.2 Structural and molecular formulae and molecular weight

$$CH_2 = CH - \overset{\overset{\displaystyle O}{\|}}{C} - O - CH_2 - CH_3$$

$C_5H_8O_2$ Mol. wt: 100.13

1.3 Chemical and physical properties of the pure substance

(a) *Description*: Colourless liquid with an acrid penetrating odour (Hawley, 1981; Windholz, 1983; National Fire Protection Association, 1984; Sax, 1984) and reported odour thresholds of 1 ppb (4 μg/m³) (Badische Corp. *et al.*, 1984) or 0.07 ppm (0.3 mg/m³) (Stahl, 1973)

(b)   *Boiling-point*: 99.8°C (Weast, 1984)

(c)   *Melting-point*: -71.2°C (Weast, 1984)

(d)   *Density*: d_4^{20} 0.9234 (Weast, 1984)

(e)   *Spectroscopy data*: Ultraviolet (Grasselli & Ritchey, 1975), infrared (Sadtler Research Laboratories, 1980; prism [1310[a]], grating [29702]), nuclear magnetic resonance (Sadtler Research Laboratories, 1980; proton [7950, 7951], C-13 [2822]) and mass spectral data (NIH/EPA Chemical Information System, 1983) have been reported.

(f)   *Solubility*: Slightly soluble in water (2 g/100 ml at 20°C); soluble in chloroform; miscible in ethanol and diethyl ether (Grasselli & Ritchey, 1975; Hawley, 1981; Windholz, 1983)

(g)   *Volatility*: Vapour pressure, 29 mm Hg at 20°C; relative vapour density (air = 1), 3.5; saturation concentration, 158 g/m³ at 20°C (Verschueren, 1983)

(h)   *Stability*: Flash-point, 15.6°C (open-cup) (Windholz, 1983; National Fire Protection Association, 1984); polymerizes easily on standing, accelerated by heat, light and peroxides; vapour forms explosive mixtures in air (Hawley, 1981; Windholz, 1983; National Fire Protection Association, 1984); can react vigorously with oxidizing materials (Sax, 1984)

(i)   *Conversion factor:* mg/m³ = 4.10 × ppm[b]

1.4 Technical products and impurities

Commercial ethyl acrylate available in the USA has the following specifications: ethyl acrylate, 99.5 wt % min; water, 0.10 wt % max; acrylic acid, 0.009 wt % max; hydroquinone monomethyl ether (MEHQ), 15-20 mg/kg (also available with 50 or 200 mg/kg MEHQ or 1000 mg/kg hydroquinone (HQ)) and substantially free of suspended matter (Celanese Chemical Co., 1984). It is also available with the following specifications: ethyl acrylate, 99.5 wt % min; water, 0.05 wt %; acidity as acrylic acid, 0.005 wt %; HQ, 10-20, 90-120, 190-220, 470-530 or 900-1100 mg/kg; MEHQ, 10-20, 20-35, 40-60, 90-120, 190-220 or 470-530 mg/kg; HQ in MEHQ-inhibited product, 1.5 mg/kg max (Union Carbide Corp., 1982).

---

[a]Spectrum number in Sadtler compilation

[b]Calculated from: mg/m³ = (molecular weight/24.45) × ppm, assuming standard temperature (25°C) and pressure (760 mm Hg)

Ethyl acrylate can undergo spontaneous polymerization. To prevent premature polymerization, inhibitors, such as HQ (see IARC, 1977) and MEHQ, are added and kept active under atmospheres containing 5-20% oxygen concentration in the vapour space. Polymerization is also inhibited by the exclusion of water and by keeping temperature below 25°C. When these precautions are taken, ethyl acrylate can be stored in tanks made of stainless-steel, aluminium or glass for up to six months. HQ and MEHQ can be removed from the ethyl acrylate prior to use in polymerization or neutralized by the addition of polymerization catalyst (Badische Corp. *et al.*, 1984).

2. Production, Use, Occurrence and Analysis

2.1 Production and use

(a)   Production

Ethyl acrylate was first prepared by Redtenbacher in 1843 by oxidizing acrolein with silver oxide, then treating the silver salt with ethyl iodide. It has been produced commercially since the early 1930s (Luskin, 1970). In the USA, a propylene oxidation process is used almost exclusively for the production of acrylic compounds. This technique, developed commercially in 1970, involves the oxidation of propylene to acrolein and the subsequent oxidation of acrolein to acrylic acid. The reactions occur in the vapour phase in shell-and-tube exchangers at near atmospheric pressure. Bismuth/cobalt oxides on silica or alumina carrier are used as catalysts for the first oxidation reaction, and a molybdenum/vanadium system for the second. The acrylic acid leaving the second reactor is absorbed with water, extracted with an organic solvent and purified by vacuum distillation (Mannsville Chemical Products Corp., 1984). The ethyl ester is formed by reacting acrylic acid with ethanol.

A technique used in the past is the modified Reppe process, in which ethyl acrylate is produced by the reaction of acetylene with nickel carbonyl (see IARC, 1976) and ethanol in the presence of an acid. In a variation of this process, a company in the Federal Republic of Germany combines acetylene, carbon monoxide and water in the presence of a nickel halide to form acrylic acid. Ethanol is used to produce the ethyl ester.

Two techniques have been developed recently for the production of acrylate esters. One involves use of organic carbonates as esterifying agents, and the other yields acrylate esters from 2-halo-1-alkenes isolated from hydrocarbon feedstocks (Haggin, 1985).

There were four major producers of ethyl acrylate in the USA in 1984. The US International Trade Commission (1984) reported production of 131 million kg in 1983.

One company in France produced 60 million kg in 1984. This company and two companies in the Federal Republic of Germany have been identified as the primary producers of ethyl acrylate in western Europe.

In Japan, about 15 million kg ethyl acrylate were used in 1982 (Anon., 1983). There are currently four major producers of ethyl acrylate in Japan.

(b) Use

Acrylic esters undergo polymerization with water to form emulsion polymers, and these are the primary form in which acrylic monomers are used. When the emulsion, or substance containing an emulsion polymer, such as paint or adhesives, is applied to a surface, the water evaporates, leaving a tough film. Acrylic emulsion polymers are used in coatings, textiles, paper, adhesives, leather, polishes and sealants (Mannsville Chemical Products Corp., 1984).

Coatings

Acrylic polymers in latex paint form a coating that is resistant to water, sunlight and weather but remains flexible at low temperatures (Union Carbide Corp., 1982). Acrylic emulsion polymers are also used as industrial finishes and in can and coil coatings.

Textiles

Acrylic resin emulsion polymers are used in textile finishing to impart texture to fabric. They can be used to improve the abrasion and dirt resistance of fabric as well as for bonding, laminating and back coating. They have been used as binders in pigments and nonwoven fabric.

Paper

Paper coated with a suspension of acrylic emulsion polymers and finely ground solids is receptive to ink and water resistant (Mannsville Chemical Products Corp., 1984). Such coatings are used most often for book and magazine stock, but also for business machine paper, folding boxboard and frozen-food packaging. These emulsions can be added to paper pulp to impart resistance to grease and oil.

Adhesives

Acrylic emulsions are used as resins in adhesives on envelopes, labels and decals (Mannsville Chemical Products Corp., 1984). Emulsion-based sealants are also used for bathtub caulk, baseboard seams and glazing; sealants with acrylic solvents are found in skylight joints, concrete roofing and exterior panel joints.

Leather

Emulsion polymers bind topcoatings to leather and prevent their migration; they are used in automotive upholstery, furniture, clothing and shoes.

Foods and cosmetics

Ethyl acrylate has been used as a fragrance additive in some soaps, detergents, creams, lotions (at levels of 0.001-0.01%) and perfumes (at levels of 0.04-0.4%) and as a synthetic fruit essence (Opdyke, 1975).

(c) Regulatory status and guidelines

Occupational exposure limits for ethyl acrylate have been set by 13 countries by regulation or recommended guideline (Table 1).

Table 1. National occupational exposure limits for ethyl acrylate[a]

Country	Year	Concentration (mg/m^3)	Interpretation[b]
Australia	1978	100	TWA
Belgium	1978	100[c]	TWA
Finland	1981	20[c]	TWA
Germany, Federal Republic of	1984	100[c]	TWA
Italy	1978	40[c]	TWA
The Netherlands	1978	100[c]	TWA
Romania	1975	50	TWA
		80	Ceiling
Sweden	1984	40[c]	TWA
Switzerland	1978	100[c]	TWA
UK	1985	100[c]	TWA
USA			
ACGIH	1984	20[c]	TWA
		100[c]	STEL
OSHA	1983	100[c]	TWA
Yugoslavia	1971	100	Ceiling

[a]From International Labour Office (1980); Työsuojeluhallitus (1981); US Occupational Safety and Health Administration (OSHA) (1983); American Conference of Governmental Industrial Hygienists (ACGIH) (1984); Arbetarskyddsstyrelsens Författningssamling (1984); Deutsches Forschungsgemeinschaft (1984); Health and Safety Executive (1985)

[b]TWA, time-weighted average; STEL, short-term exposure limit

[c]Skin notation (absorption is possible)

The Council of Europe (Conseil de l'Europe, 1981) included ethyl acetate in a list of artificial flavouring substances that may be added to foodstuffs without hazard to public health at a level of 1 ppm (mg/kg) in food and 0.2 mg/l in beverages.

The US Food and Drug Administration (1984) considers ethyl acrylate to be a 'generally recognized as safe' (GRAS) synthetic flavouring substance or food adjuvant. Ethyl acrylate polymers or copolymers are permitted as components of adhesives, resinous and polymeric coatings, paper and paperboard in contact with dry, aqueous or fatty foods, and semirigid and rigid acrylic and modified acrylic plastics. Homopolymers and acrylic copolymers of ethyl acrylate may be used as modifiers in semirigid and rigid vinyl chloride plastics.

Ethyl acrylate is classified as a hazardous waste by the US Environmental Protection Agency (1984) under the Resource Conservation and Recovery Act of 1976.

2.2 Occurrence

(a) Natural occurrence

Ethyl acrylate has been identified at low levels (0.77 mg/kg) in the volatile components of fresh pineapple (Haagen-Smit et al., 1945; Näf-Müller & Willhalm, 1971).

(b) Occupational exposure

Ethyl acrylate was detected in the air in a pilot production and processing plant at concentrations of 4-58 mg/m³ (Kuzelová et al., 1981) and in the air of the resin department of a paint manufacturing facility at concentrations of <1-24 mg/m³ (Belanger & Coye, 1981).

Mean time-weighted average (TWA) concentrations of ethyl acrylate monomer in air collected in areas near chemical reactors in a polystyrene production plant were 0.06-0.2 mg/m³ for personal breathing zone samples and 0.012-0.1 mg/m³ for work area samples. At an outdoor unloading site for lorries and containers, the TWA concentration of ethyl acrylate was as high as 230 mg/m³ (Samimi & Falbo, 1982). At a resin manufacturing plant, concentrations of 49-2750 mg/m³ ethyl acrylate monomer were measured in air emitted from a scrubber stack designed to prevent the exit of concentrations in excess of 40 mg/m³ (Jones et al., 1981).

Ethyl acrylate has been detected as a residual monomer in polyethyl acrylate (Brunn et al., 1975) and, at a concentration of 50 mg/kg, in aqueous polymer latexes used in the paper and textile industries (Bollini et al., 1975).

2.3 Analysis

Ethyl acrylate has been determined in air after adsorption onto charcoal, desorption with a solvent (carbon disulphide) and analysis by gas chromatography with flame ionization detection. This method was validated by the National Institute for Occupational Safety and Health for a range of 50-210 mg/m³ (Taylor, 1977). The same method is used to measure ethyl acrylate after personal sampling for workplace exposures using passive dosimeters (Samimi & Falbo, 1983).

Carbon dioxide laser absorption spectroscopy can be used to detect ethyl acrylate in humid air at levels down to approximately 0.08 mg/m³ (Loper et al., 1982).

3. Biological Data Relevant to the Evaluation of Carcinogenic Risk to Humans

3.1 Carcinogenicity studies in animals

(a) Oral administration

Mouse: Groups of 50 male and 50 female B6C3F$_1$ mice, seven weeks of age, received 100 or 200 mg/kg bw ethyl acrylate (purity, 99-99.5% stabilized with 15 mg/kg of the monomethyl ether of hydroquinone) in 10 ml/kg bw corn oil by gavage five times per week for 103 weeks. Similar groups of mice received corn oil only and served as vehicle controls. The experiment was terminated 104-106 weeks after the beginning of the treatment. Survival in the control, low-dose and high-dose groups was: males, 56%, 72% and 60%; females, 54%, 70% and 52%, respectively. The incidences of squamous-cell carcinomas of the forestomach in the control, low-dose and high-dose male mice were: 0/48, 2/47 and 5/50 ($p = 0.03$, Fisher exact test, high-dose $versus$ control; $p = 0.019$, Cochran-Armitage test for trend). The combined incidences of squamous-cell papillomas and carcinomas of the forestomach in the control, low-dose and high-dose groups were: males, 0/48, 5/47 and 12/50 ($p < 0.001$, high-dose $versus$ control, Fisher exact test and trend test); females, 1/50, 5/49 and 7/48 ($p = 0.026$, high-dose $versus$ control, Fisher exact and 0.022, trend test). Dose-related increases were observed in the incidence of non-neoplastic lesions (hyperkeratosis, hyperlasia and inflammation) in the forestomach [see also section 3.2(a)] in animals of each sex (National Toxicology Program, 1983).

Rat: Groups of 50 male and 50 female Fischer 344/N rats, seven weeks of age, received 100 or 200 mg/kg bw ethyl acrylate (purity, 99-99.5%, stabilized with 15 mg/kg of the monomethyl ether of hydroquinone) in 5 ml/kg bw corn oil by gavage five times per week for 103 weeks. Similar groups of rats received corn oil only and served as vehicle controls. The experiment was terminated 104-105 weeks after the beginning of the treatment. Survival in the control, low-dose and high-dose groups was: males, 82%, 64% and 68%; females, 72%, 72% and 84%. The incidences of squamous-cell carcinomas of the forestomach in the control, low-dose and high-dose male rats were: 0/50, 5/50 and 12/50 ($p < 0.001$, Fisher exact test, high-dose $versus$ control, and Cochran-Armitage test for trend). The combined incidences of squamous-cell papillomas and carcinomas of the forestomach in the control, low-dose and high-dose groups were: males, 1/50, 18/50 and 36/50 ($p < 0.001$, Fisher exact test, high-dose $versus$ control, and Cochran Armitage test for trend); females, 1/50, 6/50 and 11/50 ($p = 0.002$, Fisher exact test, high-dose $versus$ control, and Cochran-Armitage test for trend), respectively. Dose-related increases were observed in the incidence of non-neoplastic lesions (hyperkeratosis, hyperplasia and inflammation) in the forestomach [see also section 3.2(a)] in animals of each sex (National Toxicology Program, 1983).

Groups of 25 male and 25 female young Wistar rats received 0, 6-7, 60-70 or 2000 mg/l (ppm) ethyl acrylate [purity unspecified] in the drinking-water for two years. After two years of treatment, survival was: males, 52%, 48%, 60% and 72%; females, 64%, 72%, 36% and 60%, in the control, low-, mid- and high-dose groups, respectively. No treatment-related lesion was reported (Borzelleca et $al.$, 1964). [The Working Group noted the incomplete description of the findings in this study.]

(b) Skin application

$Mouse$: A group of 40 male C3H/HeJ mice, 74-79 days of age, received thrice-weekly skin applications of 25 μl undiluted ethyl acrylate (purity, >99%) on the back skin for life (approximately 23 mg per application; total dose, approximately 770 mg/kg bw). Control groups were treated either with acetone or with 0.1% 3-methylcholanthrene in acetone. The mean survival time of animals in the ethyl acrylate-treated group (408 days) did not differ significantly from that in the acetone controls (484 days). Complete necropsies were performed, and dorsal skin from all animals as well as gross lesions were examined histologically. No treatment-related tumour was observed in either ethyl acrylate- or acetone-treated mice; skin tumours (mainly squamous-cell carcinomas) were observed in 39/40 mice treated with 3-methylcholanthrene (DePass *et al.*, 1984). [The Working Group noted that no mention was made of control for possible losses of the parent compound by volatilization or polymerization.]

(c)   Inhalation exposure

Mouse: Groups of 105 female and 105 male B6C3F$_1$ mice, seven to nine weeks of age, were exposed to vapours of ethyl acrylate (purity, >99.5%) at concentrations of 100, 310 or 920 mg/m^3 [25, 75 or 225 ppm] for 6 h per day on five days per week. The treatment with the low and medium doses lasted 27 months, whereas high-dose treatment was discontinued after six months due to a significant decrease in body-weight gain. These animals were followed without further treatment for up to 27 months. Two concurrent control groups, each of 84 female and 84 male untreated mice, were used. Interim sacrifices of small groups of exposed and control animals were made at six, 12 and 18 months, such that groups of approximately 75 animals per sex in the exposed group and 60 animals per sex in the control groups were available for the full study. The mean body-weight gains of both male and female mice in the mid- and high-dose groups were significantly lower than for the control groups throughout the study. Survival in all groups was adequate for evaluation of late-appearing tumours. No treatment-related increase in the incidence of tumours was observed, with the exception of thyroid follicular adenomas, which were increased in high-dose male mice when compared to concurrent but not historical controls (2/121 in concurrent controls; 16% in historical controls; and 7/69 in high-dose males). Dose-related increases were observed in the incidence of non-neoplastic lesions of the olfactory mucosa (glandular hyperplasia and metaplasia) in animals of each sex [see also section 3.2(a)] (Miller *et al.*, 1985).

Rat: Groups of 115 female and 115 male Fischer 344 rats, seven to nine weeks of age, were exposed to vapours of ethyl acrylate (purity, >99.5%) at concentrations of 100, 310 or 920 mg/m^3 [25, 75 or 225 ppm] for 6 h per day on five days per week. The treatment with the low- and mid-doses lasted 27 months, whereas the high-dose treatment was discontinued after six months due to a significant decrease in body-weight gain. These animals were followed without further treatment for up to 27 months. Two concurrent control groups, each of 92 female and 92 male untreated rats, were used. Interim sacrifices of small groups of exposed and control rats were made after three, six, 12 and 18 months of exposure, such that 75 animals per sex in the exposed groups and 60 animals per sex in the control groups were available for the full study. The mean body-weight gains of both male and female rats in the mid- and high-dose groups were significantly lower than for the control groups throughout the study. Survival in all exposed groups was adequate for the evaluation of late-appearing tumours. No treatment-related neoplastic lesion was observed at any dose level. Dose-related increases were observed in the incidence of non-neoplastic lesions of the olfactory mucosa (glandular and basal-cell hyperplasia and metaplasia) in animals of each sex [see also section 3.2(*a*)] (Miller *et al.*, 1985).

3.2 Other relevant biological data

The toxic effects of acrylic monomers, including ethyl acrylate, have been reviewed (Autian, 1975)

(*a*)   *Experimental systems*

Toxic effects

The oral LD_{50} for ethyl acrylate (in various solvents, sometimes unspecified) in rats has been reported to range from 1 g/kg bw (Pozzani *et al.*, 1949; Paulet & Vidal, 1975; Sandmeyer & Kirwin, 1981) to 2 g/kg bw (Union Carbide Corp., 1971). The oral LD_{50} is 1.8 g/kg bw in male ddY mice (Tanii & Hashimoto, 1982) and 400 mg/kg bw in rabbits (Fassett, 1963). Intraperitoneal LD_{50}s are 450 mg/kg bw in Wistar rats (Paulet & Vidal, 1975) and 600 mg/kg bw in male ICR mice (Lawrence *et al.*, 1972). The dermal LD_{50} in rabbits has been reported to be 1.8-2 g/kg bw (undiluted) (Pozzani *et al.*, 1949; Union Carbide Corp., 1971).

LC_{50} values for 4-h exposure have been reported to range from <4100-8200 mg/m^3 (<1000-2000 ppm) in rats (Pozzani *et al.*, 1949; Fassett, 1963), from <4100-16 400 mg/m^3 (<1000-4000 ppm) in rabbits (Sandmeyer & Kirwin, 1981) and to be 3950 ppm (16 200 mg/m^3) in mice (Lomonova & Klimova, 1979).

Early studies of the inhalation toxicity of ethyl acrylate vapours in small numbers of rats, rabbits, guinea-pigs and monkeys reported signs of acute irritation in the lung and upper respiratory tract at concentrations of 1230 and 2200 mg/m^3 (300 and 540 ppm) (Pozzani *et al.*, 1949) or 4940 mg/m^3 (1204 ppm) (Treon *et al.*, 1949).

Male and female Fischer 344 rats and B6C3F1 mice exposed to 100-920 mg/m^3 (25-225 ppm) ethyl acrylate vapours for 6 h per day on five days per week for up to 27 months developed selective histopathological changes of the nasal mucosa (hyperplasia of submucosal glands and respiratory metaplasia of the olfactory epithelium) (Miller *et al.*, 1985).

Male and female Fischer 344 rats and $B6C3F_1$ mice were given 100, 200, 400, 600 or 800 mg/kg bw ethyl acrylate in corn oil by gavage. After 14 days, rats developed abdominal adhesions (at 600 and 800 mg/kg) and tissue lesions of the forestomach (at 400 mg/kg), characterized histologically as hyperkeratosis, hyperplasia and inflammation. Inflammation of the forestomach was seen in mice (at 400 and 600 mg/kg). Such lesions were not found at doses of 100 and 200 mg/kg (National Toxicology Program, 1983; Ghanayem *et al.*, 1985a,b).

Fischer 344 rats and $B6C3F_1$ mice of each sex that received 100 or 200 mg/kg bw ethyl acrylate by gavage five times per week for 103 weeks showed epithelial hyperplasia of the forestomach, usually associated with variable degrees of hyperkeratosis (see also section 3.1) (National Toxicology Program, 1983).

When applied to the skin of rabbits, ethyl acrylate caused marked local irritation, erythema, oedema and vascular damage (Treon et al., 1949).

With the guinea-pig 'maximization test' (intradermal injections of acrylate in peanut oil, acrylate in Freund's complete adjuvant (FCA) and FCA alone) and the FCA test (see Klecak et al., 1977), ethyl acrylate was shown to be a sensitizing agent (van der Walle et al., 1982). Guinea-pigs sensitized to ethyl acrylate showed cross reactions to other monoacrylates (van der Walle & Bensink, 1982).

When undiluted ethyl acrylate was applied to the skin of 40 male C3H/HeJ mice at a dose of 25 μl (23 mg/mouse per application) three times weekly for life, histological skin changes were observed, including epidermal necrosis (four animals), keratin necrosis (six animals), dermal fibrosis (six animals), hyperkeratosis (12 animals) and dermatitis (five animals) (DePass et al., 1984).

Effects on reproduction and prenatal toxicity

Groups of 10-23 pregnant Wistar rats received oral doses of 0, 25, 50, 100, 200 or 400 mg/kg bw per day ethyl acrylate [solvent unspecified] on gestation days 7-16. Maternal body weights were reduced (but not in a dose-related manner) in treated groups. The total number of resorptions was significantly increased with the three highest doses, but the number of live foetuses per litter was not significantly affected. When 50% of foetuses were examined for skeletal defects, the overall incidence of delayed ossification was found to be increased in all treated groups (Pietrowicz et al., 1980).

In an inhalation study, Murray et al. (1981) exposed pregnant Sprague-Dawley rats to 0, 205 or 615 mg/m³ (0, 50 or 150 ppm) ethyl acrylate vapour for 6 h per day on gestation days 6-15. Maternal toxicity at 615 mg/m³ (150 ppm) was reflected in reduced food consumption and body-weight gain. In the foetuses, no significant increase was seen in gross, visceral or skeletal malformations at either exposure level, although three foetuses in three litters (10% of litters) in the 615-mg/m³ (150-ppm) group had hypoplastic tail and associated skeletal defects. Historically, this defect had been noted in 1% of over 800 control litters, and the highest incidence in one control group was 7% of litters.

Absorption, distribution, excretion and metabolism

After administration of 200 mg/kg bw ethyl acrylate in corn oil by gavage to Fischer 344 rats, no trace of the compound was found in blood samples from the retro-orbital venous plexus after 15, 30 or 60 min (detection limit, 1 μg/ml); however, detectable amounts were present in the portal venous blood after 15 or 30 min (up to 27 μg/ml). This may indicate that, after absorption, ethyl acrylate is hydrolysed rapidly in the blood and/or liver and does not circulate through the body (National Toxicology Program, 1983). In-vitro experiments also indicate that ethyl acrylate binds to nonprotein sulfhydryls in erythrocytes (Miller et al., 1981).

After administration to Fischer 344 rats of 100 mg/kg bw ethyl acrylate as a 2% solution in corn oil by gavage, 30-32% of the dose remained in the stomach after 30 min and 21-27% after 2 h (National Toxicology Program, 1983). The in-vivo concentration of nonprotein sulfhydryls in the forestomach (National Toxicology Program, 1983), lungs, blood and liver (Silver & Murphy, 1978) was reduced.

Intraperitoneal injection to Wistar rats of 70 mg/kg bw ethyl acrylate (in peanut oil) resulted in the excretion of thioethers in the urine, probably as mercapturic acids or related conjugates [not identified]. Inhibition of esterases by pretreatment with tri-*ortho*-tolyl phosphate (TOTP) resulted in an approximately six-fold increase in thioether excretion after the same dose of ethyl acrylate (Delbressine, 1981). Ethyl acrylate-induced depletion of nonprotein sulfhydryls *in vivo* in rats appeared to be more pronounced after TOTP treatment (Silver & Murphy, 1978).

Nonenzymatic and enzymatic hydrolysis of ethyl acrylate to acrylic acid was demonstrated to occur *in vitro* in plasma and homogenates of rat forestomach, glandular stomach, stomach contents, liver, lung and kidney (Silver & Murphy, 1978; Miller *et al.*, 1981; National Toxicology Program, 1983).

Ethyl acrylate binds to glutathione *in vitro* both spontaneously and after catalysis by liver glutathione-*S*-transferase (Miller *et al.*, 1981).

Mutagenicity and other short-term tests

Ethyl acrylate (tested at up to 10 000 μg/plate) was not mutagenic to *Salmonella typhimurium* TA1535, TA1537, TA1538, TA98 or TA100 in the presence or absence of a metabolic system (S9) from the liver of polychlorinated biphenyl-induced rats and hamsters or phenobarbital-induced rats, when tested in liquid incubation and plate incorporation assays (Ishidate *et al.*, 1981 [details not given]; Haworth *et al.*, 1983; National Toxicology Program, 1983; Waegemaekers & Bensink, 1984). [The Working Group noted that only in the study by Waegemaekers & Bensink were the conditions used appropriate to the testing of a volatile compound.]

Ethyl acrylate did not induce sex-linked recessive lethal mutations in *Drosophila melanogaster* when injected (20 mg/ml) or administered in feed (40 000 ppm [mg/kg]) (Valencia *et al.*, 1985).

Ethyl acrylate (7.5-15 μg/ml) induced a dose-related increase in the incidence of chromosomal aberrations in cultured Chinese hamster lung cells in the absence of a metabolic system (Ishidate, 1983).

Groups of four male Balb/c mice were given two intraperitoneal injections (24 h apart) of ethyl acrylate (total dose, 225-1800 mg/kg bw), and the bone marrow was harvested 6 h after the second injection; a dose-related increase in the number of micronucleated polychromatic erythrocytes was observed (Przybojewska *et al.*, 1984).

(b) Humans

Toxic effects

Ethyl acrylate is irritating to the skin, eyes and mucous membranes of the gastrointestinal tract and respiratory system (Nemec & Bauer, 1978). A dose of 4% in petrolatum produced sensitization reactions in 10/24 volunteers; no irritation was observed in 48-h closed patch tests (Opdyke, 1975).

Prolonged exposure to 205-308 mg/m^3 (50-75 ppm) ethyl acrylate produced drowsiness, headache and nausea (Nemec & Bauer, 1978). Fourteen of 33 workers exposed over an average period of five years to 4-58 mg/m³ ethyl acrylate (and 50 mg/m³ butyl acrylate) complained of autonomic and neurotic symptoms, but electroencephalographic examination showed no organic dysfunction (Kuželová *et al.*, 1981).

Effects on reproduction and prenatal toxicity
No data were available to the Working Group.

Absorption, distribution, excretion and metabolism
No data were available to the Working Group.

Mutagenicity and chromosomal effects
No data were available to the Working Group.

3.3 Case reports and epidemiological studies of carcinogenicity to humans

No data were available to the Working Group.

4. Summary of Data Reported and Evaluation

4.1 Exposure data

Ethyl acrylate has been produced commercially since the early 1930s. Occupational exposure occurs in the manufacture of ethyl acrylate and in the manufacture and use of its emulsion polymers. It is also used as a synthetic flavouring substance and fragrance adjuvant in consumer products.

4.2 Experimental data

Ethyl acrylate was tested for carcinogenicity by gavage in mice and rats. Dose-related increases in the incidence of squamous-cell papillomas and carcinomas of the forestomach were observed in both species. Ethyl acrylate was tested by inhalation in the same strains of mice and rats; no treatment-related neoplastic lesion was observed. No treatment-related tumour was observed following skin application of ethyl acrylate for lifespan to male mice.

In one experiment in rats, oral administration of ethyl acrylate produced signs of embryotoxicity and foetotoxicity at mildly maternally toxic doses but did not increase foetal malformation. It was not embryotoxic, foetotoxic or teratogenic to rats at an airborne concentration that produced slight maternal toxicity.

Ethyl acrylate was not mutagenic to *Salmonella typhimurium* in the presence or absence of an exogenous metabolic system, nor was it mutagenic to *Drosophila melanogaster*. It induced chromosomal aberrations in Chinese hamster lung cells *in vitro* and micronuclei in the bone marrow of mice treated *in vivo*.

Overall assessment of data from short-term tests: Ethyl acrylate[a]

	Genetic activity			Cell transformation
	DNA damage	Mutation	Chromosomal effects	
Prokaryotes		−		
Fungi/ Green plants				
Insects		−		
Mammalian cells (*in vitro*)			+	
Mammals (*in vivo*)			+	
Humans (*in vivo*)				
Degree of evidence in short-term tests for genetic activity: **Limited**				Cell transformation: No data

[a]The groups into which the table is divided and the symbols '+', '−' and '?' are defined on pp. 19-20 of the Preamble; the degrees of evidence are defined on pp. 20-21.

4.3 Human data

No data were available to evaluate the reproductive effects or prenatal toxicity of ethyl acrylate to humans.

No case report or epidemiological study was available to evaluate the carcinogenicity of ethyl acrylate to humans.

4.4 Evaluation[1]

There is *sufficient evidence*[2] for the carcinogenicity of ethyl acrylate in experimental animals.

No data on humans were available.

---

[1]For definition of the italicized term, see Preamble, p. 18.

[2]In the absence of data on humans, it is reasonable, for practical purposes, to regard chemicals for which there is sufficient evidence of carcinogenicity in animals as if they presented a carcinogenic risk to humans.

5. References

American Conference of Governmental Industrial Hygienists (1984) *Threshold Limit Values for Chemical Substances and Physical Agents in the Work Environment and Biological Exposure Indices with Intended Changes for 1984-85*, Cincinnati, OH, p. 18

Anon. (1983) Acrylate ester promising. *Plast. Ind. News, 29*, 97-98

Arbetarskyddsstyrelsens Författningssamling (National Swedish Board of Occupational Safety and Health) (1984) *Hygienic Limit Values (AFS 1984:5)* (Swed.), Stockholm, p. 16

Autian, J. (1975) Structure-toxicity relationships of acrylic monomers. *Environ. Health Perspect., 11*, 141-152

Badische Corp., Celanese Chemical Co., Inc., Rohm & Haas Co. & Union Carbide Corp. (1984) *Acrylate Esters, A Guide to Safety and Handling*, Williamsburg, VA, Dallas, TX, Philadelphia, PA, Danbury, CT

Belanger, P.L. & Coye, M.J. (1981) *Health Hazard Evaluation Report No. HHE-80-68-871 Sinclair Paint Company, Los Angeles, CA (US NTIS PB82-214396)*, Washington DC, US Department of Health and Human Services, Public Health Service, Centers for Disease Control, National Institute for Occupational Safety and Health

Bollini, M., Seves, A. & Focher, B. (1975) Determination of free monomers in aqueous emulsions of synthetic polymers and copolymers (Ital.). *Textilia, 51*, 25-28

Borzelleca, J.F., Larson, P.S., Hennigar, G.R., Jr, Huf, E.G., Crawford, E.M. & Blackwell Smith, R., Jr (1964) Studies on the chronic oral toxicity of monomeric ethyl acrylate and methyl methacrylate. *Toxicol. appl. Pharmacol., 6*, 29-36

Brunn, J., Doerffel, K., Much, H. & Zimmermann, G. (1975) Ultraviolet photometric determination of residual monomer content in technical polymers of acrylic acids and acrylic acid ethyl esters (Ger.). *Plaste Kautsch., 22*, 485-486 [*Chem. Abstr., 83*, 115163m]

Celanese Chemical Co. (1984) *Ethyl Acrylate Sales Specifications (Technical Bulletin No. CCC-92)*, Dallas, TX

Conseil de l'Europe (1981) *Substances Aromatisantes et Sources Naturelles de Matières Aromatisantes* (Flavouring substances and natural occurrence of flavouring materials), Moulin-les-Metz, Maisonneuve

Delbressine, L.P.C. (1981) *Metabolic Detoxification of Olefinic Compounds*, PhD Thesis, Nijmegen, University of Nijmegen, The Netherlands, p. 99

DePass, L.R., Fowler, E.H., Meckley, D.R. & Weil, C.S. (1984) Dermal oncogenicity bioassays of acrylic acid, ethyl acrylate, and butyl acrylate. *J. Toxicol. environ. Health, 14*, 115-120

Deutsche Forschungsgemeinschaft (1984) *Maximal Concentrations in the Workplace and Biological Occupational Limit Value* (Ger.), Part XX, Weinheim, Verlag Chemie GmbH, p. 34

Fassett, D.W. (1963) *Esters.* In: Patty, F.A., ed., *Industrial Hygiene and Toxicology*, 2nd rev. ed., Vol. 2, New York, Interscience, pp. 1877-1880

Ghanayem, B.I., Maronpot, R.R. & Matthews, H.B. (1985a) Ethyl acrylate-induced gastric toxicity. I. Effect of single and repetitive dosing. *Toxicol. appl. Pharmacol.*, *80*, 323-335

Ghanayem, B.I., Maronpot, R.R. & Matthews, H.B. (1985b) Ethyl acrylate-induced gastric toxicity. II. Structure-toxicity relationships and mechanisms. *Toxicol. appl. Pharmacol.*, *80*, 336-344

Grasselli, J.G. & Ritchey, W.M., eds (1975) *CRC Atlas of Spectral Data and Physical Constants for Organic Compounds*, Vol. 4, Cleveland, OH, CRC Press, p. 314

Haagen-Smit, A.J., Kirchner, J.G., Prater, A.N. & Deasy, C.L. (1945) Chemical studies of pineapple (*Ananas sativas* Lindl). I. The volatile flavor and odor constituents of pineapple. *J. Am. chem. Soc.*, *67*, 1646-1650

Haggin, J. (1985) New Dow acrylate ester processes derive from C_1 efforts. *Chem. Eng. News*, *63*, 25-26

Hawley, G.G., ed. (1981) *The Condensed Chemical Dictionary*, 10th ed., New York, Van Nostrand Reinhold Co., pp. 422-423

Haworth, S., Lawlor, T., Mortelmans, K., Speck, W. & Zeiger, E. (1983) *Salmonella* mutagenicity test results for 250 chemicals. *Environ. Mutagenesis, Suppl. 1*, 3-142

Health and Safety Executive (1985) *Occupational Exposure Limits 1985 (Guidance Note EH 40/85)*, London, Her Majesty's Stationery Office, p. 13

IARC (1976) *IARC Monographs on the Evaluation of Carcinogenic Risk of Chemicals to Man*, Vol. 11, *Cadmium, Nickel, Some Epoxides, Miscellaneous Industrial Chemicals and General Considerations on Volatile Anaesthetics*, Lyon, pp. 75-112

IARC (1977) *IARC Monographs on the Evaluation of the Carcinogenic Risk of Chemicals to Man*, Vol. 15, *Some Fumigants, the Herbicides 2,4-D and 2,4,5-T, Chlorinated Dibenzodioxins and Miscellaneous Industrial Chemicals*, Lyon, pp. 155-175

IARC (1979) *IARC Monographs on the Evaluation of the Carcinogenic Risk of Chemicals to Humans*, Vol. 19, *Some Monomers, Plastics and Synthetic Elastomers, and Acrolein*, Lyon, pp. 57-71

International Labour Office (1980) *Occupational Exposure Limits for Airborne Toxic Substances, A Tabular Compilation of Values from Selected Countries*, 2nd (rev.) ed. (*Occupational Safety and Health Series No. 37*), Geneva, pp. 110-111

Ishidate, M., Jr and staff, eds (1983) *The Data Book of Chromosomal Aberration Tests In Vitro on 587 Chemical Substances Using a Chinese Hamster Fibroblast Cell Line (CHL Cells)*, Tokyo, The Realize Inc., p. 197

Ishidate, M., Jr, Sofuni, T. & Yoshikawa, K. (1981) Chromosomal aberration tests *in vitro* as a primary screening tool for environmental mutagens and/or carcinogens. *Gann Monogr. Cancer Res., 27,* 95-108

Jones, M.T., Pilgrim, R.C. & Murrow, P.J. (1981) *Control of acrylic monomer emissions from a process situated in a sensitive area.* In: Webb, K.A. & Smith, A.J., eds, *Proceedings of the Seventh International Clean Air Conference, Adelaide, Australia,* Ann Arbor, MI, Ann Arbor Science, pp. 809-827

Klecak, G., Geleick, H. & Frey, J.R. (1977) Screening of fragrance materials for allergenicity in the guinea pig. I. Comparison of four testing methods. *J. Soc. cosmet. Chem., 28,* 53-64

Kuželová, M., Kovařik, J., Fiedlerová, D. & Popler, A. (1981) Acrylic compounds and general health of the exposed persons (Czech.). *Pracov. Lék., 33,* 95-99

Lawrence, W.H., Bass, G.E., Purcell, W.P. & Autian, J. (1972) Use of mathematical models in the study of structure-toxicity relationships of dental compounds: I. Esters of acrylic and methacrylic acids. *J. dent. Res., 51,* 526-535

Lomonova, G.V. & Klimova, E.I. (1979) Toxicity of methyl and ethyl acrylates (Russ.). *Gig. Tr. prof. Zabol., 9,* 55-56

Loper, G.L., Sasaki, G.R. & Stamps, M.A. (1982) Carbon dioxide laser absorption spectra of toxic industrial compounds. *Appl. Optics, 21,* 1648-1653

Luskin, L.S. (1970) *Acrylic acid, methacrylic acid, and the related esters.* In: Leonard, E.C., ed., *Vinyl and Diene Monomers,* Part 1, New York, Wiley Interscience, pp. 105-203

Mannsville Chemical Products Corp. (1984) *Acrylates and Acrylic Acid (Chemical Products Synopsis),* Cortland, NY

Miller, R.R., Ayres, J.A., Rampy, L.W. & McKenna, M.J. (1981) Metabolism of acrylate esters in rat tissue homogenates. *Fundam. appl. Toxicol., 1,* 410-414

Miller, R.R., Young, J.T., Kociba, R.J., Keyes, D.G., Bodner, K.M., Calhoun, L.L. & Ayres, J.A. (1985) Chronic toxicity and oncogenicity bioassay of inhaled ethyl acrylate in Fischer 344 rats and B6C3F1 mice. *Drug chem. Toxicol., 8,* 1-42

Murray, J.S., Miller, R.R., Deacon, M.M., Hanley, T.R., Jr, Hayes, W.C., Rao, K.S. & John, J.A. (1981) Teratological evaluation of inhaled ethyl acrylate in rats. *Toxicol. appl. Pharmacol., 60,* 106-111

Näf-Müller, R. & Willhalm, B. (1971) On volatile constituents of pineapple (Ger.). *Helv. chim. Acta, 54,* 1880-1890

National Fire Protection Association (1984) *Fire Protection Guide on Hazardous Materials,* 8th ed., Quincy, MA, pp. 325M-47, 49-46 - 49-47

National Toxicology Program (1983) *NTP Technical Report on the Carcinogenesis Studies of Ethyl Acrylate (CAS No. 140-88-5) in F344/N Rats and B6C3F$_1$ Mice (Gavage Studies) (Technical Report Series No. 259),* Research Triangle Park, NC

Nemec, J. & Bauer, W., Jr (1978) *Acrylic acid and derivates.* In: Mark, H.F., Othmer, D.F., Overberger, C.G. & Seaborg, G.T., eds, *Kirk-Othmer Encyclopedia of Chemical Technology,* 3rd ed., Vol. 1, New York, John Wiley & Sons, pp. 330-354

NIH/EPA Chemical Information System (1983) *Carbon-13 NMR Spectral Search System, Mass Spectral Search System,* and *Infrared Spectral Search System,* Arlington, VA, Information Consultants

Opdyke, D.L.J. (1975) Monographs on fragrance raw materials, ethyl acrylate. *Food Cosmet. Toxicol., 13* (Suppl.), 801-802

Paulet, G. & Vidal (1975) On the toxicity of some esters acrylic and methacrylic esters of acrylamide and polyacrylamides (Fr.). *Arch. Mal. prof., 36,* 58-60

Pietrowicz, D., Owecka, A. & Barański, B. (1980) Disturbances in rat's embryonal development due to ethyl acrylate. *Zwierzeta Lab., 17,* 67-72

Pozzani, U.C., Weil, C.S. & Carpenter, C.P. (1949) Subacute vapor toxicity and range-finding data for ethyl acrylate. *J. ind. Hyg. Toxicol., 31,* 311-316

Przybojewska, B., Dziubaltowska, E. & Kowalski, Z. (1984) Genotoxic effects of ethyl acrylate and methyl acrylate in the mouse evaluated by the micronucleus test. *Mutat. Res., 135,* 189-191

Sadtler Research Laboratories (1980) *The Sadtler Standard Spectra Collection, Cumulative Index,* Philadelphia, PA

Samimi, B. & Falbo, L. (1982) Monitoring of workers exposure to low levels of airborne monomers in a polystyrene production plant. *Am. ind. Hyg. Assoc. J., 43,* 858-862

Samimi, B. & Falbo, L. (1983) Validation of Abcor (NMS) organic vapor dosimeter under various concentrations and air velocity conditions. *Am. ind. Hyg. Assoc. J., 44,* 402-408

Sandmeyer, E.E. & Kirwin, C.J., Jr (1981) *Esters.* In: Clayton, G.D. & Clayton, F.E., eds, *Patty's Industrial Hygiene and Toxicology,* 3rd rev. ed., Vol. 2A, *Toxicology,* New York, John Wiley & Sons, p. 2294

Sax, N.I. (1984) *Dangerous Properties of Industrial Materials,* 6th ed., New York, Van Nostrand Reinhold, pp. 1315-1316

Silver, E.H. & Murphy, S.D. (1978) The effect of carboxylesterase inhibition on the toxicity of methyl acrylate, ethyl acrylate and acrylic acid (Abstract No. 216). *Toxicol. appl. Pharmacol., 45,* 312-313

Stahl, W.H., ed. (1973) *Compilation of Odor and Taste Threshold Values Data (ASTM Data Series DS 48),* Philadelphia, PA, American Society for Testing and Materials, p. 32

Tanii, H. & Hashimoto, K. (1982) Structure-toxicity relationship of acrylates and methacrylates. *Toxicol. Lett., 11,* 125-129

Taylor, D.G. (1977) *NIOSH Manual of Analytical Methods,* 2nd ed., Vol. 2 (*(NIOSH) DHEW Publ. No. 77-157-B*), Washington DC, US Government Printing Office, pp. S35-1 — S35-9

Treon, J.F., Sigmon, H., Wright, H. & Kitzmiller, K.V. (1949) The toxicity of methyl and ethyl acrylate. *J. ind. Hyg. Toxicol., 31,* 317-326

Työsuojeluhallitus (National Finnish Board of Occupational Safety and Health) (1981) *Airborne Contaminants in the Workplace (Safety Bull. 3)* (Finn.), Tampere, p. 13

Union Carbide Corp. (1971) *Toxicology Studies - Ethyl Acrylate*, New York, Industrial Medicine and Toxicology Department

Union Carbide Corp. (1982) *Product Information: Ethyl, Butyl and 2-Ethylhexyl Acrylates (Technical Bulletin No. F-40252C)*, Danbury, CT

US Environmental Protection Agency (1984) Protection of environment. *US Code Fed. Regul., Title 40*, Part 261.33, p. 364

US Food and Drug Administration (1984) Food and drugs. *US Code Fed. Regul., Title 21*, Parts 172.515, 175.105, 175.300, 176.170, 176.180, 177.1010, 178.3790, pp. 49, 133, 145, 188, 198

US International Trade Commission (1984) *Synthetic Organic Chemicals, US Production and Sales, 1983 (USITC Publication 1588)*, Washington DC, US Government Printing Office, p. 258

US Occupational Safety and Health Administration (1983) *General Industry. OSHA Safety and Health Standards (29 CFR 1910) (OSHA 2206)* (rev.), Washington DC, US Government Printing Office, p. 601

Valencia, R., Mason, J.M., Woodruff, R.C. & Zimmering, S. (1985) Chemical mutagenesis testing in *Drosophila*. III. Results of 48 coded compounds tested for the National Toxicology Program. *Environ. Mutagenesis, 7*, 325-348

Verschueren, K. (1983) *Handbook of Environmental Data on Organic Chemicals*, 2nd ed., New York, Van Nostrand Reinhold, pp. 625-626

Waegemaekers, T.H.J.M. & Bensink, M.P.M. (1984) Non-mutagenicity of 27 aliphatic acrylate esters in the *Salmonella*-microsome test. *Mutat. Res., 137*, 95-102

van der Walle, H.B. & Bensink, T. (1982) Cross reaction pattern of 26 acrylic monomers on guinea pig skin. *Contact Dermatol., 8*, 376-382

van der Walle, H.B., Klecak, G., Geleick, H. & Bensink, T. (1982) Sensitizing potential of 14 mono(meth)acrylates in the guinea pig. *Contact Dermatol., 8*, 223-235

Weast, R.C., ed. (1984) *CRC Handbook of Chemistry and Physics*, 65th ed., Boca Raton, FL, CRC Press, p. C-80

Windholz, M., ed. (1983) *The Merck Index*, 10th ed., Rahway, NJ, Merck & Co., p. 546

METHYL ACRYLATE

This substance was considered by a previous Working Group, in February 1978 (IARC, 1979). Since that time, new data have become available, and these have been incorporated into the monograph and taken into consideration in the present evaluation.

1. Chemical and Physical Data

1.1 Synonyms and trade names

Chem. Abstr. Services Reg. No.: 96-33-3

Chem. Abstr. Name: 2-Propenoic acid, methyl ester

IUPAC Systematic Name: Methyl acrylate

Synonyms: Acrylic acid, methyl ester; methoxycarbonylethylene; methyl acrylate, monomer; methyl propenate; methyl propenoate; methyl prop-2-enoate; methyl-2-propenoate; propenoic acid, methyl ester

1.2 Structural and molecular formulae and molecular weight

$$CH_2 = CH - \overset{\displaystyle O}{\overset{\displaystyle \|}{C}} - O - CH_3$$

$C_2H_6O_2$ Mol. wt: 86.09

1.3 Chemical and physical properties of the pure substance

(a) *Description*: Colourless volatile liquid with an acrid odour (Hawley, 1981; Verschueren, 1983; Windholz, 1983; Sax, 1984) and odour threshold of 14 ppb (50 μg/m³) (Badische Corp. *et al.*, 1984)

(b) *Boiling-point*: 80.5°C (Weast, 1984)

(c) *Melting-point*: <-75°C (Verschueren, 1983; Weast, 1984)

(d) *Density*: d$^{20}_4$ 0.9535 (Weast, 1984)

(e) *Spectroscopy data*: Infrared (Sadtler Research Laboratories, 1980; prism [1117[a]], grating [15113]), nuclear magnetic resonance (Sadtler Research Laboratories, 1980, proton [10332], C-13 [2813]) and mass spectral data (NIH/EPA Chemical Information System, 1983) have been reported.

(f) *Solubility*: Slightly soluble in water (6 g/100 ml at 20°C); soluble in ethanol, diethyl ether, acetone and benzene (Grasselli & Ritchey, 1975; Windholz, 1983; Weast, 1984)

(g) *Volatility*: Vapour pressure, 70 mm Hg at 20°C; relative vapour density (air = 1), 3.0; saturation concentration, 319 g/m³ at 20°C (Verschueren, 1983)

(h) *Stability*: Flash-point, -2.8°C (open-cup) (Sax, 1984); polymerizes easily on standing, accelerated by heat, light and peroxides; vapour forms explosive mixtures with air (Hawley, 1981; Windholz, 1983; National Fire Protection Association, 1984); can react vigorously with oxidizing materials; dangerous when exposed to heat, spark, flame or oxidizers (Sax, 1984)

(i) *Conversion factor*: mg/m³ = 3.52 × ppm[b]

1.4 Technical products and impurities

Methyl acrylate sold commercially in the USA has the following specifications: methyl acrylate, 99.5 wt % min; water, 0.10 wt % max; acrylic acid, 0.009 wt % max; hydroquinone monomethyl ether (MEHQ), 15-20 mg/kg (also available with 50 or 200 mg/kg MEHQ or 1000 mg/kg hydroquinone (HQ)) and substantially free of suspended matter (Celanese Chemical Co., 1984).

Methyl acrylate can undergo spontaneous polymerization. To prevent premature polymerization, inhibitors, such as HQ (see IARC, 1977) and MEHQ are added and kept active under atmospheres containing 5-20% oxygen in the vapour space. Polymerization is also inhibited by the exclusion of water and by keeping temperature below 25°C. When these precautions are taken, methyl acrylate can be stored in tanks made of stainless-steel, aluminium or glass for up to six months. HQ and MEHQ inhibitors can be removed from methyl acrylate prior to its use in polymerization or neutralized by the addition of polymerization catalyst (Badische Corp. *et al.*, 1984).

---

[a]Spectrum number in Sadtler compilation

[b]Calculated from: mg/m³ = (molecular weight/24.45) × ppm, assuming standard temperature (25°C) and pressure (760 mm Hg)

2. Production, Use, Occurrence and Analysis

2.1 Production and use

(a) Production

Methyl acrylate has been produced commercially since 1944. In the USA, a propylene oxidation process is used almost exclusively for the production of acrylic compounds. This technique, developed commercially in 1970, involves the oxidation of propylene to acrolein and the subsequent oxidation of acrolein to acrylic acid. The reactions occur in the vapour phase in shell-and-tube exchangers at near atmospheric pressure. Bismuth/cobalt oxides on a silica or alumina carrier are used as catalysts for the first oxidation reaction, and a molybdenum/vanadium system for the second. The acrylic acid leaving the second reactor is absorbed with water, extracted with an organic solvent and purified by vacuum distillation (Mannsville Chemical Products Corp., 1984). The methyl ester is formed by reacting acrylic acid with methanol.

A technique used in the past is the modified Reppe process, in which methyl acrylate is produced by the reaction of acetylene with nickel carbonyl (see IARC, 1976) and methanol in the presence of an acid. In a variation of this process, acetylene, carbon monoxide and water are combined in the presence of a nickel halide to form acrylic acid. Methanol is used to produce the methyl ester.

Two techniques have been developed recently for the production of acrylate esters. One involves use of organic carbonates as esterifying agents, and the other yields acrylate esters from 2-halo-1-alkenes isolated from hydrocarbon feedstocks (Haggin, 1985).

In Japan, about 25 million kg methyl acrylate were used in 1982 and 9 million kg were exported (Anon., 1983). There are currently five major producers of methyl acrylate in Japan.

One company in France produced 20 million kg in 1984. This company and two companies in the Federal Republic of Germany have been identified as the primary producers of methyl acrylate in western Europe.

There were three major producers of methyl acrylate in the USA in 1984. About 14 million kg were produced in 1983 (Mannsville Chemical Products Corp., 1984).

(b) Use

Methyl acrylate is used primarily as a comonomer with acrylonitrile in the preparation of acrylic and modacrylic fibres. The acrylic component facilitates downstream processing, such as bulking and crimping, and increases the diffusion rate of dye into fibre. Acrylic fibres generally contain at least 85% acrylonitrile. They are used in the clothing industry for sweaters, hosiery and yarn, and in the home furnishing market for carpet, blankets and curtains. Modacrylic fibres contain more than 35% but less than 85% acrylonitrile. Because of their flame retardant properties, they are used for manufacturing children's sleepwear, draperies and curtains that must pass flame-retardant standards. Industrial applications for modacrylics include paint rollers, battery separators and protective clothing (Hobson & McPeters, 1985). Methyl acrylate has also been used in the preparation of thermoplastic coatings, adhesives and sealants and amphoteric surfactants for shampoos (US Department of Health and Human Services, 1978).

(c)   Regulatory status and guidelines

Occupational exposure limits for methyl acrylate have been set by 17 countries by regulation or recommended guideline (Table 1).

Table 1. National occupational exposure limits for methyl acrylate[a]

Country	Year	Concentration (mg/m^3)	Interpretation[b]
Australia	1978	35[c]	TWA
Belgium	1978	35[c]	TWA
Bulgaria	1971	20	Ceiling
Finland	1981	35[c]	TWA
German Democratic Republic	1979	20	TWA
		20	Ceiling
Germany, Federal Republic of	1984	35[c]	TWA
Italy	1978	20[c]	TWA
The Netherlands	1978	35[c]	TWA
Poland	1976	20[c]	Ceiling
Romania	1975	20[c]	TWA
		30	Ceiling
Sweden	1984	35[c]	TWA
Switzerland	1978	35[c]	TWA
UK	1985	35[c]	TWA
USA			
ACGIH	1984	35[c]	TWA
OSHA	1983	35[c]	TWA
USSR	1977	20	Ceiling
Yugoslavia	1971	20	Ceiling

[a]From International Labour Office (1980); Työsuojeluhallitus (1981); US Occupational Safety and Health Administration (OSHA) (1983); American Conference of Governmental Industrial Hygienists (ACGIH) (1984); Arbetarskyddsstyrelsens Författningssamling (1984); Deutsches Forschungsgemeinschaft (1984); Health and Safety Executive (1985)

[b]TWA, time-weighted average;

[c]Skin notation (absorption is possible)

Methyl acrylate polymers or copolymers are permitted by the US Food and Drug Administration (1984) as components of adhesives, resinous and polymeric coatings, paper and paperboard in contact with dry, aqueous or fatty foods, and semirigid and rigid acrylic and modified acrylic plastics.

2.2 Occurrence

(*a*) *Natural occurrence*

Methyl acrylate has been identified in the extractable volatile components of fresh pineapple purée (Näf-Müller & Willhalm, 1971)

(*b*) *Occupational exposure*

No data were available to the Working Group.

2.3 Analysis

The analytical method of the US National Institute for Occupational Safety and Health for determining methyl acrylate in air involves adsorption on charcoal, solvent desorption with carbon disulphide and analysis by gas chromatography with flame ionization detection. The useful range is reported to be 7-70 mg/m³, although levels as low as 0.09 mg/m³ have been reported in collaborative testing (Sawicki *et al.*, 1975; Taylor, 1977).

Alternate gas chromatography column packings have been recommended for improved separation from other low-molecular-weight esters (Langvardt & Ramstad, 1981); and collection of air samples on Tenax, purge-trap preconcentration, and analysis by gas chromatography/mass spectrometry have been reported to increase sensitivity (Krost *et al.*, 1982).

3. Biological Data Relevant to the Evaluation of Carcinogenic Risk to Humans

3.1 Carcinogenicity studies in animals

Inhalation exposure

Rat: In a study reported as an abstract, groups of 86 male and 86 female Sprague-Dawley rats [age unspecified] were exposed to 0, 15, 45 or 135 ppm (53, 158 or 475 mg/m³) methyl acrylate [purity unspecified] in air for 6 h per day on five days per week for two years. Interim kills [no figures provided] were performed after 12 and 18 months of exposure [survival and mode of post-mortem examination not given]. The authors stated that a dose-dependent increase could not be established for either the overall tumour incidence or for any of a variety of observed tumour types [numbers and types of tumours not given] (Klimisch & Reininghaus, 1984).

3.2 Other relevant biological data

(*a*) *Experimental systems*

The toxic effects of acrylic monomers, including methyl acrylate, have been reviewed (Autian, 1975).

Toxic effects

Oral LD_{50} values for methyl acrylate have been reported to be 826 mg/kg bw in male ddY mice (Tanii & Hashimoto, 1982), 200 mg/kg bw in rabbits (Fassett, 1963) and 227 mg/kg bw in Wistar rats (Paulet & Vidal, 1975). Intraperitoneal LD_{50}s were 254 mg/kg bw in male ICR mice (Lawrence *et al.*, 1972) and 325 mg/kg bw in Wistar rats (Paulet & Vidal, 1975); and the dermal LD_{50} (undiluted compound) in rabbits was reported to be 1240 mg/kg bw (Fassett, 1963).

Oral administration to male Fischer 344 rats of 86 and 172 mg/kg methyl acrylate in corn oil by gavage resulted in dose-dependent gastric toxicity, as judged by gross examination (increase in size of the stomach, forestomach oedema) and histopathological examination, which revealed intracellular and intercellular mucosal oedema and submucosal oedema and superficial mucosal necrosis (Ghanayem *et al.*, 1985).

In inhalation studies, 3/6 rats died after exposure for 4 h to 3500 mg/m³ (Fassett, 1963). Lomonova and Klimova (1979) reported LC_{50} values of 12 800 and 7300 mg/m³ in mice and rats, respectively [exposure period unspecified]. Inhalation of 2000 mg/m³ (578 ppm) by rabbits, guinea-pigs and rats for 7 h per day for two to seven days caused a reduction in body weight, salivation, laboured respiration and lethargy in all three species, distension of ear veins in rabbits and lachrymation in rabbits and guinea-pigs (Treon *et al.*, 1949).

Dermal application of methyl acrylate to rabbits caused marked local irritation, erythema, oedema, vascular damage and dystrophic and necrotic effects (Treon *et al.*, 1949; Suvorov, 1973).

In various tests at different dose levels in guinea-pigs, methyl acrylate was shown to induce contact sensitivity (Parker & Turk, 1983).

Effects on reproduction and prenatal toxicity

No data were available to the Working Group.

Absorption, distribution, excretion and metabolism

Autoradiography of guinea-pigs exposed dermally to 46 mg/kg bw (0.53 mmol/kg bw) 2,3-¹⁴C-methyl acrylate (undiluted) showed that the majority of the radioactivity was retained in the dermis during the first 16 h. After total penetration of the dermis, the radioactivity was seen in the subcutaneous tissues and throughout the body (Delbressine *et al.*, 1980; Seutter & Rijntjes, 1981).

Following an oral dose of 34 mg/kg bw (0.4 mmol/kg bw) 2,3-¹⁴C-methyl acrylate to guinea-pigs, autoradiography showed that the radioactivity was distributed in internal organs, especially the liver and bladder, and brain within 2 h; at 16 h it was seen only in mucous linings of the stomach, intestine and mouth epithelium. One hour after intraperitoneal injection of the same dose (no vehicle), radioactivity was concentrated in the peritoneum and liver and present in most other organs. Radioactivity quickly decreased in most organs, except the liver and bladder. After 24 and 48 h most organs had lost the radioactive material, but some was retained in mucous linings (Seutter & Rijntjes, 1981). After an intraperitoneal dose of 25 mg/kg bw (0.29 mmol/kg bw) 2,3-¹⁴C-methyl acrylate to young male guinea-pigs, 35% of the radioactivity was excreted as $^{14}CO_2$ in expired air within 8 h and 40% after

72 h (Delbressine *et al.*, 1980); 22.6% was excreted in the urine over 72 h (Seutter & Rijntjes, 1981).

Conjugation with sulfhydryl groups appears to be an important detoxification process for methyl acrylate in the guinea-pig. After oral administration of 34 mg/kg bw methyl acrylate, 11% was excreted as urinary thioether during the first 24-h period, 2.5% during the second 24-h period and 0.3% during the third. Following intraperitoneal administration (without a vehicle), these values were 16.5%, 10.7% and 2.8%, respectively (Seutter & Rijntjes, 1981). After intraperitoneal administration of 12 mg/kg bw methyl acrylate to Wistar rats, 6.6% of the dose was excreted as thioether within 24 h. Pretreatment of the animals with an esterase inhibitor, tri-*ortho*-tolylphosphate (TOTP), increased thioether excretion to 40.6% of the dose, indicating competition between nonprotein sulfhydryl conjugation and ester hydrolysis to acrylic acid. The thioethers were identified as *N*-acetyl-*S*-(2-carboxyethyl)cysteine and the corresponding monomethyl ester, with a ratio between the two metabolites of 20:1. After pretreatment with TOTP, this ratio was 1:2 (Delbressine *et al.*, 1981). In male rats exposed for 4 h to 135 (475), 370 (1300), 490 (1725) or 720 (2535) ppm (mg/m^3) methyl acrylate by inhalation, depletion of nonprotein sulfhydryl compounds was most pronounced in the lung, when compared to liver, kidney and blood (Silver & Murphy, 1981).

In vitro, the synthetic glycidic ester (i.e., the epoxide of methyl acrylate) reacted with glutathione and appeared to be a good substrate for glutathione *S*-transferase. However, after administration of methyl acrylate to Wistar rats no hydroxy mercapturic acid derived from such an epoxide has been detected. It seems unlikely, therefore, that in-vivo epoxidation of the acrylic esters occurs. Experiments with rat-liver microsomal preparations gave no indication of epoxide formation from methyl acrylate (Delbressine, 1981).

Mutagenicity and other short-term tests

Methyl acrylate (tested at up to 4700 μg/plate) was not mutagenic to *Salmonella typhimurium* TA1535, TA1537, TA1538, TA98 or TA100 in the presence or absence of a metabolic system (S9) from the liver of polychlorinated biphenyl- or phenobarbital-induced rats, when tested in both the standard plate incorporation and liquid preincubation assays (Ishidate *et al.*, 1981 [details not given]; Hachiya *et al.*, 1981; Waegemaekers & Bensink, 1984). [The Working Group noted that only in the study by Waegemaeker & Bensink were methods appropriate to the testing of a volatile compound employed.] Negative results were also reported in a spot test in *Salmonella* strains TA1535, TA1537, TA98 and TA100 (Florin *et al.*, 1980); in strain TA100, when tested at up to 3000 μg/ml in a preincubation assay with stoppered tubes (Waegemaekers & Bensink, 1984); and in strains *his* G46, *his* C3076, *his* D3052, TA1535, TA1537, TA1538, TA98 and TA100 in a plate gradient assay, both in the presence and absence of Aroclor-induced rat-liver S9 (McMahon *et al.*, 1979). Methyl acrylate was not mutagenic to *Escherichia coli* WP2 or WP2*uvr*A⁻ in a plate gradient assay, in the presence or absence of Aroclor-induced rat-liver S9 (McMahon *et al.*, 1979).

An increase in the incidence of chromosomal aberrations was observed in cultured Chinese hamster lung cells in the presence of 7.5-15 μg/ml methyl acrylate, in the absence of an exogenous metabolic system (Ishidate *et al.*, 1981, 1983).

Groups of four Balb/c mice were given two intraperitoneal injections (separated by 24 h) of methyl acrylate (total dose, 37.5-300 mg/kg bw), and the bone marrow was harvested 6 h after the second injection; a three-fold increase in the number of micronuclei was observed in polychromatic erythrocytes (Przybojewska *et al.*, 1984). Groups of four to six ddY mice were administered a single dose (250 mg/kg bw) or four doses of 125 mg/kg bw methyl acrylate by gavage, and the bone marrow was harvested 24 h after the last injection; no increase in the number of micronuclei in polychromatic erythrocytes was observed (Hachiya *et al.*, 1981). [The Working Group noted that different routes of administration were used in these two studies, and that in the latter study only a single sample was taken and no toxicity was observed with the highest dose.]

(b) Humans

Toxic effects

The toxic hazards of occupational exposure to methyl acrylate have been summarized (US Department of Health and Human Services, 1978).

Methyl acrylate is highly irritating to the skin and mucous membranes, both in the workplace and experimentally (Suvorov, 1971; Dovzhanskii, 1976; Cavelier *et al.*, 1981). It is also a recognized allergen (Khromov, 1974; Cavelier *et al.*, 1981).

A two-fold increase in the frequency of disturbances in menstrual functions was reported in 1044 female workers exposed to acrylonitrile and methyl acrylate as compared to a control group (Chobot, 1979). [The Working Group noted that deficiencies in study design made it difficult to interpret this result.]

Effects on reproduction and prenatal toxicity

No data were available to the Working Group.

Absorption, distribution, excretion and metabolism

No data were available to the Working Group.

Mutagenicity and chromosomal effects

No data were available to the Working Group.

3.3 Case reports and epidemiological studies of carcinogenicity to humans

No data were available to the Working Group.

4. Summary of Data Reported and Evaluation

4.1 Exposure data

Methyl acrylate has been available commercially since 1944. Occupational exposure may occur during its use, primarily as a comonomer with acrylonitrile in the preparation of acrylic and modacrylic fibres. No data on occupational exposure to this compound were available to the Working Group.

4.2 Experimental data

In one study reported as an abstract, in which rats were exposed to methyl acrylate by inhalation for two years, no neoplastic effect was reported.

No data were available to evaluate the reproductive effects or prenatal toxicity of methyl acrylate to experimental animals.

Methyl acrylate was not mutagenic to bacteria, in the presence or absence of an exogenous metabolic system. It induced chromosomal aberrations in Chinese hamster lung cells *in vitro* and micronuclei in the bone marrow of mice treated *in vivo*.

Overall assessment of data from short-term tests: Methyl acrylate[a]

	Genetic activity			Cell transformation
	DNA damage	Mutation	Chromosomal effects	
Prokaryotes		−		
Fungi/Green plants				
Insects				
Mammalian cells (*in vitro*)			+	
Mammals (*in vivo*)			+	
Humans (*in vivo*)				
Degree of evidence in short-term tests for genetic activity: **Limited**				Cell transformation: No data

[a]The groups into which the table is divided and the symbols '+', '−' and '?' are defined on pp. 19-20 of the Preamble; the degrees of evidence are defined on pp. 20-21.

4.3 Human data

No data were available to evaluate the reproductive effects or prenatal toxicity of methyl acrylate to humans.

No case report or epidemiological study was available to evaluate the carcinogenicity of methyl acrylate to humans.

4.4 Evaluation[1]

There is *inadequate evidence* for the carcinogenicity of methyl acrylate to experimental animals.

No data on humans were available.

In the absence of epidemiological data, no evaluation of the carcinogenicity of methyl acrylate to humans could be made.

5. References

American Conference of Governmental Industrial Hygienists (1984) *Threshold Limit Values for Chemical Substances and Physical Agents in the Work Environment and Biological Exposure Indices with Intended Changes for 1984-85*, Cincinnati, OH, p. 23

Anon. (1983) Acrylate ester promising. *Plast. Ind. News*, *29*, 97-98

Arbetarskyddsstyrelsens Författningssamling (National Swedish Board of Occupational Safety and Health) (1984) *Hygienic Limit Values (AFS 1984:5)* (Swed.), Stockholm, p. 28

Autian, J. (1975) Structure-toxicity relationships of acrylic monomers. *Environ. Health Perspect.*, *11*, 141-152

Badische Corp., Celanese Chemical Co., Inc., Rohm & Haas Co. & Union Carbide Corp. (1984) *Acrylate Esters, A Guide to Safety and Handling*, Williamsburg, VA, Dallas, TX, Philadelphia, PA, Danbury, CT

Cavelier, C., Jelen, G., Hervé-Bazin, B. & Foussereau, J. (1981) Irritation and allergy to acrylates and methacrylates. Part I. Common monoacrylates and mono-methacrylates (Fr.). *Ann. Dermatol. Venéreol. (Paris)*, *108*, 549-556

Celanese Chemical Co. (1984) *Methyl Acrylate. Sales Specifications* (*Technical Bulletin No. CCC-91*), Dallas, TX

Chobot, A.M. (1979) The menstrual function in workers of polyacrylonitrile fibre production (Russ.). *Zdravookhr. beloruss.*, *2*, 24-26

Delbressine, L.P.C. (1981) *Metabolic Detoxification of Olefinic Compounds*, PhD Thesis, Nijmegen, University of Nijmegen, The Netherlands, p. 99

Delbressine, L.P.C., Seutter, E. & Seutter-Berlage, F. (1980) Metabolism and toxicity of acrylates and methacrylates. *Br. J. Pharmacol.*, *68*, 165P-166P

---

[1]For definition of the italicized term, see Preamble, p. 18.

Delbressine, L.P.C., Seutter-Berlage, F. & Seutter, E. (1981) Identification of urinary mercapturic acids formed from arylate, methacrylate and crotonate in the rat. *Xenobiotica, 11*, 241-247

Deutsche Forschungsgemeinschaft (1984) *Maximal Concentrations in the Workplace and Biological Occupational Limit Value* (Ger.), Part XX, Weinheim, Verlag Chemie GmbH, p. 40

Dovzhanskii, I.S. (1976) Dermatosis sickness rate of workers having contact with acrylates (Russ.). *Gig. Tr. prof. Zabol., 1*, 40-41

Fassett, D.W. (1963) *Esters.* In: Patty, F.A., ed., *Industrial Hygiene and Toxicology*, 2nd rev. ed., Vol. 2, New York, Interscience, pp. 1877-1880

Florin, I., Rutberg, L., Curvall, M. & Enzell, C.R. (1980) Screening of tobacco smoke constituents for mutagenicity using the Ames' test. *Toxicology, 18*, 219-232

Ghanayem, B.I., Maronpot, R.R. & Matthews, H.B. (1985) Ethyl acrylate-induced gastric toxicity. II. Structure-toxicity elationships and mechanism. *Toxicol. appl. Pharmacol., 80*, 336-344

Grasselli, J.G. & Ritchey, W.M., eds (1975) *CRC Atlas of Spectral Data and Physical Constants for Organic Compounds*, Vol. 4, Cleveland, OH, CRC Press, p. 316

Hachiya, N., Taketani, A. & Takizawa, Y. (1981) Mutagenicity study on environmental substances. 3. Ames test and mouse bone marrow micronucleus test on acrylic resin monomer and other additives (Jpn.). *Nippon Koshu Eisei Zasshi (Jpn. J. publ. Health), 29*, 236-239

Haggin, J. (1985) New Dow acrylate ester processes derive from C_1 efforts. *Chem. Eng. News, 63*, 25-26

Hawley, G.G., ed. (1981) *The Condensed Chemical Dictionary*, 10th ed., New York, Van Nostrand Reinhold Co., p. 666

Health and Safety Executive (1985) *Occupational Exposure Limits 1985 (Guidance Note EH 40/85)*, London, Her Majesty's Stationery Office, p. 15

Hobson, P.H. & McPeters, A.L. (1985) *Acrylic and modacrylic fibers.* In: Grayson, M., ed., *Kirk-Othmer Concise Encyclopedia of Chemical Technology*, New York, John Wiley & Sons, pp. 26-29

IARC (1976) *IARC Monographs on the Evaluation of Carcinogenic Risk of Chemicals to Man*, Vol. 11, *Cadmium, Nickel, Some Epoxides, Miscellaneous Industrial Chemicals and General Considerations on Volatile Anaesthetics*, Lyon, pp. 75-112

IARC (1977) *IARC Monographs on the Evaluation of the Carcinogenic Risk of Chemicals to Man*, Vol. 15, *Some Fumigants, the Herbicides 2,4-D and 2,4,5-T, Chlorinated Dibenzodioxins and Miscellaneous Industrial Chemicals*, Lyon, pp. 155-175

IARC (1979) *IARC Monographs on the Evaluation of the Carcinogenic Risk of Chemicals to Humans*, Vol. 19, *Some Monomers, Plastics and Synthetic Elastomers, and Acrolein*, Lyon, pp. 52-71

International Labour Office (1980) *Occupational Exposure Limits for Airborne Toxic Substances, A Tabular Compilation of Values from Selected Countries*, 2nd (rev.) ed. (*Occupational Safety and Health Series No. 37*), Geneva, pp. 142-143

Ishidate, M., Jr, Sofuni, T. & Yoshikawa, K. (1981) Chromosomal aberration tests *in vitro* as a primary screening tool for environmental mutagens and/or carcinogens. *Gann Monogr. Cancer Res.*, *27*, 95-108

Ishidate, M., Jr and staff, eds (1983) *The Data Book of Chromosomal Aberration Tests In Vitro on 587 Chemical Substances Using a Chinese Hamster Fibroblast Cell Line (CHL Cells)*, Tokyo, The Realize Inc., pp. 334

Khromov, V.E. (1974) Exposure to circulating and fixed antibodies in the diagnostics of chemically-induced allergy (Russ.). *Vraceb. delo*, *12*, 115-116

Klimisch, H.-J. & Reininghaus, W. (1984) Carcinogenicity of acrylates: Long-term inhalation studies on methyl acrylate (MA) and *n*-butyl acrylate (BA) in rats (Abstract No. 211). *Toxicologist*, *4*, 53

Krost, K.J., Pellizzari, E.D., Walburn, S.G. & Hubbard, S.A. (1982) Collection and analysis of hazardous organic emissions. *Anal. Chem.*, *54*, 810-817

Langvardt, P.W. & Ramstad, T. (1981) Gas chromatography of some volatile organic compounds using Oronite NIW on Carbopack supports. *J. chromatogr. Sci.*, *19*, 536-542

Lawrence, W.H., Bass, G.E., Purcell, W.P. & Autian, J. (1972) Use of mathematical models in the study of structure-toxicity relationships of dental compounds: I. Esters of acrylic and methacrylic acids. *J. dent. Res.*, *51*, 526-535

Lomonova, G.V. & Klimova, E.I. (1979) Data on the toxicity of methyl and ethyl esters of acrylic acid (Russ.). *Gig. Tr. prof. Zabol.*, *9*, 55-56

Mannsville Chemical Products Corp. (1984) *Acrylates and Acrylic Acid* (*Chemical Products Synopsis*), Cortland, NY

McMahon, R.E., Cline, J.C. & Thompson, C.A. (1979) Assay of 855 test chemicals in ten tester strains using a new modification of the Ames test for bacterial mutagens. *Cancer Res.*, *39*, 682-693

Näf-Müller, R. & Willhalm, B. (1971) On volatile constituents of pineapple (Ger.). *Helv. chim. Acta*, *54*, 1880-1890

National Fire Protection Association (1984) *Fire Protection Guide on Hazardous Materials*, 8th ed., Quincy, MA, pp. 325M-66, 49-61

NIH/EPA Chemical Information System (1983) *Carbon-13 NMR Spectral Search System, Mass Spectral Search System, and Infrared Spectral Search System*, Arlington, VA, Information Consultants

Parker, D. & Turk, J.L. (1983) Contact sensitivity to acrylate compounds in guinea pigs. *Contact Dermatol.*, *9*, 55-60

Paulet, G. & Vidal (1975) On the toxicity of some acrylic and methacrylic esters of acrylamide and polyacrylamides (Fr.). *Arch. Mal. prof. Méd. Trav. Séc. soc.*, *36*, 58-60

Przybojewska, B., Dziubaltowska, E. & Kowalski, Z. (1984) Genotoxic effects of ethyl acrylate and methyl acrylate in the mouse evaluated by the micronucleus test. *Mutat. Res.*, *135*, 189-191

Sadtler Research Laboratories (1980) *The Sadtler Standard Spectra Collection, Cumulative Index*, Philadelphia, PA

Sawicki, E., Belsky, T., Friedel, R.A., Hyde, D.L., Monkman, J.L., Rasmussen, R.A., Ripperton, L.A. & White, L.D. (1975) Organic solvent vapors in air analytical method. *Health Lab. Sci.*, *12*, 394-402

Sax, N.I. (1984) *Dangerous Properties of Industrial Materials*, 6th ed., New York, Van Nostrand Reinhold, pp. 1794-1795

Seutter, E. & Rijntjes, N.V.M. (1981) Whole-body autoradiography after systemic and topical administration of methyl acrylate in the guinea-pig. *Arch. dermatol. Res.*, *270*, 273-284

Silver, E.H. & Murphy, S.D. (1981) Potentiation of acrylate ester toxicity by prior treatment with the carboxylesterase inhibitor triorthotolyl phosphate (TOTP). *Toxicol. appl. Pharmacol.*, *57*, 208-219

Suvorov, A.P. (1971) Results of investigating workers contacting methyl acrylate (Russ.). *Gig. Tr. prof. Zabol.*, *15*, 49-50

Suvorov, A.P. (1973) On the repeated action of low methyl acrylate concentrations on the skin (Russ.). *Farmakol. Toksikol.*, *36*, 107-109

Tanii, H. & Hashimoto, K. (1982) Structure-toxicity relationship of acrylates and methacrylates. *Toxicol. Lett.*, *11*, 125-129

Taylor, D.G. (1977) *NIOSH Manual of Analytical Methods*, 2nd ed., Vol. 2 (*DHEW (NIOSH) Publication No. 77-157-B*), Washington DC, US Government Printing Office, pp. S38-1 — S38-9

Treon, J.F., Sigmon, H., Wright, H. & Kitzmiller, K.V. (1949) The toxicity of methyl and ethyl acrylate. *J. ind. Hyg. Toxicol.*, *31*, 317-326

Työsuojeluhallitus (National Finnish Board of Occupational Safety and Health) (1981) *Airborne Contaminants in the Workplace (Safety Bull. 3)* (Finn.), Tampere, p. 19

US Department of Health and Human Services (1978) *Occupational Health Guideline for Methyl Acrylate*, US Department of Labor, Occupational Safety and Health Administration

US Food and Drug Administration (1984) Food and drugs. *US Code Fed. Regul., Title 21*, Parts 175.105, 175.300, 176.170, 176.180, 177.1010, pp. 133, 145, 176, 188, 198

US Occupational Safety and Health Administration (1983) *General Industry. OSHA Safety and Health Standards (29 CFR 1910) (OSHA 2206)* (rev.), Washington DC, US Government Printing Office, p. 601

Verschueren, K. (1983) *Handbook of Environmental Data on Organic Chemicals*, 2nd ed., New York, Van Nostrand Reinhold, p. 829

Waegemaekers, T.H.J.M. & Bensink, M.P.M. (1984) Non-mutagenicity of 27 aliphatic acrylate esters in the *Salmonella*-microsome test. *Mutat. Res.*, *137*, 95-102

Weast, R., ed. (1984) *CRC Handbook of Chemistry and Physics*, 65th ed., Boca Raton, FL, CRC Press, p. C-81

Windholz, M., ed. (1983) *The Merck Index*, 10th ed., Rahway, NJ, Merck & Co., p. 863

VINYL ACETATE

This substance was considered by a previous Working Group, in February 1978 (IARC, 1979). Since that time, new data have become available, and these have been incorporated into the monograph and taken into consideration in the present evaluation.

1. Chemical and Physical Data

1.1 Synonyms and trade names

Chem. Abstr. Services Reg. No.: 108-05-4

Chem. Abstr. Name: Acetic acid, ethenyl ester

IUPAC Systematic Name: Vinyl acetate

Synonyms: Acetic acid, ethylene ether; 1-acetoxyethylene; ethanoic acid, ethenyl ester; ethenyl acetate; ethenyl ethanoate; vinyl acetate, monomer; vinyl A monomer; vinyl ethanoate

Trade Names: Zeset T

1.2 Structural and molecular formulae and molecular weight

$$CH_2 = CH - O - \overset{\overset{\textstyle O}{\textstyle \|}}{C} - CH_3$$

$C_4H_6O_2$

Mol. wt: 86.09

1.3 Chemical and physical properties of the pure substance

(a) *Description*: Colourless liquid (Verschueren, 1983; National Fire Protection Association, 1984; Perry & Green, 1984; Sax, 1984)

(b)   *Boiling-point*: 72.2°C (Weast, 1984)

(c)   *Melting-point*: -93.2°C (Weast, 1984)

(d)   *Density*: d$^{20}_4$ 0.9317 (Weast, 1984)

(e)   *Spectroscopy data*: Ultraviolet (Grasselli & Ritchey, 1975), infrared (Sadtler Research Laboratories, 1980, prism [982[a]], grating [8112]), nuclear magnetic resonance (Sadtler Research Laboratories, 1980; proton [10345], C-13 [1841]) and mass spectral data (NIH/EPA Chemical Information System, 1983) have been reported.

(f)   *Solubility*: Slightly soluble in water (2 g/100ml at 20°C (Windholz, 1983)); soluble in diethyl ether, acetone, benzene, ethanol and chloroform (Weast, 1984); soluble in most organic solvents, including chlorinated solvents (Hawley, 1981)

(g)   *Volatility*: Vapour pressure, 115 mm Hg at 25°C (Verschueren, 1983); relative vapour density (air = 1), 3.0 (Sax, 1984); saturation conc., 398 g/m³ at 20°C (Verschueren, 1983)

(h)   *Stability*: Flash-point (closed-cup), -8°C (Buckingham, 1982; Windholz, 1983; National Fire Protection Association, 1984); polymerizes in light (Windholz, 1983); highly inflammable, may polymerize violently (Buckingham, 1982); vapour forms explosive mixtures with air (National Fire Protection Association, 1984)

(i)   *Reactivity*: Free-radical polymerization; hydrolysis catalysed by acid- or base-forming acetic acid and acetaldehyde (Daniels, 1983)

(j)   *Conversion factor*: mg/m³ = 3.52 × ppm[b]

1.4 Technical products and impurities

Various commercial grades of vinyl acetate are available in the USA, differing in the amount and type of added inhibitor. Typically, 3-5 mg/l hydroquinone (see IARC, 1977) are used if the chemical is to be stored for less than two months. For up to four months of storage, 14-17 mg/l hydroquinone are used. If indefinite storage is anticipated, then 200-300 mg/l diphenylamine are used as inhibitor (Daniels, 1983). Typical specifications for commercial vinyl acetate are as follows: appearance, clear and free of suspended matter; vinyl acetate, 99.9% min; aldehydes (as acetaldehyde), 0.01% max; acidity (as acetic acid), 0.005% max; water, 0.04% max (Celanese Chemical Co., 1984).

---

[a]Spectrum number in Sadtler compilation

[b]Calculated from: mg/m³ = (molecular weight/24.45) × ppm, assuming standard temperature (25⁰C) and pressure (760 mm Hg)

In western Europe, vinyl acetate produced by the gas-phase ethylene process has the following typical specifications: vinyl acetate, 99.9% min; ethyl acetate, 323 mg/kg (0.03%); water 240 mg/kg (0.02%); methyl acetate, 175 mg/kg (0.017%); acetaldehyde, 6 mg/kg (0.0006%); and acrolein, 1 mg/kg (0.0001%).

Typical specifications for vinyl acetate in Japan are as follows: density, 0.932-0.936; free acid (as acetic acid), 0.01% max; free aldehydes (as acetaldehyde), 0.05% max; distillation residue, 0.05% max; moisture, 0.2% max; and distillation range, 71.0-73.5°C.

2. Production, Use, Occurrence and Analysis

2.1 Production and use

(a) Production

Vinyl acetate was first produced by Klatte in 1912 as a by-product in the production of ethylidene diacetate (Matthews, 1972). The reaction was accomplished by bubbling acetylene through a mixture of anhydrous acetic acid and mercurous sulphate (Leonard, 1970). This liquid-phase process was converted to a vapour-phase process in Germany during the 1920s. By the 1940s, Germany had a yearly production volume of 12 million kg (Leonard, 1970).

The vapour-phase acetylene process accounted for most of the world production of vinyl acetate until the late 1960s (Leonard, 1970). The reaction occurs by passing acetylene and acetic acid over a catalyst bed of activated carbon saturated with zinc acetate at 180-200°C (Llewellyn & Williams, 1972). Acetylene was originally generated from calcium carbide (Leonard, 1970), then later isolated from the products of hydrocarbon cracking (Llewellyn & Williams, 1972). All US vinyl acetate plants that obtained acetylene from calcium carbide had ceased operation by 1971. Two firms recently closed plants in which acetylene was isolated for this process from hydrocarbons (Mannsville Chemical Products Corp., 1982).

The ethylene process is currently the most common method for the manufacture of vinyl acetate. It was originally developed in 1967 to allow the use of the less costly ethylene as a feedstock. In the vapour-phase ethylene process, ethylene is bubbled through acetic acid at 120°C. This stream is then passed over a catalyst bed containing palladium chloride. Two firms in the Federal Republic of Germany jointly developed an ethylene vapour-phase process utilizing 0.1-2% palladium metal or noble metal mixtures on alumina or silica beds as the catalyst (Leonard, 1970). Chemical companies in the USA and Japan also pioneered early vapour-phase technology (Daniels, 1983). A liquid-phase ethylene process was developed in 1967 by a UK firm which, at that time, operated the only ethylene-based vinyl acetate plant in the world (Leonard, 1970). The vapour-phase ethylene processes have the advantage of longer catalyst life and less corrosion (Mannsville Chemical Products Corp., 1982).

A third technique for vinyl acetate production, the acetaldehyde/acetic anhydride process, was in use in the USA until the 1960s (Mannsville Chemical Products Corp., 1982).

One US firm reacted aldehyde with acetic anhydride to yield ethylidene diacetate, which subsequently cleaves to form vinyl acetate and acetic acid (Leonard, 1970). This process may still be utilized at small plants in India, China and Mexico (Mannsville Chemical Products Corp., 1982).

Several new techniques for vinyl acetate production are being developed that utilize synthetic gas as a feed for vinyl acetate. The synthetic gas is exposed to a series of carbonylation steps to yield ethylidene diacetate, which can be converted pyrolytically to vinyl acetate and acetic acid (Mannsville Chemical Products Corp., 1982).

The US International Trade Commission reported the production of 891.8 million kg of vinyl acetate in the USA in 1983 (US International Trade Commission, 1984). Four US companies had a combined annual capacity in 1983 of 1130 million kg. Exports in that year were 268 million kg (Anon., 1984); imports were negligible (Greek, 1984).

In Canada, one firm reported a capacity of 50 million kg in January 1981. The Canadian capacity for vinyl acetate production is expected to increase to 245 million kg in 1985 (Anon., 1982). One plant in Mexico has a capacity of 27 million kg.

Western European demand for vinyl acetate was 590 million kg in 1982 (Anon., 1982). The major producers in western Europe are (in millions of kg capacity): Federal Republic of Germany (230), Spain (100), the UK (90), Italy (90), France (85) and Switzerland (6).

Five companies in Japan reported a combined capacity of 600 million kg vinyl acetate in 1981. Imports increased from 35 million kg in 1982 to approximately 50 million kg in 1983 (Anon., 1983).

(b) Use

Vinyl acetate is used primarily to produce polyvinyl acetate emulsions and polyvinyl alcohol (see IARC, 1979). These resins accounted for 75-80% of the total vinyl acetate monomer used in the USA in 1982 (Mannsville Chemical Products Corp., 1982). It is also used for the production of ethylene/vinyl acetate emulsions, vinyl chloride copolymers, polyvinyl butyral, and a small percentage for miscellaneous uses.

Polyvinyl alcohol was first developed in Germany in 1924 and became available commercially in the USA in 1939 (Cincera, 1983). It is produced by base-catalysed hydrolysis of polyvinyl acetate in the presence of methanol (Llewellyn & Williams, 1972).

Polyvinyl acetate emulsions and resins

Adhesives: The principal use of polyvinyl acetate is in adhesive emulsions ultimately used in the packaging and construction industries. Polyvinyl acetate (PVAC) homopolymers adhere well to porous surfaces, such as wood, paper, cloth and leather; they also have low viscosity and can be applied with spray guns, making them suitable as adhesives for high-speed packaging processes (Daniels, 1983). They may be used in binding paper fibres in boxboard or bag seams.

PVAC copolymers form a flexible, water-resistant film which adheres well to nonporous surfaces such as metal or plastic. The homopolymer has some degree of water resistance and can provide a suitable base for water-resistant paper adhesives used in bags and cartons.

PVAC resins containing 21-40% weight percentage vinyl acetate are commonly used in hot-melt adhesives (Daniels, 1983).

A frequent use for PVAC resins is in the production of 'white' glues, which are used in the furniture industry (Leonard, 1970). These glues contain 40-50% PVAC resin and 5% polyvinyl alcohol, which acts as a thickener.

In the construction industry, PVAC adhesives are used to smooth board seams, as a component in spackling paste and as a cement additive. The addition of PVAC to cement mortar, concrete and plaster improves the bonding and tensile strength of the material, allowing a thinner coating to be applied (Llewellyn & Williams, 1972).

PVAC are also used in the assembly of cigarette gluelines and filters.

Paints: Approximately 25% of the current US demand for PVAC emulsions is for incorporation into latex house paints (Mannsville Chemical Products Corp., 1982). Several comonomers, such as acrylic esters or ethylene, may be complexed to the vinyl acetate monomer to allow the paint to expand and contract more easily in response to temperature changes. PVAC paints are used especially for exterior applications due to their durability, permeability to moisture (which prevents blistering) and resistance to chalking (Daniels, 1983).

Textiles: PVAC emulsions are used as starch substitutes and in sizing. Copolymers of vinyl acetate are used as binders in nonwoven fabrics, such as cotton, nylon and polyester; they may also improve the snag-resistance of nylon hosiery (Llewellyn & Williams, 1972).

Paper: PVAC emulsions are used as binders in paper and paperboard coatings to impart water/grease resistance (Daniels, 1983).

Miscellaneous: PVAC is used as a chewing gum base and as an antishrinking agent for glass fibre-reinforced polyester moulding resins (Daniels, 1983).

Polyvinyl butyral

Polyvinyl butyral is produced by the reaction of polyvinyl acetate polymer with butyraldehyde (Leonard, 1970). It is used as an adhesive layer between two sheets of glass in laminated automotive and architectural safety glasses (Mannsville Chemical Products Corp., 1982). It has also been used as a protective coating, structural adhesive (Leonard, 1970), textile finish component, wash primer for steel, and in reprographics.

Ethylene-vinyl acetate copolymers

The addition of ethylene to the resin adds flexibility to the polymer (Leonard, 1970). Such elastomers are used predominantly as hot-melt adhesives, flexible films and in coating applications. Heat and oil resistance can be imparted to specially moulded rubbers by ethylene-vinyl acetate copolymers that contain more than 50% vinyl acetate monomer (Mannsville Chemical Products Corp., 1982).

Polyvinyl chloride copolymers

Polymers that contain approximately 13% vinyl acetate are used as resins for vinyl floor tiles and for phonograph records. A small percentage of vinyl chloride-vinyl acetate copolymers are used for coatings, injection mouldings and rigid sheet production (Mannsville Chemical Products Corp., 1982).

(c) *Regulatory status and guidelines*

Occupational exposure limits to vinyl acetate have been set by by 13 countries by regulation or recommended guideline (Table 1).

Table 1. National occupational exposure limits for vinyl acetate[a]

Country	Year	Concentration (mg/m³)	Interpretation[b]
Australia	1978	30	TWA
Belgium	1978	30	TWA
Finland	1981	30	TWA
		60	STEL
Germany, Federal Republic of	1984	35	TWA
The Netherlands	1978	30	TWA
Poland	1976	10	Ceiling
Romania	1975	50	TWA
		100	Ceiling
Sweden	1984	35	TWA
		50	STEL
Switzerland	1978	35	TWA
UK	1985	30	TWA
		60	STEL
USA			
ACGIH	1984	30	TWA
		60	STEL
NIOSH	1978	15	Ceiling
USSR	1977	10	Ceiling
Yugoslavia	1971	10	Ceiling

[a]From National Institute for Occupational Safety and Health (NIOSH) (1978); International Labour Office (1980); Työsuojeluhallitus (1981); American Conference of Governmental Industrial Hygienists (ACGIH) (1984); Arbetarskyddsstyrelsens Författningssamling (1984); Deutsche Forschungsgemeinschaft (1984); Health and Safety Executive (1985)

[b]TWA, time-weighted average; STEL, short-term exposure limit

Polyvinyl acetate has been approved for use by the US Food and Drug Administration (1984) as components of surfaces in contact with food, including adhesives, resinous and polymeric coatings, components of paper or paperboard in contact with dry, fatty or aqueous foods, constituents of cellophane, and textiles and textile fibres. Vinyl acetate-vinyl chloride copolymer resins are approved for use as components in resinous and polymeric coatings, cellophane and acrylic and modified acrylic plastics. Copolymers of ethylene-vinyl acetate-vinyl alcohol are approved for use in articles in contact with food, with limitations on thickness based on polymer composition. Ethylene-vinyl acetate copolymers may also be used in this way.

Vinyl acetate-crotonic acid copolymer, the surface of polyolefin films that is in contact with food, may be used as a coating (US Food and Drug Administration, 1984).

2.2 Occurrence

(a) Natural occurrence

With the exception of an isolated report of the occurrence in trace quantities in plants (Spence & Tucknott, 1983), it is not known whether vinyl acetate occurs as a natural product.

(b) Occupational exposure

Occupational exposure to vinyl acetate occurs primarily among workers engaged in monomer production and polymerization operations, primarily *via* inhalation of the vapour and skin contact with both vapour and liquid. The National Institute for Occupational Safety and Health (1978) estimated that 70 000 workers are potentially exposed to vinyl acetate in the USA. Residual levels of monomer in the polymer range up to 5 g/kg (Daniels, 1983).

Vinyl acetate has been detected at 50 mg/l in waste-water effluent from a polyvinyl acetate plant (Stepanyan *et al.*, 1970). In a vinyl acetate production plant, air concentrations ranged from non-detectable to 173 mg/m^3, with a mean of 30 mg/m^3. During hopper cleaning, short-term concentrations as high as 1150 mg/m^3 were measured (Deese & Joyner, 1969). Air levels have also been detected in various paint, adhesive production and polymerization plants (Table 2).

(c) Air

Ambient air levels of 0.25 to 2 mg/m^3 were detected in Houston, Texas, USA (Gordon & Meeks, 1975), and a level of 0.5 mg/m^3 was detected near a waste disposal site in Edison, NJ, USA (Pellizzari, 1982).

2.3 Analysis

Selected methods for the analysis of vinyl acetate in various matrices are identified in Table 3.

The analytical method of the US National Institute for Occupational Safety and Health for determining vinyl acetate in air has been validated over the range 8-210 mg/m^3 for a 1.5-l air sample drawn through a sampling tube containing 300 mg Chromosorb 107 sorbent. The lowest quantifiable level is reported to be 0.5 μg per sampling tube, or approximately 0.3 mg/m^3 in air (Taylor, 1978; Foerst & Teass, 1980).

Table 2. Occupational exposures to vinyl acetate in various industries

Industry	Type of sample	Concentration (mg/m³ air)	Reference
Vinyl acetate production	personal	1.4-17	National Institute for Occupational Safety and Health (1978)
Vinyl acetate production and polymerization	personal	0-173	Deese & Joyner (1969)
Polymer adhesive manufacture	personal	<0.4-18	Boxer & Reed (1983)
Latex paint manufacture	personal area	<6.7-126 <4.2-36.6	Belanger & Coy (1981)
Vinyl copolymer production	area	9.73-11.48	Jedrychowski et al. (1979)
Vinyl acetate production	area	0.63-4.29	Jedrychowski et al. (1979)
Polyvinyl acetate production	area	1.17-1.40	Jedrychowski et al. (1979)

Table 3. Methods for the analysis of vinyl acetate[a]

Sample matrix	Sample preparation	Assay procedure[a]	Limit of detection	Reference
Air	Adsorb on Chromosorb 107; desorb into a sample reservoir (heat purging with helium); inject aliquot from reservoir onto GC	GC/FID	0.3 mg/m³	Taylor (1978); Foerst & Teass (1980)
	Adsorb on charcoal inhibited with hydroquinone; desorb by solvent extraction (carbon disulphide with 2% acetone); inject aliquot	GC/FID	1.3 mg/m³	Kimble et al. (1982)
	Adsorb onTenax-GC; desorb (heat), purge (helium), trap (liquid nitrogen-cooled nickel capillary); vaporize (heat, helium) directly onto capillary GC column	GC/MS	0.5 μg/m³[b]	Krost et al. (1982); Pellizzari (1982)
Water	Purge (nitrogen); trap (OV-1/Tenax-GC/silica gel); desorb as vapour (heat purging with nitrogen) directly onto GC column	GC/MS	1 μg/l	Spingarn et al. (1982)

[a]Abbreviations: GC/FID, gas chromatography/flame ionization detection; GC/MS, gas chromatography/mass spectrometry

[b]The only concentration reported in ambient air samples (Pellizzari, 1982)

Trapping of airborne vinyl acetate on activated charcoal and solvent desorption have also been reported, but early studies suggested a lack of stability of adsorbed vinyl acetate and a decreasing desorption efficiency at lower air concentrations (Foerst & Teass, 1980; Sidhu, 1981). More recently, charcoal inhibited with hydroquinone and preceded in the sampling tube by calcium sulphate (drying agent) has been reported to be a reliable and sensitive sampling procedure over the range 7-28 mg/m³. The lower limit of detection for an 18-l air sample is 1.3 mg/m³ (Kimble, 1981; Kimble et al., 1982).

Analysis of Tenax-trapped samples by GC/MS has been recommended for more complex matrices, such as air in the vicinity of chemical waste dumps (Pellizzari, 1982).

In water samples, the purge-trap technique using 3% OV-1 on Chromosorb W/Tenax-GC/silica gel with analysis by GC/MS has been recommended for vinyl acetate at levels down to 1 μg/l (Spingarn et al., 1982). The method is based on the US Environmental Protection Agency Method 624, although vinyl acetate is not specifically listed for this method (US Environmental Protection Agency, 1984).

3. Biological Data Relevant to the Evaluation of Carcinogenic Risk to Humans

3.1 Carcinogenicity studies in animals

(a) Oral administration

Rat: Groups of 20 male and 20 female Fischer F344 rats, seven to eight weeks of age, received 0 (controls), 1000 or 2500 mg/l vinyl acetate (with no significant impurities) in the drinking-water for 100 weeks and were then observed for the rest of their lifetime (maximum, 130 weeks). At that time, survival in males and females was: controls, 7/20 and 5/20; 1000 mg/l, 8/20 and 11/20; 2500 mg/l, 6/20 and 11/20, respectively. Increases in the incidences of liver neoplastic nodules (0 control, 4 low-dose and 2 high-dose males; 0 control, 0 low-dose and 6 high-dose females [$p < 0.01$]), of uterine adenocarcinomas (0 control, 1 low-dose and 5 high-dose females [$p < 0.024$]) and polyps (0 control, 3 low-dose, and 5 high-dose females), and thyroid C-cell adenomas (0 control, 2 low-dose and 5 high-dose females [p = 0.024]) were observed in the treated groups. No malignant neoplasm was found in the liver (Lijinsky & Reuber, 1983). [The Working Group noted the small number of animals used, that histopathological examination was limited to gross lesions and major organs only, that the animals received less than the nominal doses of the compound due to the instability of vinyl acetate in the drinking-water, and the lack of characterization of the decomposition products.]

(b) Inhalation exposure

Rat: A group of 96 Sprague-Dawley rats [sex unspecified] was exposed for 4 h per day on five days per week for 52 weeks to the maximum tolerated concentration, 8.8 g/m³ (2500 ppm), of vinyl acetate in air. No tumour was reported to have occurred during 135 weeks. Early mortality was high: only 49 animals survived for 26 or more weeks (Maltoni & Lefemine, 1974; Maltoni et al., 1974; Maltoni & Lefemine, 1975). [The Working Group was unable to evaluate the significance of the results due to the poor survival of the animals and because the time of death of animals that lived longer than 26 weeks was not indicated.]

(c)   Carcinogenicity of metabolites

There is *sufficient evidence* for the carcinogenicity of acetaldehyde to experimental animals (IARC, 1985).

3.2 Other relevant biological data

(a)   Experimental systems

Toxic effects

The oral LD_{50} of vinyl acetate in rats was 2.9 g/kg bw; the LD_{50} in rabbits by skin application was more than 5 g/kg bw (Union Carbide Corp., 1958).

Data on acute inhalation toxicity indicate an LC_{50} of 13 000 mg/m³ (3680 ppm) for rats and 5150 mg/m³ (1460 ppm) for mice after a 4-h exposure (Union Carbide Corp., 1973). Other values after a 4-h exposure were reported to be 14 000 mg/m³ (4000 ppm) in rats (Carpenter et al., 1949; National Institute for Occupational Safety and Health, 1978), 21 800 mg/m³ (6200 ppm) in guinea-pigs, 5400 mg/m³ (1530 ppm) in mice and 8800 mg/m³ (2500 ppm) in rabbits (National Institute for Occupational Safety and Health, 1978).

Following exposure for 6 h per day on five days per week over a four-week period, signs of irritation of the respiratory tract were observed in mice exposed to concentrations of 520 mg/m³ (150 ppm) and in rats exposed to 1760 mg/m³ (500 ppm). Exposure of both species to 3500 mg/m³ (1000 ppm) for 6 h per day on six days per week over three months caused a retardation in weight gain; no specific damage to parenchymal organs was noted (Hazleton Laboratories Europe, 1979; Owen, 1983). In another study, exposure of rats to 7000 mg/m³ (2000 ppm) vinyl acetate for 6 h per day over a three-week period resulted in irritation of the eyes and nose and respiratory difficulty (Gage, 1970).

Oral administration of 100 or 200 mg/kg bw vinyl acetate twice daily to newborn rats for three weeks and subsequent administration of phenobarbital in the drinking-water for eight weeks did not induce ATPase-deficiency or γ-glutamyltranspeptidase-positive foci in the liver (Laib & Bolt, 1986).

Effects on reproduction and prenatal toxicity

No published data were available to the Working Group

Absorption, distribution, excretion and metabolism

Unlike the other vinylic monomers, the biological effects of vinyl acetate could be due to its hydrolysis to acetaldehyde rather than to epoxidation of the vinyl moiety. Rats exposed to vinyl acetate exhaled acetaldehyde (see IARC, 1985) as a result of hydrolysis by esterases (Filov, 1959; Simon et al., 1985a). When mice were exposed to ¹⁴C-vinyl acetate, the radioactivity excretion pattern was similar to that observed with ^{14}C-acetaldehyde. In both cases, the majority of radioactivity was exhaled as $^{14}CO_2$ (Hazleton Laboratories Europe, 1979).

In vitro, vinyl acetate is metabolized mainly by hydrolysis to acetaldehyde and acetic acid. Esterases present in whole blood or plasma of rats and mice and those present in the liver and lung catalyse this reaction (Hazleton Laboratories Europe, 1979; Simon *et al.*, 1985a). Characterization of the kinetic parameters of esterases from different tissues revealed that hepatic microsomes from rats and purified carboxyl esterase from porcine liver display the highest activities (Simon *et al.*, 1985a).

Rat-liver supernatant catalyses conjugation of vinyl acetate with glutathione (Boyland & Chasseaud, 1967). Accordingly, administration of vinyl acetate at doses of about 500 mg/kg bw has led to a slight reduction in hepatic glutathione levels in rats and some other species (Boyland & Chasseaud, 1970; Holub & Tarkowski, 1982).

A slight, but dose-dependent decrease in hepatic microsomal cytochrome P-450 was reported in rats exposed for six months to 10-500 mg/m³ (2.9-143 ppm) vinyl acetate (Holub, 1983).

When male and female Fischer 344 rats and male Wistar rats were given ^{14}C-vinyl acetate orally or by inhalation for 4 h, radioactivity was incorporated metabolically into hepatic DNA, but no specific alkylation product could be detected (Simon *et al.*, 1985b).

Mutagenicity and other short-term tests

Vinyl acetate vapour (tested at up to 2% v/v for various periods) was not mutagenic to *Salmonella typhimurium* TA1530 or TA100 in the presence or absence of a metabolic system (S9) from the liver of phenobarbital-induced mice (Bartsch *et al.*, 1979); liquid vinyl acetate (tested at up to 1000 μg/plate) was not mutagenic to strains TA1535, TA1537, TA1538, TA98 or TA100 in the presence or absence of S9 from the liver of Aroclor- or methylcholanthrene-induced rats or Aroclor-induced hamsters or of S13 from mouse liver, when tested in liquid preincubation and plate incorporation assays (McCann *et al.*, 1975; Dahl *et al.*, 1978; Lijinsky & Andrews, 1980) and in the spot test (Florin *et al.*, 1980).

Treatment of isolated human lymphocytes and whole-blood cultures with vinyl acetate for 48 h induced dose-related and statistically significant increases in sister chromatid exchanges (0.1-1 mM) and chromosomal aberrations (0.125-2 mM). The effect was greater in lymphocytes than in whole blood. The authors attributed this to inactivation of the active species by red-blood cells. Sister chromatid exchanges were also induced in cultured Chinese hamster ovary cells treated with 0.125-1 mM vinyl acetate for 24 h, in the absence of an exogenous metabolic system (Norppa *et al.*, 1985; Jantunen *et al.*, 1986).

It was reported in an abstract that vinyl acetate enhanced the transformation of Syrian hamster embryo cells by adenovirus SA7 (Casto *et al.*, 1977).

There is *sufficient evidence* of the genetic activity of acetaldehyde in short-term tests (IARC, 1985).

(b)   *Humans*

Toxic effects

The toxic effects of vinyl acetate have been reviewed (National Institute for Occupational Safety and Health, 1978).

Exposure of four volunteers to increasing concentrations of vinyl acetate indicated that irritation of the mucous membranes of the throat can occur with concentrations as low as 20 ppm (69 mg/m^3), and eye irritation at 72 ppm (250 mg/m^3) (National Institute for Occupational Safety and Health, 1978). Deese and Joyner (1969) reported that levels of 76 mg/m^3 (22 ppm) produced eye and throat irritation.

Dermal contact with vinyl acetate may produce irritation, with blister formation (National Institute for Occupational Safety and Health, 1978).

Impairment of ventilatory function and symptoms of chronic bronchitis have been reported among workers in polyvinyl acetate plants exposed to up to 40 ppm (140 mg/m^3), with a frequency related to degree and length of exposure; however, the workers were also exposed to other chemicals, such as various aldehydes and vinyl copolymers (Amatouni & Aharonian, 1979; Jedrychowkski *et al.*, 1979; Amatouni & Aharonian, 1980; Aharonian & Amatouni, 1982).

Among 558 workers employed in a plant where polyvinyl acetate was produced, liver function changes were reported in the 'majority' of the workers in the main production departments. 'Neurological disorders' were reported to occur five times more frequently among workers in the vinyl acetate department than in an unspecified control group; no increase was noted in workers in other departments. Overall, 25% of the production workers had some kind of skin disorder (Nargizyan *et al.*, 1978). [The Working Group noted the incomplete reporting of the findings.]

Effects on reproduction and prenatal toxicity
No data were available to the Working Group.

Absorption, distribution, excretion and metabolism
As plasma from human subjects converts vinyl acetate to acetaldehyde and acetic acid, it is assumed that metabolism of the compound in humans follows the same metabolic pathways as in animals (Simon *et al.*, 1985a).

Mutagenicity and chromosomal effects
No data were available to the Working Group.

3.3 Case reports and epidemiological studies of carcinogenicity to humans

In an attempt to identify the specific exposure associated with an excess lung cancer risk noted previously in a US synthetic chemicals plant, Waxweiler *et al.* (1981) considered 19 chemicals, one of which was vinyl acetate. Company personnel assigned a rank of exposure to vinyl acetate (from 0 to 5) to each job in the plant for each year since its start in 1942.

These exposure data were then linked with detailed, individual work histories so as to obtain for each of the 4806 male workers ever employed in the plant an estimate of his exposure to vinyl acetate; 'doses' were calculated by multiplying the exposure rank of a job by the number of days worked at that job. Cumulative 'doses' for 45 workers who died from lung cancer during the study period (1942-1973) were then compared with expected 'doses' based on the cumulative exposure of subcohorts of fellow workers matched individually to the cases by year of birth and age when hired into the plant. This comparison failed to suggest any specific association between exposure to vinyl acetate in the plant and excess lung cancer risk.

4. Summary of Data Reported and Evaluation

4.1 Exposure data

Vinyl acetate has been available commercially since the 1920s. It is currently used to produce polyvinyl acetate and polyvinyl alcohol, which are formulated in latex paints and glues. Occupational exposure to vinyl acetate occurs primarily during monomer production, polymerization operations and product formulation.

4.2 Experimental data

Administration of vinyl acetate in the drinking-water to rats was associated with an increased incidence of uterine adenocarcinomas; however, the lesions could not be linked specifically to treatment with vinyl acetate.

No data were available to evaluate the reproductive effects or prenatal toxicity of vinyl acetate to experimental animals.

Vinyl acetate was not mutagenic to *Salmonella typhimurium* in the presence or absence of an exogenous metabolic system. It induced sister chromatid exchanges and chromosomal aberrations *in vitro* in human lymphocytes and whole-blood cultures, and in Chinese hamster ovary cells.

4.3 Human data

No data were available to evaluate the reproductive effects or prenatal toxicity of vinyl acetate to humans.

The increased lung cancer risk observed in a synthetic chemical plant could not be associated specifically with exposure to vinyl acetate.

Overall assessment of data from short-term tests: Vinyl acetate[a]

	Genetic activity			Cell transformation
	DNA damage	Mutation	Chromosomal effects	
Prokaryotes		−		
Fungi/Green plants				
Insects				
Mammalian cells (*in vitro*)			+	
Mammals (*in vivo*)				
Humans (*in vivo*)				
Degree of evidence in short-term tests for genetic activity: **Inadequate**				Cell transformation: No adequate data

[a]The groups into which the table is divided and the symbols '+', '−' and '?' are defined on pp. 19-20 of the Preamble; the degrees of evidence are defined on pp. 20-21.

4.4 Evaluation[1]

There is *inadequate evidence* for the carcinogenicity of vinyl acetate to experimental animals.

There is *inadequate evidence* for the carcinogenicity of vinyl acetate to humans.

In the absence of adequate epidemiological data, no evaluation of the carcinogenicity of vinyl acetate to humans could be made.

5. References

Aharonian, Z.P. & Amatouni, V.G. (1982) Significance of the production risk factor in the development of chronic bronchitis and disturbance of the ventilatory function of the lungs in persons exposed to vinyl acetate and its derivatives (Russ.). *Zh. eksp. Klin. Med.*, 22, 151-155

---

[1]For definition of the italicized terms, see Preamble, pp. 18 and 22.

Amatouni, V.G. & Aharonian, Z.P. (1979) The state of the function of external respiration in persons occupied in the production of vinyl acetate and its derivatives (Russ.) *Zh. eksp. Klin. Med.*, *19*, 72-78

Amatouni, V.G. & Aharonian, Z.P. (1980) Chronic bronchitis and pulmonary function in workers of a polyvinyl acetate factory (Russ.). *Gig. Tr. Prof. Zabol.*, *2*, 14-16

American Conference of Governmental Industrial Hygienists (1984) *Threshold Limit Values for Chemical Substances and Physical Agents in the Work Environment and Biological Exposure Indices with Intended Changes for 1984-85*, Cincinnati, OH, p. 33

Anon. (1982) Vinyl acetate demand. *Chem. Mark. Rep.*, *221*, 7, 25

Anon. (1983) VAC import rise. *Plast. Ind. News*, *29*, 66

Anon. (1984) A big trade setback for US producers. *Chem. Week*, *134*, 24-27

Arbetarskyddsstyrelsens Författningssamling (National Swedish Board of Occupational Safety and Health) (1984) *Hygienic Limit Values (AFS 1984:5)* (Swed.), Stockholm, p. 34

Bartsch, H., Malaveille, C., Barbin, A. & Planche, G. (1979) Mutagenic and alkylating metabolites of halo-ethylenes, chlorobutadienes and dichlorobutenes produced by rodent or human liver tissues. Evidence for oxirane formation by P450-linked microsomal mono-oxygenases. *Arch. Toxicol.*, *41*, 249-277

Belanger, P.L. & Coy, M.Y. (1981) *Health Hazard Evaluation Report No. HHE-80-68-871, Sinclair Paint Company, Los Angeles, CA (US NTIS PB82-214396)*, Cincinnati, OH, National Institute for Occupational Safety and Health

Boxer, P.A. & Reed, L.D. (1983) *Health Hazard Evaluation Report No. HETA-82-051-1269, National Starch & Chemical, Meredosia, IL* (US NTIS PB84-209923), Cincinnati, OH, National Institute for Occupational Safety and Health

Boyland, E. & Chasseaud, L.F. (1967) Enzyme-catalyzed conjugations of glutathione with unsaturated compounds. *Biochem. J.*, *104*, 95-102

Boyland, E. & Chasseaud, L.F. (1970) The effect of some carbonyl compounds on rat liver glutathione levels. *Biochem. Pharmacol.*, *19*, 1526-1528

Buckingham, J., ed. (1982) *Dictionary of Organic Compounds*, 5th ed., Vol. 3, New York, Chapman and Hall, pp. 2487-2488 [E-00514]

Carpenter, C.P., Smyth, H.F., Jr. & Pozzani, U.C. (1949) The assay of acute vapor toxicity, and the grading and interpretation of results on 96 chemical compounds. *J. ind. Hyg. Toxicol.*, *31*, 343-346

Casto, B.C., Meyers, J. & DiPaolo, J.A. (1977) Assay of industrial chemicals in Syrian hamster cells for enhancement of viral transformation (Abstract No. 617). *Proc. Am. Assoc. Cancer Res.*, *18*, 155

Celanese Chemical Co. (1984) *Vinyl Acetate: Sales Specifications (Tech. Bull. No. CCC-90)*, Dallas, TX

Cincera, D.L. (1983) *Vinyl polymers (vinyl chloride)*. In: Mark, H.F., Othmer, D.F., Overberger, C.G. & Seaborg, G.T., eds, *Kirk-Othmer Encyclopedia of Chemical Technology*, 3rd ed., Vol. 23, New York, John Wiley & Sons, pp. 848-865

Dahl, G.A., Miller, J.A. & Miller, E.C. (1978) Vinyl carbamate as a promutagen and a more carcinogenic analog of ethyl carbamate. *Cancer Res.*, *38*, 3793-3804

Daniels, W. (1983) *Vinyl polymers (acetate)*. In: Mark, H.F., Othmer, D.F., Overberger, C.B. & Seaborg, G.T., eds, *Kirk-Othmer Encyclopedia of Chemical Technology*, 3rd ed., Vol. 23, New York, John Wiley & Sons, pp. 817-847

Deese, D.E. & Joyner, R.E. (1969) Vinyl acetate: A study of chronic human exposure. *Am. ind. Hyg. Assoc. J.*, *30*, 449-457

Deutsche Forschungsgemeinschaft (1984) *Maximal Concentrations in the Workplace and Biological Occupational Limit Value* (Ger.), Part XX, Weinheim, Verlag Chemie GmbH, p. 55

Filov, V.A. (1959) The fate of complex esters of vinyl alcohol and fatty acid in the body (Russ.). *Gig. Tr. prof. Zabol.*, *3*, 42-46

Florin, I., Rutberg, L., Curvall, M., Enzell, C.R. (1980) Screening of tobacco smoke constitutents for mutagenicity using Ames' test. *Toxicology*, *18*, 219-232

Foerst, D.L. & Teass, A.W. (1980) *A sampling and analytical method for vinyl acetate*. In: Dollberg, D.B. & Zerstuyft, A.W., eds, *Analytical Technics in Occupational Health Chemistry* (*ACS Symposium Series No. 120*), Washington DC, American Chemical Society, pp. 169-184

Gage, J.C. (1970) The subacute inhalation toxicity of 109 industrial chemicals. *Br. J. ind. Med.*, *27*, 1-18

Gordon, S.J. & Meeks, S.A. (1975) *A study of gaseous pollutants in the Houston, Texas area*. In: *Dispersion and Control of Atmospheric Emissions and New Energy Sources — Pollution Potential* (*AIChE Symposium Series, 73*), New York, American Institute of Chemical Engineers, pp. 84-94

Grasselli, J.G. & Ritchey, W.M., eds (1975) *CRC Atlas of Spectral Data and Physical Constants for Organic Compounds*, Vol. 2, Cleveland, OH, CRC Press, Inc., p. 79

Greek, B.F. (1984) Phenol, vinyl acetate face tightening supply. *Chem. Eng. News*, *62*, 10, 12

Hawley, G.G., ed. (1981) *The Condensed Chemical Dictionary*, 10th ed., New York, Van Nostrand Reinhold Co., p. 1084

Hazleton Laboratories Europe (1979) *Vinyl acetate. Unpublished reports Nos 1910-51/8, 2511-51/11-14, 1835-51/3, 1884-51/3, 2286-51/5, 2303-51/5. Compilation of data.* In: Henschler, D., ed., *Gesundheitsschädliche Arbeitsstoffe, Toxikologischarbeitsmedizinische Begründungen von MAK-Werten*, Weinheim, Verlag Chemie

Health and Safety Executive (1985) *Occupational Exposure Limits 1985 (Guidance Note EH 40/85)*, London, Her Majesty's Stationery Office, p. 21

Holub, J. (1983) Influence of vinyl acetate on the activity of microsomal enzymes in the liver of rats (Pol.). *Przegl. Lék.*, *40*, 515-516

Holub, J. & Tarkowski, S. (1982) Hepatic content of free sulfhydryl compounds in animals exposed to vinyl acetate. *Int. Arch. occup. environ. Health, 51*, 185-189

IARC (1977) *IARC Monographs on the Evaluation of the Carcinogenic Risk of Chemicals to Man*, Vol. 15, *Some Fumigants, the Herbicides 2,4-D and 2,4,5-T, Chlorinated Dibenzodioxins and Miscellaneous Industrial Chemicals*, Lyon, pp. 155-175

IARC (1979) *IARC Monographs on the Evaluation of the Carcinogenic Risk of Chemicals to Humans*, Vol. 19, *Some Monomers, Plastics, and Synthetic Elastomers, and Acrolein*, Lyon, pp. 341-366

IARC (1985) *IARC Monographs on the Evaluation of the Carcinogenic Risk of Chemicals to Humans*, Vol. 36, *Allyl Compounds, Aldehydes, Epoxides and Peroxides*, Lyon, pp. 101-132

International Labor Office (1980) *Occupational Exposure, Limits for Airborne Toxic Substances (Occupational Safety and Health Series No. 37)*, Geneva, pp. 214-215

Jantunen, K., Mäki-Paakkanen, J. & Norppa, H. (1986) Induction of chromosome aberrations by styrene and vinylacetate in cultured human lymphocytes: Dependence on erythrocytes. *Mutat. Res., 159*, 109-116

Jedrychowski, W., Prochowska, K., Garlińska, J. & Bruzgielewicz, J. (1979) The occurrence of chronic nonspecific diseases of respiratory tract in workers of vinyl resins establishment (Pol.). *Przegl. Lék., 36*, 679-682

Kimble, H.J. (1981) Analysis of vinyl acetate. *US Patent No. 4292042 to Union Carbide Corp.*

Kimble, H.J., Ketcham, N.H., Kuryla, W.C., Neff, J.E. & Patel, M.A. (1982) A solid sorbent tube for vinyl acetate monomer that eliminates the effect of moisture in environmental sampling. *Am. ind. Hyg. Assoc. J., 43*, 137-144

Krost, K.J., Pellizzari, E.D., Walburn, S.G. & Hubbard, S.A. (1982) Collection and analysis of hazardous organic emissions. *Anal. Chem., 54*, 810-817

Laib, R.J. & Bolt, H.M. (1986) On the question of the carcinogenicity of vinyl acetate (Ger.). *Verh. Dtsch. Ges. Arbeitsmed., 25* (in press)

Leonard, E.C. (1970) *Vinyl acetate.* In: Leonard, E.C., ed., *Vinyl and Diene Monomers*, Part 1, New York, Wiley Interscience, pp. 263-328

Lijinsky, W. & Andrews, A.W. (1980) Mutagenicity of vinyl compounds in *Salmonella typhimurium. Teratog. Carcinog. Mutagenesis, 1*, 259-267

Lijinsky, W. & Reuber, M.D. (1983) Chronic toxicity studies of vinyl acetate in Fischer rats. *Toxicol. appl. Pharmacol., 68*, 43-53

Llewellyn, I. & Williams H. (1972) *Vinyl acetate homopolymers and copolymers.* In: Matthews, G., ed., *Vinyl and Allied Polymers,* Vol. 2, Cleveland, OH, CRC Press, Inc., pp. 362-385

Maltoni, C. & Lefemine, G. (1974) Carcinogenicity bioassays of vinyl chloride. I. Research plan and early results. *Environ. Res., 7*, 387-405

Maltoni, C. & Lefemine, G. (1975) Carcinogenicity bioassays of vinyl chloride: Current results. *Ann. NY Acad. Sci., 246*, 195-218

Maltoni, C., Lefemine, G., Chieco, P. & Carretti, D. (1974) Vinyl chloride carcinogenesis: Current results and perspectives. *Med. Lav.*, *65*, 421-444

Mannsville Chemical Products Corp. (1982) *Vinyl Acetate (Chemical Products Synopsis)*, Cortland, NY

Matthews, G., ed. (1972) *Vinyl and Allied Polymers*, Vol. 2, Cleveland, OH, CRC Press, Inc., p. 9

McCann, J., Choi, E., Yamasaki, E. & Ames, B.N. (1975) Detection of carcinogens as mutagens in the *Salmonella*/microsome test: Assay of 300 chemicals. *Proc. natl Acad. Sci. USA*, *72*, 5135-5139

Nargizyan, G.A., Oganesyan, T.A., Organesyan, L.T. & Grigoryan, A.V. (1978) Occupational disease in the principal chemical industries of the Armenian SSR (Russ.). *Zh. eksp. Klin. Med.*, *18*, 101-104

National Fire Protection Association (1984) *Fire Protection Guide on Hazardous Materials*, 8th ed., Quincy, MA, pp. 325M-93, 49-92 - 49-93

National Institute for Occupational Safety and Health (1978) *Criteria for a Recommended Standard for Occupational Exposure to Vinyl Acetate (DHEW (NIOSH) Pub. No. 78-205)*, Cincinnati, OH

NIH/EPA Chemical Information System (1983) *Carbon-13 NMR Spectral Search System, Mass Spectral Search System,* and *Infrared Spectral Search System*, Arlington, VA, Information Consultants, Inc.

Norppa, H., Yursi, F., Pfäffli, P., Mäki-Paakkanen, J. & Järventaus, H. (1985) Chromosome damage induced by vinyl acetate through in vitro formation of acetaldehyde in human lymphocytes and Chinese hamster ovary cells. *Cancer Res.*, *45*, 4816-4821

Owen, P.E. (1983) Vinyl acetate - Three month inhalation toxicity study in the rat and mouse (Abstract). *Human Toxicol.*, *2*, 416

Pellizzari, E.D. (1982) Analysis for organic vapor emissions near industrial and chemical waste disposal sites. *Environ. Sci. Technol.*, *16*, 781-785

Perry, R.H. & Green, D.W., eds (1984) *Perry's Chemical Engineers' Handbook*, 6th ed., New York, McGraw-Hill, p. 3-44

Sadtler Research Laboratories (1980) *The Sadtler Standard Spectra Collection, Cumulative Index*, Philadelphia, PA

Sax, N.I. (1984) *Dangerous Properties of Industrial Materials*, 6th ed., New York, Van Nostrand Reinhold Co., p. 85

Sidhu, K.S. (1981) Determination of vinyl acetate in air by gas chromatography. *J. appl. Toxicol.*, *1*, 300-302

Simon, P., Filser, J.G. & Bolt, H.M. (1985a) Metabolism and pharmacokinetics of vinyl acetate. *Arch. Toxicol.*, *57*, 19-23

Simon, P., Ottenwälder, H. & Bolt, H.M. (1985b) Vinyl acetate: DNA-binding assay *in vivo*. *Toxicol. Lett.*, *27*, 115-120

Spence, R.-M. & Tucknott, O.G. (1983) The examination of the headspace volatiles of watercress. *J. Sci. Food Agric.*, *34*, 768-772

Spingarn, N.E., Northington, D.J. & Pressely, T. (1982) Analysis of volatile hazardous substances by GC/MS. *J. chromatogr. Sci.*, *20*, 286-288

Stepanyan, I.S., Padaryan, G.M., Airapetyan, L.K. & Maslyukova, D.F. (1970) Ionization-chromatographic method for determining some components of waste waters from the plant 'Polivinilatsetat' (Russ.). *Prom. Arm.*, *9*, 76-78 [*Chem. Abstr.*, *74*, 90928p]

Taylor, D.G. (1978) *NIOSH Manual of Analytical Methods*, 2nd ed., Vol. 4 (*DHEW (NIOSH) Publ. No. 78-175*), Washington, DC, US Government Printing Office, pp. 278-1 -278-8

Työsuojeluhallitus (National Finnish Board of Occupational Safety and Health) (1981) *Airborne Contaminants in the Workplace* (Safety Bull. 3) (Finn.), Tampere, p. 27

Union Carbide Corp. (1958) *Toxicology Studies — Vinyl Acetate, H.Q.*, New York, Industrial Medicine and Toxicology Department

Union Carbide Corp. (1973) *Vinyl Acetate — Single Animal Inhalation and Human Sensory Response* (*Special Report 36-72*), Danbury, CT

US Environmental Protection Agency (1984) Guidelines establishing test procedures for the analysis of pollutants under the Clean Water Act (40 CFR 136) Purgeables (US EPA Method 624). *Fed. Regist.*, *49*, 43373-43384

US Food and Drug Administration (1984) Food and drugs. *US Code Fed. Regul.*, *Title 21*, Parts 175.105, 175.300, 175.350, 176.170, 176.180, 177.1010, 177.1200, 177.1350, 177.1360, 177.1670, 177.2260, 177.2800, 178.3910, pp. 133, 145, 160, 180, 189, 199, 211, 225, 255, 271, 289, 348

US International Trade Commission (1984) *Synthetic Organic Chemicals, US Production and Sales, 1983* (*USITC Publication 1588*), Washington DC, US Government Printing Office, p. 258

Verschueren, K. (1983) *Handbook of Environmental Data on Organic Chemicals*, 2nd ed., New York, Van Nostrand Reinhold Co., pp. 1184-1185

Waxweiler, R.J., Smith, A.H., Falk, H. & Tyroler, H.A. (1981) Excess lung cancer risk in a synthetic chemicals plant. *Environ. Health Perspect.*, *41*, 159-165

Weast, R.C., ed. (1984) *CRC Handbook of Chemistry and Physics*, 65th ed., Boca Raton, FL, CRC Press, p. C-570

Windholz, M., ed. (1983) *The Merck Index*, 10th ed., Rahway, NJ, Merck & Co., p. 1429

VINYL BROMIDE

This substance was considered by a previous Working Group, in February 1978 (IARC, 1979). Since that time, new data have become available, and these have been incorporated into the monograph and taken into consideration in the present evaluation.

1. Chemical and Physical Data

1.1 Synonyms and trade names

Chem. Abstr. Services Reg. No.: 593-60-2
Chem. Abstr. Name: Ethene, bromo-
IUPAC Systematic Name: Bromoethylene
Synonym: NCI-C50373

1.2 Structural and molecular formulae and molecular weight

$$CH_2 = CH - Br$$

C_2H_3Br

Mol. wt: 106.96

1.3 Chemical and physical properties of the pure substance

(a) *Description*: Gas under normal atmospheric conditions, colourless liquid under pressure; has a characteristic pungent odour (Ethyl Corp., 1980; Hawley, 1981)

(b) *Boiling-point*: 15.8°C (Weast, 1984)

(c) *Melting-point*: -139.5°C (Weast, 1984)

(d) *Density*: d_4^{20} 1.4933 (Weast, 1984); 1.522 at 20°C (Ethyl Corp., 1980)

(e)   *Spectroscopy data*: Infrared (Pouchert, 1981 [56D]), nuclear magnetic resonance (Pouchert, 1983 [86C]) and mass spectral data (NIH/EPA Chemical Information System, 1983) have been reported.

(f)   *Solubility*: Insoluble in water (Sax, 1984); soluble in ethanol, diethyl ether, acetone, benzene and chloroform (Grasselli & Ritchey, 1975; Weast, 1984)

(g)   *Volatility*: Vapour pressure, 895 mm Hg at 20°C (Ramey & Lini, 1971); relative vapour density, 3.7 (Ethyl Corp., 1980)

(h)   *Stability*: Polymerizes rapidly in sunlight (Buckingham, 1982); can react vigorously with oxidizing materials (Sax, 1984)

(i)   *Conversion factor*: $mg/m^3 = 4.37 \times ppm^a$

1.4 Technical products and impurities

Vinyl bromide is sold commercially in the USA in oxygen-free containers; shipping containers are normally under positive pressure because the vapour pressure of vinyl bromide is so high. In addition to precautions used to minimize contact with oxygen, peroxides and other free-radical initiators that cause polymerization, inhibitors are also added to the product.

Product specifications for polymerization-grade vinyl bromide are as follows: vinyl bromide content, 99.8 wt % min (exclusive of inhibitor); appearance, clear and free of suspended matter; water, 100 mg/kg max; nonvolatile matter (including inhibitor), 500 mg/kg max; inhibitor (hydroquinone methyl ether), 175-225 mg/kg (Ethyl Corp., 1980).

2. Production, Use, Occurrence and Analysis

2.1 Production and use

(a)   *Production*

Vinyl bromide can be produced by the catalytic addition of hydrogen bromide to acetylene in the presence of mercury and/or copper halide catalysts or by partial dehydrobromination of ethylene dibromide with alcoholic potassium hydroxide (Ramey & Lini, 1971).

---

[a]Calculated from: mg/m^3 = (molecular weight/24.45) × ppm, assuming standard temperature (25°C) and pressure (760 mm Hg)

Vinyl bromide was first produced in the USA in 1968, and in 1982 production exceeded 2.3 million kg (Benya *et al.*, 1982). At one time, two US firms were known to produce vinyl bromide (US Environmental Protection Agency, 1980), but in 1985 only one US producer was identified. No data were available on the quantities of vinyl bromide produced in 1983. In Japan, two major companies produced vinyl bromide in 1981, but production figures were not available.

(b) Use

Vinyl bromide is used as an intermediate in organic synthesis and in the manufacture of polymers, copolymers, flame retardants, pharmaceuticals and fumigants (Ethyl Corp., 1980).

There has been little interest in the homopolymer of vinyl bromide in view of its thermal and photolytic instability. Vinyl bromide is used primarily in polymers as a flame retardant in the production of modacrylic fibres for carpet-backing material. It has also been used in small quantities as a comonomer with acrylonitrile in the production of fabrics and fabric blends to be used in sleepwear (mostly for children) and home furnishings. It is also copolymerized with vinyl acetate and maleic anhydride to produce granular products. Vinyl bromide-vinyl chloride copolymers are used for preparing films, for laminating fibres and as rubber substitutes (Larsen, 1980). Vinyl bromide is also used in leather and fabricated metal products (National Institute for Occupational Safety and Health, 1978).

(c) Regulatory status and guidelines

Occupational exposure limits for vinyl bromide have been set by six countries by regulation or recommended guideline (Table 1).

The US National Institute for Occupational Safety and Health (1978, 1983) has recommended that exposure to vinyl halides be restricted to the lowest possible level, with the eventual goal of zero exposure.

2.2 Occurrence

(a) Natural occurrence

It is not known whether vinyl bromide occurs as a natural product.

(b) Occupational exposure

On the basis of results from the National Occupational Hazards Survey, a 'probable estimate' of 26 000 US workers potentially exposed to vinyl bromide was calculated (National Institute for Occupational Safety and Health, 1978).

Median 8-h time-weighted average exposures at a vinyl bromide manufacturing plant ranged from 0.4 to 27.5 mg/m^3, depending on the job and area surveyed. Personal air samples showed that a plant operator was exposed to 0.4-1.7 mg/m^3, a lab technician to 1.3-2.2 mg/m^3 and two loading crewmen to 5.2 and 27.5 (1-h sample) mg/m^3 (Bales, 1978; Oser, 1980).

Table 1. National occupational exposure limits for vinyl bromide[a]

Country	Year	Concentration (mg/m^3)	Interpretation[b]
Australia	1978	1100	TWA
Belgium	1978	1100	TWA
Finland	1981	20	TWA
The Netherlands	1978	1100	TWA
UK	1985	20	TWA
USA			
ACGIH	1984	20	TWA
NIOSH	1984	4	TWA
OSHA	1978	4	TWA
		20	Ceiling

[a]From National Institute for Occupational Safety and Health (NIOSH) (1978); International Labour Office (1980); Työsuojeluhallitus (1981); NIOSH (1983); American Conference of Governmental Industrial Hygienists (ACGIH) (1984); Health and Safety Executive (1985)

[b]TWA, time-weighted average

(c)   Air

Sampling conducted in and around two communities in Arkansas, USA, where bromine industries were sited led to the identification of vinyl bromide in air, but the actual levels detected were not reported (DeCarlo, 1979).

2.3 Analysis

Selected methods for the analysis of vinyl bromide in air are given in Table 2.

The analytical method of the US National Institute for Occupational Safety and Health for determination of vinyl bromide by gas chromatography/flame ionization detection has been validated over the range 1.3-56 mg/m^3 (Spafford & Dillon, 1981; Taylor, 1981). The estimated limit of detection for vinyl bromide by the gas chromatography/mass spectrometric method developed by Pellizzari et al. (1978) for environmental monitoring is 10^3-10^5 lower, although no specific range is given.

Table 2. Methods for the analysis of vinyl bromide in air[a]

Sample preparation	Assay procedure[a]	Limit of detection	Reference
Adsorb (charcoal tube); desorb (ethanol)	GC/FID	1.3 mg/m³	Spafford & Dillon (1981); Taylor (1981)
Adsorb (charcoal tube); desorb (heat), purge (helium), dry (calcium sulphate tube) and adsorb (Tenax tube); desorb (thermal) and trap (liquid nitrogen); vaporize (heat) onto capillary GC column	GC/MS	8 ng/m³	Pellizzari et al. (1978)
Adsorb (Tenax-GC); desorb (heat), purge (helium), trap (liquid nitrogen cooled nickel capillary); vaporize (heat) directly onto capillary GC column	GC/MS	250 ng/m³	Pellizzari et al. (1978); Krost et al. (1982)

[a]Abbreviations: GC/FID, gas chromatography/flame ionization detection; GC/MS, gas chromatography/mass spectrometry

3. Biological Data Relevant to the Evaluation of Carcinogenic Risk to Humans

3.1 Carcinogenicity studies in animals[1]

(a) Skin application

Mouse: A group of 30 female ICR/Ha Swiss mice received topical applications of 15 mg vinyl bromide [purity unspecified] in 0.1 ml acetone thrice weekly for 60 weeks. No skin tumour was observed. In a two-stage skin carcinogenesis study to test for initiating activity, further groups of 30 mice received a single application of vinyl bromide followed by thrice-weekly applications for 60 weeks of 2.5 μg 12-0-tetradecanoylphorbol 13-acetate (TPA) in 0.1 ml acetone, a single application of 7,12-dimethylbenz[a]anthracene followed by treatment with TPA (positive controls), treatment with TPA only, or no treatment at all (160 mice). One of 30 mice treated with vinyl bromide followed by TPA developed a skin papilloma at 412 days; one skin carcinoma occurred among the 30 TPA-treated controls

[1]The Working Group was aware of recently completed studies on repeated subcutaneous injection of vinyl bromide to mice (IARC, 1984).

after 44 days; no skin tumour developed in the 160 untreated controls within 420 days; and the positive-control group showed the expected high number of skin tumours (Van Duuren, 1977). [The Working Group noted that sites other than the skin were not examined, and that the test material was volatile.]

(b)   Inhalation exposure

Rat: Groups of 120 male and 120 female Sprague-Dawley rats, nine to ten weeks of age, were exposed to 10, 50, 250 or 1250 ppm (44, 219, 1093 or 5875 mg/m³) vinyl bromide (purity, 99.9%; 0.02% hydroquinone methyl ether as stabilizer, as well as 0.03% ethylene oxide, 0.0007% acetylene, 0.008% aldehydes and ketones) in air for 6 h per day on five days per week for 104 weeks, at which time they were sacrificed. In the group exposed to 1250 ppm, exposure was terminated at 72 weeks because about 50% of animals had died, and the remainder were sacrificed. A group of 144 male and 144 female rats served as untreated controls. Average survival time was not stated. Treatment-related increases in the incidences of liver angiosarcoma were observed in all treated groups: males: 0/144 controls, 7/120 at 10 ppm ($p < 0.025$); 36/120 at 50 ppm ($p < 0.001$); 61/120 at 250 ppm ($p < 0.001$) and 43/120 at 1250 ppm ($p < 0.001$); females: 1/144, 10/120, 50/120, 61/120 and 41/120, respectively ($p < 0.001$ for all groups). In addition, increases were observed in the incidences of squamous-cell carcinoma of the Zymbal gland: males, 2/142, 1/99, 1/112, 13/114 ($p < 0.005$) and 35/116 ($p < 0.005$); females, 0/139, 0/99, 3/113, 2/119 and 11/114 ($p < 0.001$), neoplastic nodules and hepatocellular carcinoma: males, 4/143, 5/103, 10/119, 13/120 ($p < 0.025$) and 5/119; females: 7/142, 18/101 ($p < 0.005$), 12/113, 21/118 ($p < 0.005$) and 9/112 in treated animals compared to controls (Benya *et al.*, 1982).

(c)   Subcutaneous administration

Mouse: A group of 30 female ICR/Ha Swiss mice was injected subcutaneously with 25 mg/animal vinyl bromide in 0.05 ml trioctanoin once weekly for 48 weeks and observed up to 420 days. No local tumour was seen in treated mice, nor in 30 mice given 48 weekly injections of trioctanoin alone, nor in 60 untreated controls observed up to 420 days (Van Duuren, 1977). [The Working Group noted that examination of the animals for pathological lesions was limited to the injection site.]

3.2 Other relevant biological data

(a)   Experimental systems
Toxic effects

The oral LD_{50} of vinyl bromide given as a 50% solution in corn oil was approximately 500 mg/kg bw in male rats. No histopathological change was found in rats exposed for 7 h to 110 000 mg/m³ (25 000 ppm) (Leong & Torkelson, 1970).

In subacute inhalation studies, rats were exposed to 44 000 mg/m³ (10 000 ppm) vinyl bromide in air for 7 h per day on five days a week for four weeks; and rats, rabbits and monkeys were exposed to 1100 or 2200 mg/m³ (250 or 500 ppm) vinyl bromide for 6 h a day on five days a week for six months. No significant change was detected in food consumption, haematology, gross pathology or histopathology (Leong & Torkelson, 1970).

The hepatoxicity of vinyl bromide in rats is enhanced by pretreatment with poly-chlorinated biphenyls. Aroclor 1254-pretreated rats exposed by inhalation for 4 h to 44 000 mg/m^3 (10 000 ppm) vinyl bromide showed increases in serum alanine-α-ketoglutarate transaminase and serum sorbitol dehydrogenase, and histological signs of liver damage. The enhancement was more pronounced in fasted than in fed rats (Conolly & Jaeger, 1977; Conolly et al., 1978).

Newborn Wistar rats exposed to 8800 mg/m^3 (2000 ppm) vinyl bromide for 8 h per day on five days per week for 8-15 weeks developed ATPase-deficient foci in the liver, but to an extent about ten-fold lower than was seen after similar exposure to vinyl chloride (Bolt et al., 1979, 1982). [See also section 3.1.]

Effects on reproduction and prenatal toxicity

No data were available to the Working Group.

Absorption, distribution, excretion and metabolism

Inhalation pharmacokinetics of vinyl bromide have been studied in rats (Filser & Bolt, 1979, 1981; Gargas & Andersen, 1982). The compound was readily taken up by the lung and, at equilibrium, showed an 11-fold accumulation in the entire organism compared to the concentration in the gas phase. Metabolism was saturable at exposure concentrations of over 250 mg/m^3 (55 ppm) (Filser & Bolt, 1979) and was associated with the release of bromide into the plasma (Gargas & Andersen, 1982). Nonvolatile bromide levels in the blood increased with duration of exposure to vinyl bromide in rats, rabbits and monkeys (Leong & Torkelson, 1970).

It was reported in an abstract that pretreatment of rats with phenobarbital accelerated the release of bromide from vinyl bromide in animals exposed to 88 000 mg/m^3 (20 000 ppm) vinyl bromide for 5 h per day, once, twice or for five or ten consecutive days (VanStee et al., 1977).

When a mixture of vinyl bromide in air was passed through a mouse-liver microsomal system, a volatile alkylating metabolite was formed, as demonstrated by trapping with 4-(4-nitrobenzyl)pyridine (Barbin et al., 1975; Bartsch et al., 1976, 1979). Results of experiments in vitro indicate that the primary metabolite formed by mixed-function oxidases from vinyl bromide is 2-bromoethylene oxide, while the rearrangement product of the latter, 2-bromoacetaldehyde, might be the major alkylating agent bound to protein (Guengerich et al., 1981). Irreversible protein binding of metabolites of [1,2-^{14}C]-vinyl bromide has been established both with rat-liver microsomes in vitro (Bolt et al., 1978) and in rats in vivo (Bolt et al., 1980).

A comparative study using isolated rat hepatocytes and hepatic sinusoidal cells revealed that the metabolism of vinyl bromide to reactive metabolites was confined primarily to hepatocytes (Ottenwälder & Bolt, 1980).

When incubated with liver microsomes from phenobarbital-treated rats, vinyl bromide alkylates the prosthetic group (haem) of cytochrome P-450. The alkylated moiety has been identified as the dimethyl ester of N-(2-oxoethyl)protoporphyrin IX (Ortiz de Montellano *et al.*, 1982).

Incubation of [1,2-^{14}C]-vinyl bromide with rat-liver microsomes and RNA resulted in alkylation of RNA and formation of 1,N^6-ethenoadenosine and 3,N^4-ethenocytidine. The same alkylation products occurred in the hepatic RNA of rats exposed to the radioactive compound (Ottenwälder *et al.*, 1979).

Like other halogenated C_1 and C_2 compounds that are transformed to reactive metabolites, vinyl bromide alters rat intermediary metabolism, leading to increased exhalation of acetone (Filser *et al.*, 1982).

Exposure of rats to 87 400 mg/m^3 (20 000 ppm) vinyl bromide for 4 h per day for ten days caused a decrease in hepatic cytochrome P-450 (Drew *et al.*, 1976).

Mutagenicity and other short-term tests

Vinyl bromide (0.2-20% v/v in air for various time periods) was mutagenic to *Salmonella typhimurium* TA1530 and TA100 in the presence or absence of a metabolic system (S9) from the liver of Aroclor-induced rats or phenobarbital-induced mice or humans (Bartsch, 1976; Bartsch *et al.*, 1976 (Abstract), 1979; Lijinsky & Andrews, 1980).

(*b*)   *Humans*

Toxic effects

Short-term inhalation of high concentrations of vinyl bromide [levels not given] is reported to cause loss of consciousness. Skin and eye contact with liquid vinyl bromide produced irritation and caused a 'frost-bite' type of burn (Fawcett, 1976; Benya *et al.*, 1982).

Effects on reproduction and prenatal toxicity
No data were available to the Working Group.

Absorption, distribution, excretion and metabolism
No data were available to the Working Group.

Mutagenicity and chromosomal effects
No data were available to the Working Group.

3.3 Case reports and epidemiological studies of carcinogenicity to humans

No data were available to the Working Group.

4. Summary of Data Reported and Evaluation

4.1 Exposure data

Vinyl bromide has been available commercially since 1968. Occupational exposure may occur during the production of vinyl bromide and its polymers.

4.2 Experimental data

Vinyl bromide was tested in female mice by skin application and by subcutaneous injection, and in rats by inhalation exposure. In the inhalation study in rats, there was a dose-related increase in the incidence of liver angiosarcomas and Zymbal gland carcinomas; an increased incidence of liver neoplastic nodules and hepatocellular carcinoma was also noted. In the limited studies in mice by skin application and subcutaneous administration, no local tumour was observed.

No data were available to evaluate the reproductive or prenatal toxicity of vinyl bromide to experimental animals.

Vinyl bromide was mutagenic to *Salmonella typhimurium* in the presence or absence of an exogenous metabolic system.

Overall assessment of data from short-term tests: Vinyl bromide[a]

	Genetic activity			Cell transformation
	DNA damage	Mutation	Chromosomal effects	
Prokaryotes		+		
Fungi/Green plants				
Insects				
Mammalian cells (*in vitro*)				
Mammals (*in vivo*)				
Humans (*in vivo*)				
Degree of evidence in short-term tests for genetic activity: **Inadequate**				Cell transformation: No data

[a]The groups into which the table is divided and the symbol '+' are defined on pp. 19-20 of the Preamble; the degrees of evidence are defined on pp. 20-21.

4.3 Human data

No data were available to evaluate the reproductive effects or prenatal toxicity of vinyl bromide to humans.

No case report or epidemiological study was available to evaluate the carcinogenicity of vinyl bromide to humans.

4.4 Evaluation[1]

There is *sufficient evidence*[2] for the carcinogenicity of vinyl bromide to experimental animals.

No data on humans were available.

5. References

American Conference of Governmental Industrial Hygienists (1984) *Threshold Limit Values for Chemical Substances and Physical Agents in the Work Environment and Biological Exposure Indices with Intended Changes for 1984-85*, Cincinnati, OH, pp. 33, 42

Bales, R.E. (1978) *Vinyl Fluoride and Vinyl Bromide Industrial Hygiene Survey Report (DHEW (NIOSH) Pub. No. 79-111; US NTIS PS80-190150)*, Cincinnati, OH, National Institute for Occupational Safety and Health

Barbin, A., Brésil, H., Croisy, A., Jacquignon, P., Malaveille, C., Montesano, R. & Bartsch, H. (1975) Liver-microsome-mediated formation of alkylating agents from vinyl bromide and vinyl chloride. *Biochem. biophys. Res. Commun., 67*, 596-603

Bartsch, H. (1976) *Mutagenicity tests in chemical carcinogenesis.* In: Rosenfeld, C. & Davis, W., eds, *Environmental Pollution and Carcinogenic Risks (IARC Scientific Publications No. 13)*, Lyon, International Agency for Research on Cancer, pp. 229-240

Bartsch, H., Malaveille, C., Barbin, A., Planche, G. & Montesano, R. (1976) Alkylating and mutagenic metabolites of halogenated olefins produced by human and animal tissues (Abstract no. 67). *Proc. Am. Assoc. Cancer Res., 17*, 17

Bartsch, H., Malaveille, C., Barbin, A. & Planche, G. (1979) Mutagenic and alkylating metabolites of halo-ethylenes, chlorobutadienes and dichlorobutenes produced by rodent or human liver tissues. Evidence for oxirane formation by P450-linked microsomal mono-oxygenases. *Arch. Toxicol., 41*, 249-277

Benya, T.J., Busey, W.M., Dorato, M.A. & Berteau, P.E. (1982) Inhalation carcinogenicity bioassay of vinyl bromide in rats. *Toxicol. appl. Pharmacol., 64*, 367-379

Bolt, H.M., Filser, J.G. & Hinderer, R.K. (1978) Rat liver microsomal uptake and irreversible protein binding of [1,2-^{14}C]-vinyl bromide. *Toxicol. appl. Pharmacol., 44*, 481-489

---

[1]For definition of the italicized term, see Preamble, p. 18.

[2]In the absence of adequate data in humans, it is reasonable, for practical purposes, to regard chemicals for which there is sufficient evidence of carcinogenicity in animals as if they represented a carcinogenic risk to humans.

Bolt, H.M., Laib, R.J. & Stöckle, G. (1979) Formation of pre-neoplastic hepatocellular foci by vinyl bromide in newborn rats. *Arch. Toxicol.*, *43*, 83-84

Bolt, H.M., Filser, J.G., Laib, R.J. & Ottenwälder, H. (1980) Binding kinetics of vinyl chloride and vinyl bromide at very low doses. *Arch. Toxicol.*, *Suppl. 3*, 129-142

Bolt, H.M., Laib, R.J. & Filser, J.G. (1982) Reactive metabolites and carcinogenicity of halogenated ethylenes. *Biochem. Pharmacol.*, *31*, 1-4

Buckingham, J., ed. (1982) *Dictionary of Organic Compounds*, 5th ed., Vol. 1, New York, Chapman and Hall, p. 799 [B-02403]

Conolly, R.B. & Jaeger, R.J. (1977) Acute hepatotoxicity of ethylene and halogenated ethylenes after PCB pretreatment. *Environ. Health Perspect.*, *21*, 131-135

Conolly, R.B., Jaeger, R.J. & Szabo, S. (1978) Acute hepatotoxicity of ethylene, vinyl fluoride, vinyl chloride, and vinyl bromide after Aroclor 1254 pretreatment. *Exp. mol. Pharmacol.*, *28*, 25-33

DeCarlo, V.J. (1979) Studies on brominated chemicals in the environment. *Ann. N.Y. Acad. Sci.*, *320*, 678-681

Drew, R.T., Patel, J.M. & van Stee, E.W. (1976) The effects of vinyl bromide exposure in rats pretreated with phenobarbital or diethylmaleate (Abstract No. 204). *Toxicol. appl. Pharmacol.*, *37*, 176-177

Ethyl Corp. (1980) *Vinyl Bromide (Technical Bulletin IC-74)*, Baton Rouge, LA

Fawcett, H.H. (1976) *Investigation of Agents Which Are Newly Suspected As Occupational Health Hazards. Vinyl Halides (Vinyl Fluoride and Vinyl Bromide)*, Rockville, MD, Tracor Jitco, Inc., pp. 9-12

Filser, J.G. & Bolt, H.M. (1979) Pharmacokinetics of halogenated ethylenes in rats. *Arch. Toxicol.*, *42*, 123-136

Filser, J.G. & Bolt, H.M. (1981) Inhalation pharmacokinetics based on gas uptake studies. I. Improvement of kinetic models. *Arch. Toxicol.*, *47*, 279-292

Filser, J.G., Jung, P. & Bolt, H.M. (1982) Increased acetone exhalation induced by metabolites of halogenated C_1 and C_2 compounds. *Arch. Toxicol.*, *49*, 107-116

Gargas, M.L. & Andersen, M.E. (1982) Metabolism of inhaled brominated hydrocarbons: Validation of gas uptake results by determination of a stable metabolite. *Toxicol. appl. Pharmacol.*, *66*, 55-68

Grasselli, J.G. & Ritchey, W.M., eds (1975) *CRC Atlas of Spectral Data and Physical Constants for Organic Compounds*, Vol. 3, Cleveland, OH, CRC Press, Inc., p. 279

Guengerich, F.P., Mason, P.S., Stott, W.T., Fox, T.R. & Watanabe, P.G. (1981) Roles of 2-haloethylene oxides and 2-haloacetaldehydes derived from vinyl bromide and vinyl chloride in irreversible binding to protein and DNA. *Cancer Res.*, *41*, 4391-4398

Hawley, G.G., ed. (1981) *The Condensed Chemical Dictionary*, 10th ed., New York, Van Nostrand Reinhold Co., p. 1084

Health and Safety Executive (1985) *Occupational Exposure Limits 1985 (Guidance Note EH 40/85)*, London, Her Majesty's Stationery Office, p. 9

IARC (1979) *IARC Monographs on the Evaluation of the Carcinogenic Risk of Chemicals to Humans*, Vol. 19, *Some Monomers, Plastics and Synthetic Elastomers, and Acrolein*, Lyon, pp. 367-375

IARC (1984) *Information Bulletin on the Survey of Chemicals Being Tested for Carcinogenicity*, No. 11, Lyon, p. 191

International Labour Office (1980) *Occupational Exposure Limits for Airborne Toxic Substances, A Tabular Compilation of Values from Selected Countries*, 2nd (rev.) ed. (*Occupational Safety and Health Series No. 37*), Geneva, pp. 214-215

Krost, K.J., Pellizzari, E.D., Walburn, S.G. & Hubbard, S.A. (1982) Collection and analysis of hazardous organic emissions. *Anal. Chem.*, *54*, 810-817

Larsen, E.R. (1980) *Halogenated flame retardants*. In: Mark, H.F., Othmer, D.F., Overberger, C.G. & Seaborg, G.T., eds, *Kirk-Othmer Encyclopedia of Chemical Technology*, 3rd ed., Vol. 10, New York, John Wiley & Sons, pp. 373-395

Leong, B.K.J. & Torkelson, T.R. (1970) Effects of repeated inhalation of vinyl bromide in laboratory animals with recommendations for industrial handling. *Am. ind. Hyg. Assoc.*, *31*, 1-11

Lijinsky, W. & Andrews, A.W. (1980) Mutagenicity of vinyl compounds in *Salmonella typhimurium*. *Teratog. Carcinog. Mutagenesis*, *1*, 259-267

National Institute for Occupational Safety and Health (1978) *Vinyl Halides Carcinogenicity* (*Current Intelligence Bulletin No. 28; DHEW (NIOSH) Pub. No. 79-102*), Cincinnati, OH

National Institute for Occupational Safety and Health (1983) *NIOSH Recommendations for Occupational Health Standards* (*CDC MMWR Suppl., Vol. 32, No. 1S*), Cincinnati, OH

NIH/EPA Chemical Information System (1983) *Carbon-13 NMR Spectral Search System, Mass Spectral Search System* and *Infrared Spectral Search System*, Arlington, VA, Information Consultants, Inc.

Ortiz de Montellano, P.R., Kunze, K.L., Beilan, H.S. & Wheeler, C. (1982) Destruction of cytochrome P-450 by vinyl fluoride, fluoroxene, and acetylene. Evidence for a radical intermediate in olefin oxidation. *Biochemistry*, *21*, 1331-1339

Oser, J.L. (1980) Extent of industrial exposure to epidhlorohydrin, vinyl fluoride, vinyl bromide and ethylene dibromide. *Am. ind. Hyg. Assoc. J.*, *41*, 463-468

Ottenwälder, H. & Bolt, H.M. (1980) Metabolic activation of vinyl chloride and vinyl bromide by isolated hepatocytes and hepatic sinusoidal cells. *J. environ. Pathol. Toxicol.*, *4*, 411-417

Ottenwälder, H., Laib, R.J. & Bolt, H.M. (1979) Alkylation of RNA by vinyl bromide metabolites *in vitro* and *in vivo*. *Arch. Toxicol.*, *41*, 279-286

Pellizzari, E.D., Zweidinger, R.A. & Erickson, M.D. (1978) *Environmental Monitoring Near Industrial Sites: Brominated Chemicals, Part II: Appendix (EPA-560/6-78-002A; US NTIS PB-286483)*, Prepared for the US Environmental Protection Agency by Research Triangle Institute, Research Triangle Park, NC

Pouchert, C.J., ed. (1981) *The Aldrich Library of Infrared Spectra*, 3rd ed., Milwaukee, WI, Aldrich Chemical Co., p. 56

Pouchert, C.J., ed. (1983) *The Aldrich Library of NMR Spectra*, 2nd ed., Vol. 1, Milwaukee, WI, Aldrich Chemical Co., p. 86

Ramey, K.C. & Lini, D.C. (1971) *Vinyl bromide polymers*. In: Bikales, N.M., ed., *Encyclopedia of Polymer Science and Technology*, Vol. 14, New York, Wiley Interscience, pp. 273-281

Sax, N.I. (1984) *Dangerous Properties of Industrial Materials*, 6th ed., New York, Van Nostrand Reinhold Co., pp. 2726-2727

Spafford, R.B. & Dillon, H.K. (1981) *Analytical Methods Evaluation and Validation for Vinylidene Fluoride, Vinyl Bromide, Vinyl Fluoride, Benzenethiol, and n-Octanethiol: Research Report for Vinyl Bromide* (*US NTIS PB83-133447*). Prepared for the National Institute for Occupational Safety and Health by Southern Research Institute, Birmingham, AL

Taylor, D.G. (1981) *NIOSH Manual of Analytical Methods*, Vol. 7 (*DHHS (NIOSH) Pub. No. 82-100*), Washington DC, US Government Printing Office, pp. 349-1 — 349-9

Työsuojeluhallitus (National Finnish Board of Occupational Safety and Health) (1981) *Airborne Contaminants in the Workplace (Safety Bulletin 3)* (Finn.), Tampere, p. 27

US Environmental Protection Agency (1980) *TSCA Chemical Assessment Series, Chemical Hazard Information Profiles (CHIPS), August 1976 — August 1978* (*EPA-560/11-80-011*), Washington DC, Office of Pesticides and Toxic Substances, pp. 277-289

US International Trade Commission (1984) *Synthetic Organic Chemicals, US Production and Sales, 1983* (*USITC Publication 1588*), Washington DC, US Government Printing Office

Van Duuren, B.L. (1977) Chemical structure, reactivity, and carcinogenicity of halohydrocarbons. *Environ. Health Perspect.*, *21*, 17-23

VanStee, E.W., Patel, J.M., Gupta, B.N. & Drew, R.T. (1977) Consequences of vinyl bromide debromination in the rat (Abstract no. 105). *Toxicol. appl. Pharmacol.*, *41*, 175

Weast, R.C., ed. (1984) *CRC Handbook of Chemistry and Physics*, 65th ed., Boca Raton, FL, CRC Press, Inc., p. C-270

VINYL FLUORIDE

1. Chemical and Physical Data

1.1 Synonyms and trade names

Chem. Abstr. Services Reg. No.: 75-02-5
Chem. Abstr. Name: Ethene, fluoro-
IUPAC Systematic Name: Fluoroethylene
Synonyms: Monofluoroethylene; VF; vinyl fluoride, monomer

1.2 Structural and molecular formulae and molecular weight

$$CH_2 = CH - F$$

C_2H_3F Mol. wt: 46.05

1.3 Chemical and physical properties of the pure substance

(a)   *Description*: Colourless gas with an ethereal odour (Brasure, 1980; Sax, 1984)

(b)   *Boiling-point*: -72.2°C (Weast, 1984)

(c)   *Melting-point*: -160.5°C (Weast, 1984)

(d)   *Density*: Liquid density, 0.620 g/cm³ at 25°C (Brasure, 1980)

(e)   *Spectroscopy data*: Infrared (Sadtler Research Laboratories, 1980; prism [30864[a]], grating [48458P]) and mass spectral data (NIH/EPA Chemical Information System, 1983) have been reported.

---

[a]Spectrum number in Sadtler compilation

(f)   *Solubility*: Insoluble in water; soluble in ethanol and diethyl ether (Hawley, 1981; Sax, 1984, Weast, 1984); soluble in acetone (Weast, 1984)

(g)   *Volatility*: Vapour pressure, 25 atm (19 000 mg Hg) at 21°C (Brasure, 1980)

(h)   *Stability*: Polymerizes freely; forms explosive mixtures with air (Buckingham, 1982); ignites in presence of heat or sources of ignition (Sax, 1984)

(i)   *Conversion factor*: mg/m³ = 1.88 × ppm[a]

1.4 Technical products and impurities

Vinyl fluoride is not available commercially in bulk quantities, although it is produced and used internally by one company in the USA (US Environmental Protection Agency, 1981). It is relatively unreactive, in comparison to other monomers, and requires high pressure, temperatures of 60-140°C and free radical catalysts for polymerization. However, for storage purposes, stabilizers such as terpenes (D-limonene) are added to prevent spontaneous polymerization (Cohen & Kraft, 1971; Grayson, 1985). Vinyl fluoride is available with a purity of 99% (Weiss, 1980)

2. Production, Use, Occurrence and Analysis

2.1 Production and use

(a)   *Production*

Vinyl fluoride is produced by the addition of hydrogen fluoride to acetylene in the presence of mercury catalysts. In another method, 1,1-difluoroethane (also formed by the addition of hydrogen fluoride to acetylene) is pyrolysed to vinyl fluoride. Vinyl fluoride has been produced in the USA since 1962 (US Environmental Protection Agency, 1980). No data were available on the quantities of vinyl fluoride produced in 1983.

(b)   *Use*

Vinyl fluoride is used to produce polyvinyl fluoride and other fluoropolymers. Since vinyl fluoride is less reactive than vinyl chloride, free-radical polymerization with peroxide-type catalysts requires high pressures (4350-14500 psi; 300-1000 atm) and moderate

---

[a]Calculated from: mg/m³ = (molecular weight/24.45) × ppm, assuming standard temperature (25°C) and pressure (760 mm Hg)

temperatures (60-140°C) (Grayson, 1985). The introduction of commercial polyvinyl fluoride by E.I. duPont de Nemours, Inc. in 1962 (US Environmental Protection Agency, 1980) was aided by the development of a Ziegler-Natta catalyst that allowed polymerization at lower temperatures and pressures (Cohen & Kraft, 1971).

Homopolymers and copolymers made from vinyl fluoride show exceptional resistance to chemical attack and water absorption. They are quite stable at relatively high temperatures and are highly stable when exposed to sunlight. Polyvinyl fluoride is used as a protective and decorative surface for building panels and sidings, as a protective cover for pipes (Cohen & Kraft, 1971) and electrical equipment (US Environmental Protection Agency, 1980), for insulating storage tanks, as a top coat on wall coverings, on interior finish in commercial aeroplanes, and as a surface for highway markers. Polyvinyl fluoride film does not fracture when the material to which it is bonded expands or contracts (Cohen & Kraft, 1971).

(c) Regulatory status and guidelines

The US National Institute for Occupational Safety and Health (1978, 1983) has recommended that exposure to vinyl halides be restricted to the minimum detectable level, with the eventual goal of zero exposure. It has recommended an exposure limit of 2 mg/m^3 as an eight-hour time-weighted average, with a ceiling value of 10 mg/m^3 for any 15-min sampling period.

2.2 Occurrence

(a) Natural occurrence

It is not known whether vinyl fluoride occurs as a natural product.

(b) Occupational exposure

Surveys made at a vinyl fluoride manufacturing plant and a vinyl fluoride polymerization plant (Table 1) showed that exposure levels for production and control operations were generally <4 mg/m^3, while exposures associated with polymer operations ranged from 2-9 mg/m^3, with a time-weighted average of 3.6 mg/m^3 (Bales, 1978; Oser, 1980).

2.3 Analysis

Vinyl fluoride has been determined in workplace air (1-9 mg/m^3) by collection in poly(tetrafluoroethylene) bags and analysis by gas chromatography (Bales, 1978).

Table 1. Occupational exposures to vinyl fluoride at manufacturing and polymerization plants[a]

Industry	Job classification	Type of sample	Concentration (mg/m^3)[b]
Manufacturing	Plant operator	Personal	<4
	Control room	Area	<4
	Plant operator (start-up)	Personal	40
Polymerization	Polymer operator	Personal	2-8
	Supervisor	Area	2-4
	Pumproom	Area	9

[a]From Bales (1978); Oser (1980)

[b]Eight-hour time-weighted average samples

3. Biological Data Relevant to the Evaluation of Carcinogenic Risk to Humans

3.1 Carcinogenicity studies in animals

No data on the carcinogenicity of vinyl fluoride were available to the Working Group.

3.2 Other relevant biological data

(a) Experimental systems

Toxic effects

The available data indicate that the acute inhalation toxicity of vinyl fluoride in rats and mice cannot be determined due to the occurrence of asphyxia (Lester & Greenberg, 1950; Kopečný et al., 1964; Clayton, 1967).

Rats pretreated with Aroclor 1254 for three consecutive days and then exposed to 18 000 mg/m^3 (10 000 ppm) vinyl fluoride for 4 h had significantly increased serum levels of alanine-α-ketoglutarate transaminase and histological signs of acute hepatotoxicity (Conolly et al., 1978).

Newborn Wistar rats exposed to 4000 mg/m^3 (2100 ppm) vinyl fluoride for 8 h per day on five days per week for 4-14 weeks developed ATPase-deficient foci in the liver (Bolt et al., 1981), but to an extent about 20-fold lower than was seen after similar exposure to vinyl chloride (Bolt *et al.*, 1979). This may be attributable to the slower metabolism of vinyl fluoride under inhalation conditions.

Effects on reproduction and prenatal toxicity
No data were available to the Working Group.

Absorption, distribution, excretion and metabolism
In rats, vinyl fluoride was readily taken up *via* the pulmonary route and, at equilibrium, reached a concentration in the entire organism which was 90% of that in the gas phase. Metabolism was saturable after exposure to concentrations greater than 140 mg/m^3 (75 ppm) (Filser & Bolt, 1979, 1981) and was associated with the release of fluoride into the urine (Dilley *et al.*, 1974). The rate of metabolism was much slower than that of vinyl chloride or vinyl bromide under similar exposure conditions (Filser & Bolt, 1979).

When incubated with liver microsomes from phenobarbital-treated rats, vinyl fluoride alkylates the prosthetic group (haem) of cytochrome P-450. The alkylated moiety has been identified as the dimethyl ester of *N*-(2-oxoethyl)protoporphyrin IX (Ortiz de Montellano *et al.*, 1982).

Like other halogenated C_1 and C_2 compounds that are transformed to reactive metabolites, vinyl fluoride causes changes in rat intermediary metabolism which lead to increased exhalation of acetone (Filser *et al.*, 1982).

Mutagenicity and other short-term tests
No data were available to the Working Group.

(*b*) *Humans*
No data were available to the Working Group.

3.3 Case reports and epidemiological studies of carcinogenicity to humans

No data were available to the Working Group.

4. Summary of Data Reported and Evaluation

4.1 Exposure data

Vinyl fluoride has been produced commercially since 1962 by a single company, as an intermediate, for use within the company. It is used to produce polyvinyl fluoride and other fluoropolymers. Occupational exposure is limited to the manufacture of the monomer and its conversion polymers.

4.2 Experimental data

No data were available to evaluate the carcinogenicity, reproductive effects or prenatal toxicity of vinyl fluoride to experimental animals or the activity of vinyl fluoride in short-term tests.

4.3 Human data

No data were available to evaluate the reproductive effects or prenatal toxicity of vinyl fluoride to humans.

No case report or epidemiological study was available to evaluate the carcinogenicity of vinyl bromide to humans.

4.4 Evaluation

No data were available to evaluate the carcinogenicity of vinyl fluoride to experimental animals or to humans.

5. References

Bales, R.E. (1978) *Vinyl Halides Carcinogenicity (Current Intelligence Bulletin No. 28; DHEW (NIOSH) Pub. No. 79-102)*, Cincinnati, OH, National Institute for Occupational Safety and Health

Bolt, H.M., Laib, R.J. & Stöckle, G. (1979) Formation of pre-neoplastic hepatocellular foci by vinyl bromide in newborn rats. *Arch. Toxicol.*, *43*, 83-84

Bolt, H.M., Laib, R.J. & Klein, K.-P. (1981) Formation of pre-neoplastic hepatocellular foci by vinyl fluoride in newborn rats. *Arch. Toxicol.*, *47*, 71-73

Brasure, D.E. (1980) *Polyvinyl fluoride*. In: Mark, H.F., Othmer, D.F., Overberger, C.B. & Seaborg, G.T., eds, *Kirk-Othmer Encyclopedia of Chemical Technology*, 3rd ed., Vol. 11, New York, John Wiley & Sons, pp. 57-64

Buckingham, J., ed. (1982) *Dictionary of Organic Compounds*, 5th ed., Vol. 3, New York, Chapman and Hall, p. 2649 [F-00396]

Clayton, J.W., Jr (1967) Fluorocarbon toxicity and biological action. *Fluorine Chem. Rev.*, *1*, 197-252

Cohen, F.S. & Kraft, P. (1971) *Vinyl fluoride polymers.* In: Bikales, N.M., ed., *Encyclopedia of Polymer Science and Technology*, Vol. 14, New York, Wiley Interscience, pp. 522-540

Conolly, R.B., Jaeger, R.J. & Szabo, S. (1978) Acute hepatotoxicity of ethylene, vinyl fluoride, vinyl chloride, and vinyl bromide after Aroclor 1254 pretreatment. *Exp. mol. Pharmacol.*, *28*, 25-33

Dilley, J.V., Carter, V.L., Jr & Harris, E.S. (1974) Fluoride ion excretion by male rats after inhalation of one of several fluoroethylenes or hexafluoropropene. *Toxicol. appl. Pharmacol.*, *27*, 582-590

Filser, J.G. & Bolt, H.M. (1979) Pharmacokinetics of halogenated ethylenes in rats. *Arch. Toxicol.*, *42*, 123-136

Filser, J.G. & Bolt, H.M. (1981) Inhalation pharmacokinetics based on gas uptake studies. I. Improvement of kinetic models. *Arch. Toxicol.*, *47*, 279-292

Filser, J.G., Jung, P. & Bolt, H.M. (1982) Increased acetone exhalation induced by metabolites of halogenated C_1 and C_2 compounds. *Arch. Toxicol.*, *49*, 107-116

Grayson, M., ed. (1985) *Kirk-Othmer Concise Encyclopedia of Chemical Technology*, New York, John Wiley & Sons, pp. 516-517

Hawley, G.G., ed. (1981) *The Condensed Chemical Dictionary*, 10th ed., New York, Van Nostrand Reinhold Co., p. 1086

Kopečný, J., Lúčanská, N., Šipka, F., Černý, E. & Ambros, D. (1964) Toxicity of vinyl fluoride (Pol.). *Pracov. Lék.*, *16*, 310-311

Lester, D. & Greenberg, L.A. (1950) Acute and chronic toxicity of some halogenated derivatives of methane and ethane. *Arch. ind. Hyg. occup. Med.*, *2*, 335-344

National Institute for Occupational Safety and Health (1978) *Vinyl Fluoride and Vinyl Bromide Industrial Hygiene Survey Report* (*DHEW (NIOSH) Pub. No. 79-111; US NTIS PB80-190150*), Cincinnati, OH, pp. 13-18

National Institute for Occupational Safety and Health (1983) NIOSH recommendations for occupational health standards. *Morb. Mortal. Wkly Rep.*, *32*, *Suppl.*, 22S

NIH/EPA Chemical Information System (1983) *Carbon-13 NMR Spectral Search System, Mass Spectral Search System* and *Infrared Spectral Search System*, Arlington, VA, Information Consultants, Inc.

Ortiz de Montellano, P.R., Kunze, K.L., Beilan, H.S. & Wheeler, C. (1982) Destruction of cytochrome P-450 by vinyl fluoride, fluroxene, and acetylene. Evidence for a radical intermediate in olefin oxidation. *Biochemistry*, *21*, 1331-1339

Oser, J.L. (1980) Extent of industrial exposure to epichlorohydrin, vinyl fluoride, vinyl bromide and ethylene dibromide. *Am. ind. Hyg. Assoc. J.*, *41*, 463-468

Sadtler Research Laboratories (1980) *The Sadtler Standard Spectra Collection, Cumulative Index*, Philadelphia, PA

Sax, N.I. (1984) *Dangerous Properties of Industrial Materials*, 6th ed., New York, Van Nostrand Reinhold, Co., p. 2730

US Environmental Protection Agency (1980) *TSCA Chemical Assessment Series, Chemical Information Profiles (CHIPs), August 1976 — August 1978 (EPA-560/11-80-011)*, Washington DC, Office of Pesticides and Toxic Substances, pp. 277-289

US Environmental Protection Agency (1981) Fluoroalkenes; response to the interagency testing committee. *Fed. Regist.*, *46*, 53704-53708

US International Trade Commission (1984) *Synthetic Organic Chemicals, US Production and Sales, 1983 (USITC Publication 1588)*, Washington DC, US Government Printing Office

Weast, R.C., ed. (1984) *CRC Handbook of Chemistry and Physics*, 65th ed., Boca Raton, FL, CRC Press, p. C-571

Weiss, G., ed. (1980) *Hazardous Chemicals Data Book*, Park Ridge, NJ, Noyes Data Corp., p. 913

1,3-BUTADIENE

1. Chemical and Physical Data

1.1 Synonyms and trade names

Chem. Abstr. Services Reg. No.: 106-99-0
Chem. Abstr. Name: 1,3-Butadiene
IUPAC Systematic Name: 1,3-Butadiene
Synonyms: Biethylene; bivinyl; butadiene; butadiene (VAN); buta-1,3-diene; α, γ-butadiene; *trans*-butadiene; divinyl; erythrene; NCI-C50602; pyrrolylene; vinylethylene

1.2 Structural and molecular formulae and molecular weight

$$CH_2 = CH - CH = CH_2$$

C_4H_6 Mol. wt: 54.09

1.3 Chemical and physical properties of the pure substance

(a) *Description*: Colourless mildly aromatic gas; easily liquefied (Hawley, 1981; Verschueren, 1983; Perry & Green, 1984; Sax, 1984)

(b) *Boiling-point*: -4.4°C (Weast, 1984)

(c) *Melting-point*: -108.9°C (Weast, 1984)

(d) *Density*: d_4^{20} 0.6211 (Weast, 1984)

(e) *Spectroscopy data*: Ultraviolet (Grasselli & Ritchey, 1975), infrared (Sadtler Research Laboratories, 1980; prism [893[a]], grating [36758]), nuclear magnetic resonance and mass spectral data (NIH/EPA Chemical Information System, 1983) have been reported.

---

[a]Spectrum number in Sadtler compilation

(f) *Solubility*: Very slightly soluble in water (0.23 g/ 100 g at 0°C; 0.19 g/ 100 g at 50°C); soluble in ethanol, diethyl ether, benzene and organic solvents; very soluble in acetone (Grasselli & Ritchey, 1975; Hawley, 1981; Klein, 1981; Windholz, 1983)

(g) *Volatility*: Vapour pressure, 1840 mm Hg at 21°C (Sax, 1984); 760 mm Hg at -4.5°C (Weast, 1984); relative vapour density (air = 1), 1.87 (Verschueren, 1983)

(h) *Stability*: Flash-point, -76°C; very reactive; may form acrolein and peroxides upon exposure to air; can react with oxidizing materials (Parsons & Wilkins, 1976; Kirshenbaum, 1978; Sax, 1984); polymerizes readily, particularly if oxygen is present (Hawley, 1981); forms explosive mixtures with air (National Fire Protection Association, 1984)

(i) *Conversion factor*: mg/ m³ = 2.21 × ppm[a]

1.4 Technical products and impurities

1,3-Butadiene is available commercially as a liquefied gas under pressure. The polymerization grade has a minimum purity of 99% with acetylene as an impurity in the ppm range. Isobutene, 1-butene, butane and *cis*-2- and *trans*-2-butene have been detected in pure-grade butadiene (Miller, 1978).

1,3-Butadiene is stabilized with hydroquinone (see IARC, 1977), catechol (see IARC, 1977), *tert*-butylcatechol or aliphatic mercaptans (Kirshenbaum, 1978; Windholz, 1983).

2. Production, Use, Occurrence and Analysis

2.1 Production and use

(a) *Production*

1,3-Butadiene was first produced in the late 1800s by the pyrolysis of petroleum hydrocarbons (Kirshenbaum, 1978). Commercial production started in the 1930s.

1,3-Butadiene is manufactured either as a co-product of the steam cracking of naphtha to yield ethylene or through the catalytic dehydrogenation of *n*-butane or *n*-butene (Mannsville Chemical Products Corp., 1983). Its isolation as a co-product represented 20% of US production in 1970 (Miller, 1978), but this method now accounts for most of the current 1,3-butadiene output, due in part to an increased demand for ethylene (Anon., 1985).

---

[a]Calculated from: mg/ m³ = (molecular weight/ 24.45) × ppm, assuming standard temperature (25°C) and pressure (760 mm Hg)

Western European and Japanese chemical manufacturers also utilize naphtha steam cracking techniques as the primary means of producing 1,3-butadiene (Kirshenbaum, 1978).

The dehydrogenation of *n*-butane, known as the Houdry process, and the oxidative dehydrogenation of *n*-butene are currently less significant methods for the commercial production of 1,3-butadiene. The Houdry process involves passing a preheated butane feed stream over a fixed-bed reactor containing a chromia-alumina catalyst. In oxidative dehydrogenation, a process used since 1965, a mixture of butenes, air and steam is exposed to a catalytic matrix at approximately 500-600°C (Miller, 1978). The hydrogen released in this dehydrogenation step combines with oxygen in an exothermic reaction, which increases the energy efficiency of the manufacturing process (Mannsville Chemical Products Corp., 1983). The dehydrogenation method has been phased out in recent years, but was responsible for producing approximately 50-100% of the US 1,3-butadiene supply between 1960 and 1977 (Miller, 1978). Reflecting this trend, three US plants with a total capacity of 272.7 million kg were closed in 1982 (Mannsville Chemical Products Corp., 1983).

The crude C_4 fraction obtained by naphtha steam cracking and the products of butane/butene dehydrogenation contain hydrocarbons with boiling-points similar to that of 1,3-butadiene; these include isobutylene, 1- and 2-butene and *n*-butane (Kirshenbaum, 1978). This similarity prevents the use of simple distillation techniques to separate 1,3-butadiene from the C_4 hydrocarbon mixture. An extractive distillation process is used which selectively alters the volatility of the components in the distillate and ultimately permits the 1,3-butadiene to be removed and purified. The solvents employed for this technique include acetonitrile, furfural, dimethylformamide, dimethylacetamide and methyl pyrrolidinone. The cuprous ammonium acetate system has also proven to be useful as a selective extraction recovery process (Miller, 1978; Mannsville Chemical Products Corp., 1983).

An estimated 3.57 million tonnes of 1,3-butadiene were produced worldwide in 1983 (Anon., 1984a).

1,3-Butadiene remains a major industrial commodity in the USA, ranking 36th among all chemicals produced in 1983 (Anon., 1984b). Eleven major US producers with 16 plant locations produced 1.04 million tonnes in 1983 (Anon. 1984a). The US imported approximately 400 000 tonnes of butadiene in 1983, accounting for roughly one-third of total US consumption (Anon., 1984c). The US Department of Commerce reported that the majority of the 1,3-butadiene was imported from The Netherlands and the UK, with lesser amounts imported from Italy, France, Finland and Belgium (Leviton, 1983). The USA, in turn, exported 43 900 tonnes of 1,3-butadiene in 1983 (Anon., 1984c).

In western Europe, where 1,3-butadiene is derived almost exclusively as a co-product, 1.5 million tonnes were produced in 1983, from a combined capacity of 2.58 million tonnes. During the same period, 36 000 tonnes were imported and 329 000 tonnes were exported. In 1983 the Federal Republic of Germany had six companies with a total annual capacity of 653 000 tonnes; five French firms reported a combined capacity of 355 000 tonnes; Italy, The Netherlands and Spain had three plants each with total capacities of 325 000, 430 000 and 190 000 tonnes, respectively; production capacity in Belgium was 140 000 tonnes; that in Finland, 20 000 tonnes; that in Portugal, 42 000 tonnes; and that in Sweden, 25 000 tonnes.

1,3-Butadiene production in Japan in 1983 was 556 000 tonnes (Anon., 1984c) by seven major domestic producers. Of the 44 200 tonnes of 1,3-butadiene imported to Japan in 1983, about half came from Singapore and the remainder from sources in Europe and Taiwan.

In 1983, Canada produced 133 000 tonnes and Mexico, 18 500 tonnes (Anon., 1984b).

(b) Use

Synthetic polymeric elastomers, such as styrene-butadiene and polybutadiene rubber, constitute the largest use of 1,3-butadiene monomer. An estimated 50% of the 1,3-butadiene produced in the USA is used in the production of styrene-butadiene rubber and 22% of the total supply for polybutadiene production. Other applications for 1,3-butadiene include chloroprene/neoprene rubber (6%), nitrile rubber (3%), hexamethylenediamine (9%), acrylonitrile-butadiene-styrene resins (5%) and miscellaneous uses (5%) (Mannsville Chemical Products Corp., 1983).

Styrene-butadiene rubber

Worldwide annual production of styrene-butadiene rubber (SBR) and latex has fallen from a peak in 1978 of 3.34 million tonnes to a level in 1982 of 2.5 million tonnes; total use in 1984 is expected to be 2.75 million tonnes (Greek, 1984). In the US, SBR production in 1983 was 880 000 tonnes (US International Trade Commission, 1984), 64% less than the 1978 level (US International Trade Commission, 1979).

Approximately 74% of the total SBR produced in North America is used to manufacture tyres (Greek, 1984); the remainder is used mainly for hoses, belts (Leviton, 1983) and gaskets (Mansville Chemical Products Corp., 1983).

SBR formulations generally contain a ratio of 77:23 butadiene:styrene. The polymer contains trace amounts of *tert*-dodecyl mercaptan, ferrous sulphate, potassium pyrophosphate and resin acid soap (Miller, 1978).

Polybutadiene rubber

About 85% of the polybutadiene produced in North America is used in tyre manufacture (Greek, 1984) and is blended with SBR to provide better resilience and heat resistance (Miller, 1978). The commercial grade of polybutadiene contains primarily the *cis*-1,4-isomer (Greek, 1984).

The total global production of polybutadiene was approximately 832 000 tonnes in 1982, to which US manufacturers contributed 288 million kg (Greek, 1984). Like SBR, small amounts of polybutadiene are used in high-impact resins (Miller, 1978), hoses, belts, seals and gaskets (Leviton, 1983).

Nitrile rubber

Nitrile rubber, a copolymer of acrylonitrile and 1,3-butadiene, accounts for about 3% of the total US 1,3-butadiene supply (Miller, 1978). It is used in applications which require resistance to oils, gasoline and heat (Mannsville Chemical Products Corp., 1983), such as hoses, seals, gaskets and adhesives (Leviton, 1983); the oil resistance is imparted by the acrylonitrile component (Miller, 1978). Nitrile latex is used to produce oil-resistant textile and paper products (Mannsville Chemical Products Corp., 1983).

Worldwide nitrile rubber production in 1982 was reported to be 182 000 tonnes, of which 45 000 tonnes were produced in the USA (Greek, 1984).

Acrylonitrile-butadiene-styrene resins

Acrylonitrile-butadiene-styrene (ABS) resins are created when styrene and acrylonitrile monomers are grafted onto a polybutadiene rubber. They are used for their high impact resistance in the production of piping (29%), appliances (18%), automotive components (18%), business machines and telephones (5%), luggage (6%), and recreational vehicles (8%) (Miller, 1978).

US production of ABS terpolymer resins was 479 000 tonnes in 1983 (US International Trade Commission, 1984).

Hexamethylenediamine

A nonelastomeric utilization of 1,3-butadiene is in the production of adiponitrile, which is hydrogenated to form hexamethylenediamine (Miller, 1978). The latter is a precursor of Nylon 6/6 and Nylon 6/12 used in carpet material. Approximately 187 000 tonnes 1,3-butadiene were used for adiponitrile production in the USA in 1981 (Leviton, 1983).

A plant in France produces adiponitrile with an annual capacity of 104 000 tonnes per year (Miller, 1978).

Miscellaneous uses

1,3-Butadiene is used in the production of impact modifiers, such as methyl methacrylate-butadiene-styrene terpolymers, which are used in polyvinyl chloride plastics and in the packaging and construction industries (Miller, 1978). US imports of these resins were 12.7 million kg in 1983 (Anon, 1984c).

A small amount of 1,3-butadiene is used for conversion to cyclododecatriene, a precursor of Nylon 12, Nylon 6/12 and Qiana® nylon fibre. A similar butadiene oligomer, cyclooctadiene, is a monomer in the ethylene-propylene terpolymer (Nordel®). A US company had the capacity to produce 54.5 million kg of this terpolymer in 1975 (Miller, 1978).

Other minor uses of 1,3-butadiene are in the manufacture of elastomers, other resins, chemical intermediates, pesticides and fungicides (Miller, 1978).

(c) Regulatory status and guidelines

Occupational exposure limits to 1,3-butadiene are set by 15 countries by regulation or recommended guidelines (Table 1).

The US Food and Drug Administration (1984) has approved the use of polymers or copolymers of 1,3-butadiene as components of articles in contact with food as pressure-sensitive adhesives, resinous or polymeric coatings and rubber articles intended for repeated use.

2.2 Occurrence

(a) Natural occurrence

It is not known whether 1,3-butadiene occurs as a natural product.

Table 1. National occupational exposure limits for 1,3-butadiene[a]

Country	Year	Concentration (mg/m³)	Interpretation[b]
Australia	1978	2200	TWA
Belgium	1978	2200	TWA
Bulgaria	1971	100	Ceiling
Czechoslovakia	1976	500	TWA
		2500	Ceiling
Finland	1981	2200	TWA
German Democratic Republic	1979	500	TWA
	1978	1500	Ceiling
Italy	1978	1000	TWA
The Netherlands	1978	2200	TWA
Poland	1976	100	Ceiling
Romania	1975	1500	TWA
		2000	Ceiling
Switzerland	1978	2200	TWA
UK	1985	2200	TWA
		2750	Ceiling
USA			
ACGIH	1984	2200[c]	TWA
		2750	STEL
OSHA	1983	2200	TWA
NIOSH	1984	2200	TWA
USSR	1977	100	Ceiling
Yugoslavia	1971	500	Ceiling

[a]From International Labour Office (1980); Työsuojeluhallitus (1981); US Occupational Safety and Health Administration (OSHA) (1983); American Conference of Governmental Industrial Hygienists (ACGIH) (1984); National Institute for Occupational Safety and Health (NIOSH) (1984); Health and Safety Executive (1985)

[b]TWA, time-weighted average; STEL, short-term exposure limit

[c]With notice of an intended change to 22 mg/m³

(b)   Occupational exposure

The National Institute for Occupational Safety and Health (1984) estimated that 65 000 workers are potentially exposed to 1,3-butadiene in the USA. Potential exposure is greatest during operations involving production and polymerization. Unreacted 1,3-butadiene monomer has been quantified in SBR latex (mean, 11.8 μg/g; no. of samples, 463), in SBR dry rubber (<0.1-1.4 μg/g; no. of samples, 8), in SBR oil extended (<0.1-1.5 μg/g; no. of samples, 5), in SBR black masterbatch (1.0-1.6 μg/g; no. of samples, 6), in polybutadiene (<0.1 μg/g; no. of samples, 4) and in nitrile rubber (<0.1-1.3 μg/g; no. of samples, 8) (International Institute of Synthetic Rubber Producers, 1984).

Exposure to 1,3-butadiene in 11 North American polymer plants in 1976 to 1981 is summarized in Table 2, giving the percentage of 8-h time-weighted average personal samples containing the indicated concentration ranges for various work categories (International Institute of Synthetic Rubber Producers, 1984). Data on 1,3-butadiene exposure were derived primarily from the SBR industry, the primary user of 1,3-butadiene.

Table 3 summarizes exposures in various synthetic rubber and plastics industries.

(c)   Air

1,3-Butadiene has been detected in urban air at an average concentration of 0.002 μg/m^3 (Natusch, 1978). In the USA, combined levels of 1,3-butadiene and 2-butene were 5.9-24.4 ppb (0.01-0.05 mg/m^3) in Tulsa, OK (Arnts & Meeks, 1981) and 0-0.019 ppm (0-0.042 mg/m^3) in Houston, TX (Siddiqi & Worley, 1977). Levels of 1,3-butadiene were 0.004 mg/m^3 in Denver, CO, and <0.001-0.028 mg/m^3 in various cities in Texas (Hunt *et al.*, 1984); urban air in the Los Angeles/Riverside, CA, area contained levels as high as 0.02 mg/m^3 (Parsons & Wilkins, 1976).

(d)   Food

Levels of <0.2 μg/kg 1,3-butadiene were found in retail soft margarine; the plastic tubs containing the margarine contained <5-310 μg/kg (Startin & Gilbert, 1984).

(e)   Water

1,3-Butadiene has been detected in drinking-water in the USA (US Environmental Protection Agency, 1978; Kraybill, 1980).

(f)   Miscellaneous

1,3-Butadiene has been detected in cigarette smoke (0.001-0.003 cm^3/'puff'), gasoline vapour (2 μg/m^3) (Parsons & Wilkins, 1976), automobile exhaust (22-44 mg/m^3) (Neligan, 1962) and smoke generated during house fires (up to 33 mg/m^3) (Berg *et al.*, 1978).

2.3 Analysis

Selected methods for the analysis of 1,3-butadiene in various matrices are listed in Table 4.

The analytical method of the US National Institute for Occupational Safety and Health for 1,3-butadiene in air (Taylor, 1977) has been validated over the range of the occupational exposure limit (1065-4590 mg/m^3) and can be extended to lower concentrations (200 mg/m^3 or less) if the charcoal desorption efficiency is adequate. Thermal desorption of the 1,3-butadiene from charcoal has been suggested as an alternative to solvent extraction (Coker, 1977). Other sampling and analysis methods with much lower limits of detection have been developed (see Table 4). Capillary columns have been used successfully for the analysis of 1,3-butadiene in complex hydrocarbon mixtures (Schneider *et al.*, 1978; Hutte *et al.*, 1984).

Table 2. Occupational exposure to 1,3-butadiene in 11 North American polymer plants, 1976-1981[a]

Work category	No. of samples	Ppm [mg/m³] 1,3-butadiene							
		0-500 [0-11.05]	5.01-10.00 [11.07-22.1]	10.01-25.00 [22.12-52.25]	25.01-50.00 [55.27-110.5]	50.01-100.00 [110.52-221]	100.01-200.00 [221.02-442]	200.01-500.00 [442.02-1105]	500.01-1000.00 [1105.2-2210]
Tank car loaders/unloaders	259	108	13	32	43	37	19	7	
Percent		41.7	5.0	12.4	16.6	14.3	7.3	2.7	
Vessel cleaners	331	320	7	3	1				
Percent		96.7	2.1	0.9	0.3				
Charge solution make-up	118	108	7	2	1				
Percent		91.5	5.9	1.7	0.9				
Reactor operators	427	348	32	18	13	12	4		
Percent		81.5	7.5	4.2	3.1	2.8	0.9		
Stripping-column operators	367	256	31	47	19	11	2		1
Percent		69.8	8.4	12.8	5.2	3.0	0.5		0.3
Coagulation operators	525	497	13	12	3				
Percent		94.6	2.5	2.3	0.6				
Dryer operators	325	323	1	1					
Percent		99.4	0.3	0.3					
Baler and packing operators	247	244	1	1	1				
Percent		98.0	0.4	1.2	0.4				
Warehousemen	112	112							
Percent		100.0							
Laboratory analysts	330	252	37	24	6	5	2	2	
Percent		76.4	11.2	7.3	1.8	1.5	0.6	0.6	
Maintenance crafts	517	456	24	19	9	7		2	
Percent		88.2	4.6	3.7	1.7	1.4		0.4	
Foremen and leadmen	128	119	4	1	2	2			
Percent		92.9	3.1	0.8	1.6	1.6			
Waste treatment	80	78	1	1					
Percent		97.6	1.2	1.2					
Total	3766	3221	171	161	98	74	27	11	3
Percent		85.5	4.5	4.3	2.6	2.0	0.7	0.3	0.1

[a]From International Institute of Synthetic Rubber Producers (1984)

[b]8-h time-weighted personal samples

Table 3. Occupational exposure to 1,3-butadiene in rubber and plastics industries

Industry[a]	Job classification	Concentration (mg/m³ air)[b]	Reference
SBR manufacture	Production	2-44	Meinhardt et al. (1978); Crandall et al. (1981)
	Polymerization	1	Checkoway & Williams (1982)
	Supervisory	2.2	Meinhardt et al. (1978)
	Tank farm	1-55	Crandall et al. (1981); Checkoway & Williams (1982)
	Maintenance	0.5-17	Meinhardt et al. (1978); Crandall et al. (1981); Checkoway & Williams (1982)
	Laboratory	3-73	Meinhardt et al. (1978); Crandall et al. (1981)
	General production	13-88	Jones (1981)
	Workplace environment (two plants)	3 and 30	Meinhardt et al. (1982)
	Miscellaneous	0.2-3.6	Meinhardt et al. (1978); Checkoway & Williams (1982)
ABS fabrication	Plastic moulding of aircraft parts	1.5-3	Burroughs (1979)
	Injection moulding	<0.05	National Institute for Occupational Safety and Health (1980)
Polybutadiene rubber manufacture			Rubber Manufacturers' Association (1984)
Warehouse	Banbury operator	0.02	
	Put-up batcher	0.02	
	Mill tender	0.03	
	Mill tender	0.02	
Break-down mill	Break-down mill	ND (<0.04) and 0.04	
	Blender mill	ND and 0.07	
	Feed mill	ND and 0.04	
	Calender	ND and 0.11	
	Curing presses	ND and 0.04	
Tyre plants (processing SBR and polybutadiene rubbers)	Area samples - unspecified	ND (<0.04) - 0.6	Rubber Manufacturers' Association (1984)

[a]SBR, styrene-butadiene rubber; ABS, acrylonitrile-butadiene-styrene

[b]Time-weighted averages or mean values

Table 4. Methods for the analysis of 1,3-butadiene

Sample matrix	Sample preparation	Assay procedure[a]	Limit of detection	Reference
Air	Adsorb (charcoal); extract (carbon disulphide)	GC/FID	200 mg/m³	Taylor (1977)
	Collect air sample in evacuated vessel or Tedlar bag; concentrate by freeze-trapping in alumina-filled precolumn (liquid oxygen temperature); flash evaporate (150°C) onto GC column	GC/FID	0.2-1 μg/m³	Lonneman et al. (1974); Lonneman (1977); Lonneman et al. (1978); Schneider et al. (1978)
	Adsorb (Tenax-TA); desorb (250°C) onto GC column	GC/FID	0.02 μg/m³	Hutte et al. (1984)
Foods and plastic food packaging material	Dissolve (N,N-dimethyl-acetamide) or melt; inject headspace sample	GC/MS-SIM	~1 μg/kg	Startin & Gilbert (1984)

[a]Abbreviations: GC/FID, gas chromatography/flame ionization detection; GC/MS-SIM, gas chromatography/mass spectrometry with single-ion monitoring

3. Biological Data Relevant to the Evaluation of Carcinogenic Risk to Humans

3.1 Carcinogenicity studies in animals

Inhalation exposure

Mouse: Groups of 50 male and 50 female B6C3F$_1$ mice, eight to nine weeks of age, were exposed to 625 or 1250 ppm (1380 or 2760 mg/m³) 1,3-butadiene (minimum purity, >98.9%) for 6 h per day on five days per week for 61 weeks. An equal number of untreated animals (sham exposed in chambers) served as controls. The study was terminated after 61 weeks because of a high incidence of lethal neoplasms in the exposed animals; survivors were: males — 49/50 controls, 11/50 low-dose and 7/50 high-dose; females — 46/50 controls, 14/50 low-dose and 30/50 high-dose. Haemangiosarcomas originating in the heart with metastases to various organs were found in: males — 0/50 controls, 16/49 ($p < 0.001$) low-dose and 7/49 ($p = 0.006$) high-dose; females — 0/50 controls, 11/48 ($p < 0.001$) low-dose and 18/49 ($p < 0.001$) high-dose (Fisher exact test). [The Working Group noted that the incidence of haemangiosarcomas of the heart in historical controls was 1/2372 in males and 1/2443 in females.] Other types of neoplasms for which the incidences were increased in animals of each sex (Fisher exact test) were malignant lymphomas: males —0/50 controls, 23/50 ($p < 0.001$) low-dose and 29/50 ($p < 0.001$) high-dose; females —1/50 controls, 10/49 ($p = 0.003$) low-dose and 10/49 ($p = 0.003$) high-dose; alveolar bronchiolar adenomas or carcinomas of the lung: males — 2/50 controls, 14/49 ($p < 0.001$) low-dose and 15/49 ($p < 0.001$) high-dose; females — 3/49 controls, 12/48 ($p = 0.01$) low-dose and 23/49 ($p < 0.001$) high-dose; papillomas or carcinomas of the forestomach: males — 0/49 controls, 7/40 ($p = 0.003$) low-dose and 1/44 ($p = 0.473$) high-dose; females — 0/49 controls, 5/42 ($p = 0.018$) low-dose and 10/49 ($p < 0.001$) high-dose. Tumours that occurred with a statistically significantly increased incidence in females only included hepatocellular adenoma or carcinoma of the liver: 0/50 controls, 2/47 ($p = 0.232$) low-dose and 5/49 ($p = 0.027$) high-dose; acinar-cell carcinoma of the mammary gland: 0/50 controls, 2/49 low-dose and 6/49 ($p = 0.012$) high-dose; granulosa-cell tumours of the ovary: 0/49 controls, 6/45 ($p = 0.01$) low-dose and 12/48 ($p < 0.001$) high-dose (National Toxicology Program, 1984; Huff *et al.*, 1985).

Rat: In a study reported only in an abstract, rats exposed by inhalation to 0, 1000 or 8000 ppm (2210 or 17 689 mg/m³) 1,3-butadiene showed dose-related increases in the incidences of common and uncommon tumour types [not identified] (Owen *et al.*, 1985). [The Working Group noted that insufficient details were reported.]

3.2 Other relevant biological data

(a) Experimental systems

Toxic effects

LC_{50} values for 1,3-butadiene were reported to be 270 000 mg/m³ (122 170 ppm) in mice exposed for 2 h and 285 000 mg/m³ (129 000 ppm) in rats exposed for 4 h; after 1 h of exposure, rats were in a state of deep narcosis (Shugaev, 1969). Oral LD_{50} values of 5.5 g/kg bw for rats and 3.2 g/kg bw for mice have been reported (National Toxicology Program, 1984).

In rats exposed to 1-2200 mg/m³ (0.45-1000 ppm), morphological changes were observed in liver, kidney, spleen, nasopharynx and heart [details not given]. Changes in the immune status and alterations in nervous system function have also been observed (Crouch *et al.*, 1979).

Groups of 24 rats were exposed to 1300-14 800 mg/m³ (600-6700 ppm) 1,3-butadiene for 7.5 h per day on six days per week for eight months; no adverse effect was noted except for a slight retardation in growth with the highest concentration (Carpenter *et al.*, 1944). Rats exposed to 2200-17700 mg/m³ (1000-8000 ppm) 1,3-butadiene for 6 h per day on five days per week for 13 weeks showed no treatment-related effect other than increased salivation in females; in particular, there was no change in gonadal weight or histology (Crouch *et al.*, 1979).

B6C3F1 mice exposed to 625 or 1250 ppm (1380 or 2760 mg/m³) 1,3-butadiene for 6 h per day on five days per week for 61 weeks (for details, see section 3.1) showed atrophy of the ovary and testis, atrophy and metaplasia of the nasal and respiratory epithelium, hyperplasia of the forestomach epithelium and liver necrosis (National Toxicology Program, 1984).

Effects on reproduction and prenatal toxicity

Fertility was reported to be unimpaired in mating studies in rats, guinea-pigs and rabbits exposed to 1300, 5000 or 14 800 mg/m³ (600, 2300 or 6700 ppm) 1,3-butadiene by inhalation for 7.5 hours per day on six days per week for eight months (Carpenter *et al.*, 1944). [The Working Group noted the incomplete reporting of this study.]

No published studies on teratogenicity were available to the Working Group.

Absorption, distribution, excretion and metabolism

Male Sprague-Dawley rats were exposed in closed inhalation chambers to various initial concentrations of 1,3-butadiene to study the pharmacokinetic behaviour of the compound. Analysis of the resulting concentration decline curves of 1,3-butadiene in the gas phase revealed that its metabolism was saturable. Below 1800-2200 mg/m³ (800-1000 ppm), 1,3-butadiene was metabolized according to first-order kinetics; at higher exposure concentrations, a maximal metabolic rate of 220 μmol/h per kg bw was observed, and this was enhanced by pretreatment with Aroclor 1254 (Bolt *et al.*, 1984).

1,3-Butadiene is converted to 1,2-epoxybutene (vinyl oxirane) by mixed-function oxidases in rat liver microsomes *in vitro*. Pretreatment of rats with phenobarbital increased enzyme activity (Malvoisin *et al.*, 1979; Bolt *et al.*, 1983). 1,2-Epoxybutene is further metabolized to 1,2:3,4-diepoxybutane (see IARC, 1976) and 3-butene-1,2 diol; the latter product is metabolized by mixed-function oxidases to 3,4-epoxy-1,2-butanediol (see Fig. 1) (Malvoisin & Roberfroid, 1982).

1,2-Epoxybutene is present in the expired air of rats exposed to 1,3-butadiene (Bolt *et al.*, 1983). When male Sprague-Dawley rats were exposed in closed exposure chambers to concentrations higher than 2200 mg/m³ (1000 ppm) 1,3-butadiene, which stimulates the maximum possible metabolic rate, about 8.8 mg/m³ (4 ppm) 1,2-epoxybutene were measured in the gas phase under steady-state conditions. Kinetic analysis revealed that only 29% of the total amount of 1,3-butadiene metabolized under these conditions was available systemically as 1,2-epoxybutene. This was considered to be related to a first-pass metabolism of the 1,2-epoxybutene originating in the liver (Filser & Bolt, 1984).

Mutagenicity and other short-term tests

1,3-Butadiene (purity, 99.5%) at concentrations of 4-32% was mutagenic to *Salmonella typhimurium* TA1530 in the presence of a metabolic system (S9) from the livers of Aroclor- or phenobarbital-induced rats (de Meester *et al.*, 1980). It was not mutagenic in this strain in plate incorporation and liquid preincubation assays [doses not reported] (Poncelet *et al.*, 1980). Although 1,3-butadiene had previously been reported to be mutagenic to strains TA1530 and TA1535 in the absence of S9 (de Meester *et al.*, 1978), this activity was

Fig. 1. Possible pathways for metabolism of 1,3-butadiene by rat liver microsomes[a]

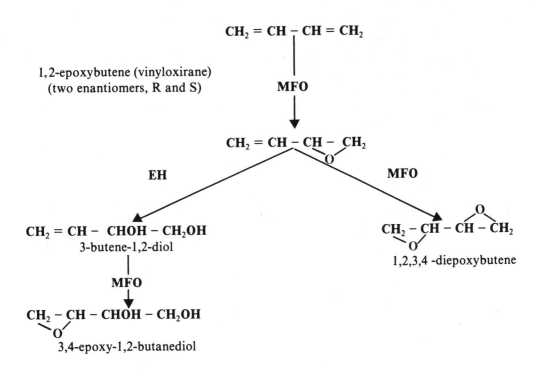

[a]From Malvoisin and Roberfroid (1982); MFO, mixed-function oxidases; EH, epoxide hydrolase

subsequently attributed to cross-contamination by volatile mutagenic metabolites formed on plates containing S9 (Duverger *et al.*, 1981).

Mutagenicity of metabolites

1,2-Epoxybutene was mutagenic to *S. typhimurium* TA1530, TA1535 and TA100, but not to TA1537, TA1538 or TA98 (de Meester *et al.*, 1978; Gervasi *et al.*, 1985). It was reported to be mutagenic to *Escherichia coli* WP2 uvrA in the absence of an exogenous metabolic system [details not given] (Hemminki *et al.*, 1980).

1,2:3,4-Diepoxybutane induced prophage in *Bacillus megaterium*, *Pseudomonas pyocyanea* (Lwoff, 1953) and *Escherichia coli* k-12 (Heinemann & Howard, 1964). It was mutagenic to *S. typhimurium* TA1535 (0.01-0.1 ul/plate) (McCann *et al.*, 1975; Rosenkranz & Poirier, 1979) and TA100 (2-15 mM) (Gervasi *et al.*, 1985) in the absence of a metabolic system. At concentrations of 0.05-1 mM, 1,2:3,4-diepoxybutane induced streptomycin resistance in fluctuation tests with *Klebsiella pneumoniae*, in the absence of a metabolic system (Voogd *et al.*, 1981).

It induced reverse mutations in *Schizosaccharomyces pombe* (Clarke & Loprieno, 1965) and in B and B/r strains of *E. coli* after treatment for 1 h at 37°C with 0.01 M and 0.02 M aqueous solutions, respectively (Glover, 1956). Reverse mutations were also induced in the adenine-requiring mutant 38701 of *Neurospora crassa* after treatment with a 0.2 M solution (Kölmark & Westergaard, 1953).

1,2:3,4-Diepoxybutane induced mitotic gene conversions in *Saccharomyces cerevisiae* D4 after 5 h of treatment with a 0.005 M solution (Zimmermann, 1971) and mitotic recombination in *S. cerevisiae* D81 (Zimmermann & Vig, 1975) and D3 (Simmon, 1979). It induced nuclear point mutations, but not cytoplasmic mutations in *S. cerevisiae* (0.4%, 15-60 min) (Polakowska & Putrament, 1979). At a concentration of 0.013%, it induced dose-related increases in mitotic crossing-over, mitotic gene conversion and reverse mutation in *S. cerevisiae* D7 (Sandhu *et al.*, 1984). 1,2:3,4-Diepoxybutane (0-50 mM) induced reverse mutations in spheroplasts of *N. crassa* (Pope *et al.*, 1984).

In *Drosophila melanogaster*, 1,2:3,4-diepoxybutane induced sex-linked recessive lethal mutations, visible mutations, semi-lethal mutations (Bird & Fahmy, 1953), translocations (Watson, 1972) and minute mutations (Fahmy & Fahmy, 1970). 1,2:3,4-Diepoxybutane given in the diet (0.1%) to larvae of *D. melanogaster* induced somatic recombination and point mutations in surviving adults (Graf *et al.*, 1983). The compound induced sex-linked recessive lethal mutations in adult *D. melanogaster* fed 2 mM in the diet for 48 h (Sankaranarayanan *et al.*, 1983).

A group of three male Swiss-Webster mice received 444 mg/kg bw 1,2:3,4-diepoxybutane intramuscularly in an intraperitoneal host-mediated assay employing reverse mutation in *S. typhimurium* TA1530 and TA1538 and mitotic recombination in *S. cerevisiae* D3. Positive results were obtained only with strain TA1530 (Simmon *et al.*, 1979).

1,2:3,4-Diepoxybutane (3×10^{-7} and 3×10^{-6} M) induced a dose-related increase in sister chromatid exchanges in cultured Chinese hamster ovary cells (Perry & Evans, 1975). Concentrations of 0.1-0.5 µg/ml induced a dose-related increase in sister chromatid exchanges in cultured lymphocytes from normal donors and from patients with a variety of solid tumours (Wiencke *et al.*, 1982).

1,2:3,4-Diepoxybutane (0.01 µg/ml for six days) induced chromosomal damage in early-passage, cultured human fibroblasts from patients with Fanconi's anaemia (Auerbach & Wolman, 1976) and in fibroblasts from heterozygotes for Fanconi's anaemia (Auerbach & Wolman, 1978). Treatment with concentrations of 0.001-0.1 µg/ml for 24 h induced dose-related increases in chromosomal damage in cultured lymphoblastoid cell lines from normal individuals and from patients with Fanconi's anaemia (homo- and heterozygotes), ataxia telangiectasia and xeroderma pigmentosum (Cohen *et al.*, 1982). 1,2:3,4-Diepoxybutane (0.01 µg/ml) induced chromosomal aberrations but not sister chromatid exchange in cultured lymphocytes from homo- (FA/FA) and heterozygotes (FA/+) for Fanconi's anaemia (Porfirio *et al.*, 1983).

Groups of intact and partially-hepatectomized Swiss-Webster mice received single intraperitoneal injections (10-291 µmol/kg bw, three mice per group) of 1,2:3,4-diepoxybutane (purity, 97%). Significant, dose-related increases in sister chromatid exchanges were seen in bone-marrow and alveolar macrophages of both intact and partially-hepatectomized mice and in the regenerating liver of hepatectomized mice (Conner *et al.*, 1983).

(b) Humans

Toxic effects

The toxic effects of combined exposures to 1,3-butadiene and other agents (e.g., styrene, chloroprene, hydrogen sulphide, acrylonitrile) have been reviewed (Parsons & Wilkins, 1976). Concentrations of several thousand ppm 1,3-butadiene cause irritation to skin, eyes, nose and throat (Carpenter *et al.*, 1944; Wilson *et al.*, 1948; Parson & Wilkins, 1976).

Several studies have been reported on the effects of occupational exposure to 1,3-butadiene, mainly from the USSR. Few are substantiated by details on the atmospheric concentration or duration of exposure, and control data are not generally provided. The effects reported include haematological disorders (Batkina, 1966; Volkova & Bagdinov, 1969), liver enlargement and 'liver and bile-duct diseases' (Volkova & Bagdinov, 1969), kidney malfunctions, laryngotracheitis, upper-respiratory-tract irritation, conjunctivitis, gastritis, various skin disorders and a variety of neuraesthenic symptoms (Parsons & Wilkins, 1976).

Checkoway and Williams (1982) reported slight changes in haematological indices among eight workers exposed to about 20 ppm (44.2 mg/m^3) 1,3-butadiene, 14 ppm (59.5 mg/m^3) styrene and 0.03 ppm (0.1 mg/m^3) benzene, relative to those among 145 workers exposed to less than 2 ppm (4.4 and 8.5 mg/m^3, respectively) 1,3-butadiene and styrene and less than 0.1 ppm (0.3 mg/m^3) benzene. [The Working Group considered that these changes cannot be indicative of an effect on the bone marrow.]

Effects on reproduction and prenatal toxicity
No data were available to the Working Group.

Absorption, distribution, excretion and metabolism
No data were available to the Working Group.

Mutagenicity and chromosomal effects
No data were available to the Working Group.

3.3 Case reports and epidemiological studies of carcinogenicity to humans

Epidemiological evaluation of a possible carcinogenic effect of 1,3-butadiene is complicated by mixed exposures.

A retrospective cohort study (Meinhardt *et al.*, 1982) was conducted in two styrene-butadiene rubber producing facilities (plants A and B) in eastern Texas on ~~1656~~ (plant A) *1662* and 1094 (plant B) white males who had been employed for at least six months (total, 53 929 person-years at risk). The only environmental samples were taken at the time of the study;

mean exposures to 1,3-butadiene were 1.24 ppm at plant A (standard deviation, SD, 1.20) (2.74 mg/m³) and 13.5 ppm at plant B (SD, 30) (30 mg/m³); those for styrene were 0.94 ppm (SD, 1.23) (4 mg/m³) and 1.99 ppm (SD, 3.00) (8.5 mg/m³), respectively; traces of benzene were also detected in plant A. The follow-up period lasted from 1943 to 1976 (plant A) and from 1950 to 1976 (plant B). [The Working Group considered that in view of the changes that can occur in processes and environmental conditions of an industry with time, the environmental sampling is probably not representative.] The standardized mortality ratio (SMR) for all causes of death was 80 for workers in plant A. Nine deaths from cancer of the lymphatic and haematopoietic tissues occurred in the cohort employed at plant A between January 1943 and March 1976 (5.79 expected), giving a SMR of 155 (not significant). However, further analysis showed that these nine cases were employed between January 1943 and December 1945, for which time period the expected number was 4.25, giving a statistically significant SMR of 212. The SMR for leukaemias was 278. No other excess of cancer was found. Exposure to 1,3-butadiene for workers employed at plant B in 1976 was ten-fold that at plant A. The SMR for all causes of death was 66. No excess cancer mortality was found, but the numbers observed were low. (> the SMRs were not statistically significant

A number of studies have investigated the mortality of workers engaged in the rubber industry (Andjelkovic et al., 1976; McMichael et al., 1976; Monson & Nakano, 1976; Andjelkovic et al., 1977), where there is potential exposure to 1,3-butadiene, among other chemicals, and several have shown elevated SMRs for cancers at various sites. All of these studies are described in detail in previous IARC Monographs volumes (IARC, 1979, 1982). In only one study (McMichael et al., 1976) was exposure to styrene-butadiene specified. This report suggested an association between lymphatic and haematopoietic malignancy and work in the styrene-butadiene rubber manufacture department of a rubber plant. The age-adjusted ratios of rates of exposure were 4.4 for those exposed for more than two years and 5.6 for those exposed for more than five years. This association was not seen in workers in any other department, nor for cancer at any other site.

4. Summary of Data Reported and Evaluation

4.1 Exposure data

Large-scale commercial production of 1,3-butadiene was begun in the 1930s. Occupational exposure to this compound occurs during the manufacture of the monomer and its use in the production of polybutadiene rubber, styrene-butadiene rubber, acrylonitrile-butadiene-styrene polymers and other polymers. 1,3-Butadiene has also been measured at low levels in ambient urban air.

4.2 Experimental data

1,3-Butadiene was tested for carcinogenicity in mice by inhalation. It was carcinogenic to animals of both sexes, producing an unusual neoplasm of the heart, the incidence of which was dose-related in females. It also produced tumours at several other sites, including lung, stomach, liver, mammary gland and the lymphatic system in a dose-related manner.

The data available to the Working Group were inadequate to evaluate the reproductive and prenatal toxicity of 1,3-butadiene to experimental animals.

1,3-Butadiene was mutagenic to *Salmonella typhimurium* in the presence of an exogenous metabolic system. A metabolite, 1,2-epoxybutene, identified *in vivo*, was also mutagenic to bacteria.

Overall assessment of data from short-term tests: 1,3-Butadiene[a]

	Genetic activity			Cell transformation
	DNA damage	Mutation	Chromosomal effects	
Prokaryotes		+		
Fungi/Green plants				
Insects				
Mammalian cells (*in vitro*)				
Mammals (*in vivo*)				
Humans (*in vivo*)				
Degree of evidence in short-term tests for genetic activity: **Inadequate**				Cell transformation: No data

[a]The groups into which the table is divided and the symbol '+' are defined on pp. 19-20 of the Preamble; the degrees of evidence are defined on pp. 20-21.

4.3 Human data

No data were available to evaluate the reproductive effects or prenatal toxicity of 1,3-butadiene to humans.

The available studies provide some evidence of an association between an excess of leukaemias and lymphomas and work in an environment with mixed exposure to 1,3-butadiene and other chemicals, especially styrene and possibly benzene. The mixed exposure patterns typical of the rubber industry render it impossible to single out 1,3-butadiene as a specific causative agent.

4.4 Evaluation[1]

There is *sufficient evidence*[2] for the carcinogenicity of 1,3-butadiene in experimental animals.

There is *inadequate evidence* for the carcinogenicity of 1,3-butadiene in humans.

5. References

American Conference of Governmental Industrial Hygienists (1984) *Threshold Limit Values for Chemical Substances and Physical Agents in the Work Environment and Biological Exposure Indices with Intended Changes for 1984-85*, Cincinnati, OH, pp. 11, 36, 41

Andjelkovic, D., Taulbee, J. & Symons, M. (1976) Mortality experience of a cohort of rubber workers, 1964-1973. *J. occup. Med., 18*, 387-394

Andjelkovic, D., Taulbee, J., Symons, M. & Williams, T. (1977) Mortality of rubber workers with reference to work experience. *J. occup. Med., 19*, 397-405

Anon. (1984a) Butadiene imports weaken price/supply shortfalls in the late 1980's. *Chem. Mark. Rep., 225*, 3,17

Anon. (1984b) Facts and figures for the chemical industry. *Chem. Eng. News, 62*, 33-74

Anon. (1984c) A big trade setback for US producers. *Chem. Week, 134*, 24-27

Anon. (1985) Butadiene. *Chem. Eng. News*, 25 March, 25

Arnts, R.R. & Meeks, S.A. (1981) Biogenic hydrocarbon contribution to the ambient air of selected areas. *Atmos. Environ., 15*, 1643-1651

Auerbach, A.D. & Wolman, S.R. (1976) Susceptibility of Fanconi's anaemia fibroblasts to chromosome damage by carcinogens. *Nature, 261*, 494-496

Auerbach, A.D. & Wolman, S.R. (1978) Carcinogen-induced chromosome breakage in Fanconi's anaemia heterozygous cells. *Nature, 271*, 69-70

Batkina, I.P. (1966) Maximum permissible concentration of divinyl vapors in factory air. *Hyg. Sanit., 31*, 334-338

Berg, S., Frostling, H. & Jacobsson, S. (1978) *Chemical analysis of fire gases with gas chromatography-mass spectrometry*. In: *Proceedings of an International Symposium on the Control of Air Pollution in the Work Environment, 1977*, Part 1, Stockholm, Arbetarskyddsfonden, pp. 309-321

---

[1]For definitions of the italicized terms, see Preamble, pp. 18 and 22.

[2]In the absence of adequate data in humans, it is reasonable, for practical purposes, to regard chemicals for which there is sufficient evidence of carcinogenicity in animals as if they represented a carcinogenic risk to humans.

Bird, M.J. & Fahmy, O.G. (1953) Cytogenetic analysis of the action of carcinogens and tumour inhibitors in *Drosophila melanogaster*. I. 1,2:3,4-Diepoxybutane. *Proc. R. Soc. B.*, *140*, 556-578

Bolt, H.M., Schmiedel, G., Filser, J.G., Rolzhäuser, H.P., Lieser, K., Wistuba, D. & Schurig, V. (1983) Biological activation of 1,3-butadiene to vinyl oxirane by rat liver microsomes and expiration of the reactive metabolite by exposed rats. *J. Cancer Res. clin. Oncol.*, *106*, 112-116

Bolt, H.M., Filser, J.G. & Störmer, F. (1984) Inhalation pharmacokinetics based on gas uptake studies. V. Comparative pharmacokinetics of ethylene and 1,3-butadiene in rats. *Arch. Toxicol.*, *55*, 213-218

Burroughs, G.E. (1979) *Health Hazard Evaluation Determination. Report No. 78-110-585. Piper Aircraft Corporation, Vero Beach, FL (NTIS PB80-196702)*, Cincinnati, OH, National Institute for Occupational Safety and Health

Carpenter, C.P., Shaffer, C.B., Weil, C.S. & Smyth, H.F., Jr (1944) Studies on the inhalation of 1:3-butadiene; with a comparison of its narcotic effect with benzol, toluol and styrene, and a note on the elimination of styrene by the human. *J. ind. Hyg. Toxicol.*, *26*, 69-78

Checkoway, H. & Williams, T.M. (1982) A hematology survey of workers at a styrene-butadiene synthetic rubber manufacturing plant. *Am. ind. Hyg. Assoc. J.*, *43*, 164-169

Clarke, C.H. & Loprieno, N. (1965) The influence of genetic background on the induction of methionine reversions by diepoxybutane in *Schizosaccharomyces pombe*. *Microbiol. Genet. Bull.*, *22*, 11-12

Cohen, M.M., Fruchtman, C.E., Simpson, S.J. & Martin, A.O. (1982) The cytogenetic response of Fanconi's anemia lymphoblastoid cell lines to various clastogens. *Cytogenet. Cell Genet.*, *34*, 230-240

Coker, D.T. (1977) Heat desorption of vapour-trapping tubes. *Proc. analyt. Div. chem. Soc.*, *14*, 108-109

Conner, M.K., Luo, J.E. & de Gotera, O.G. (1983) Induction and rapid repair of sister-chromatid exchanges in multiple murine tissues *in vivo* by diepoxybutane. *Mutat. Res.*, *108*, 251-263

Crandall, M.S., Young, R.J. & Blade, L.M. (1981) *In-depth Industrial Hygiene Composite Report on Exposure to Styrene and Butadiene at Two Styrene-Butadiene Rubber Processing Plants (NTIS PB82-151390)*, Cincinnati, OH, Industrial Hygiene Section, Industrywide Studies Branch, Division of Surveillance, Hazard Evaluations and Field Studies, National Institute for Occupational Safety and Health

Crouch, C.N., Pullinger, D.H. & Gaunt, I.F. (1979) Inhalation toxicity studies with 1,3-butadiene. 2. 3 Month toxicity study in rats. *Am. ind. Hyg. Assoc. J.*, *40*, 796-802

Duverger, M., Lambotte, M., Malvoisin, E., de Meester, C., Poncelet, F. & Mercier, M. (1981) Metabolic activation and mutagenicity of 4 vinylic monomers (vinyl chloride, styrene, acrylonitrile, butadiene). *Toxicol. Eur. Res.*, *3*, 131-140

Fahmy, O.G. & Fahmy, M.J. (1970) Gene elimination in carcinogenesis: Reinterpretation of the somatic mutation theory. *Cancer Res., 30*, 195-205

Filser, J.G. & Bolt, H.M. (1984) Inhalation pharmacokinetics based on gas uptake studies. VI. Comparative evaluation of ethylene oxide and butadiene monoxide as exhaled reactive metabolites of ethylene and 1,3-butadiene in rats. *Arch. Toxicol., 55*, 219-223

Gervasi, P.G., Citti, L., Del Monte, M., Longo, V. & Benetti, D. (1985) Mutagenicity and chemical reactivity of epoxidic intermediates of the isoprene metabolism and other structurally related compounds. *Mutat. Res., 156*, 77-82

Glover, S.W. (1956) A comparative study of induced reversions in *Escherichia coli*. In: *Genetic Studies with Bacteria (Carnegie Institution of Washington Publication 612)*, Washington DC, Carnegie Institution, pp. 121-136

Graf, U., Juon, H., Katz, A.J., Frei, H.J. & Würgler, F.E. (1983) A pilot study on a new *Drosophila* spot test. *Mutat. Res., 120*, 233-239

Grasselli, J.G. & Ritchey, W.M., eds (1975) *CRC Atlas of Spectral Data and Physical Constants for Organic Compounds*, Vol. 2, Cleveland, OH, CRC Press, Inc., p. 565

Greek, B.F. (1984) Elastomers finally recover growth. *Chem. Eng. News, 62*, 35-56

Hawley, G.G., ed. (1981) *The Condensed Chemical Dictionary*, 10th ed., New York, Van Nostrand Reinhold, p. 156

Health and Safety Executive (1985) *Occupational Exposure Limits (Guidance Note EH 40/85)*, London, Her Majesty's Stationery Office, p. 9

Heinemann, B. & Howard, A.J. (1964) Induction of lambda bacteriophage in *Escherichia coli* as a screening test for potential antitumor agents. *Appl. Microbiol., 12*, 234-239

Hemminki, K., Falck, K. & Vainio, H. (1980) Comparison of alkylation rates and mutagenicity of directly acting industrial and laboratory chemicals. Epoxides, glycidyl ethers, methylating and ethylating agents, halogenated hydrocarbons, hydrazine derivatives, aldehydes, thiuram and dithiocarbamate derivatives. *Arch. Toxicol., 46*, 277-285

Huff, J.E., Melnick, R.L., Solleveld, H.A., Haseman, J.K., Powers, M. & Miller, R.A. (1985) Multiple organ carcinogenicity of 1,3-butadiene in B6C3F$_1$ mice after 60 weeks of inhalation exposure. *Science, 227*, 548-549

Hunt, W.F., Jr, Faoro, R.B. & Duggan, G.M. (1984) *Compilation of Air Toxic and Trace Metal Summary Statistics (EPA-450/4-84-015)*, Research Triangle Park, NC, US Environmental Protection Agency, Office of Air and Radiation, Office of Air Quality Planning and Standards, pp. 4, 101

Hutte, R.S., Williams, E.J., Staehelin, J., Hawthorne, S.B., Barkley, R.M. & Sievers, R.E. (1984) Chromatographic analysis of organic compounds in the atmosphere. *J. Chromatogr., 302*, 173-179

IARC (1976) *IARC Monographs on the Evaluation of Carcinogenic Risk of Chemicals to Man*, Vol. 11, *Cadmium, Nickel, Some Epoxides, Miscellaneous Industrial Chemicals, and General Considerations on Volatile Anaesthetics*, Lyon, pp. 115-121

IARC (1977) *IARC Monographs on the Evaluation of the Carcinogenic Risk of Chemicals to Man*, Vol. 15, *Some Fumigants, the Herbicides 2,4-D and 2,4,5-T, Chlorinated Dibenzodioxins and Miscellaneous Industrial Chemicals*, Lyon, pp. 155-175

IARC (1979) *IARC Monographs on the Evaluation of the Carcinogenic Risk of Chemicals to Humans*, Vol. 28, *The Rubber Industry*, Lyon, pp. 192-198

IARC (1982) *IARC Monographs on the Evaluation of the Carcinogenic Risk of Chemicals to Humans*, Suppl. 4, *Chemicals, Industrial Processes and Industries Associated with Cancer in Humans (IARC Monographs Volumes 1 to 29)*, Lyon, pp. 144-145

International Institute of Synthetic Rubber Producers (1984) *Comments Upon the EPA TSCA 4(f) Listing of 1,3-Butadiene*, Houston, TX

International Labour Office (1980) *Occupational Exposure Limits for Airborne Toxic Substances, A Tabular Compilation of Values from Selected Countries*, 2nd (rev.) ed. (*Occupational Safety and Health Series No. 37*), Geneva, pp. 56-57

Jones, B. (1981) Worker exposure to selected synthetic rubber chemicals: A·field comparison of two sampling methods. *Ann. Am. Conf. gov. ind. Hyg.*, *1*, 249-252

Kirshenbaum, I. (1978) *Butadiene*. In: Mark, H.F., Othmer, D.F., Overberger, C.G. & Seaborg, G.T., eds, *Kirk-Othmer Encyclopedia of Chemical Technology*, 3rd ed., Vol. 4, New York, John Wiley & Sons, pp. 313-337

Klein, A. (1981) *Latex technology*. In: Mark, H.F., Othmer, D.F., Overberger, C.G. & Seaborg, G.T., eds, *Kirk-Othmer Encyclopedia of Chemical Technology*, 3rd ed., Vol. 14, New York, John Wiley & Sons, p. 83

Kölmark, G. & Westergaard, M. (1953) Further studies on chemically induced reversions at the adenine locus of *Neurospora*. *Hereditas*, *39*, 209-223

Kraybill, H.F. (1980) Evaluation of public health aspects of carcinogenic/mutagenic biorefractories in drinking water. *Prev. Med.*, *9*, 212-218

Leviton, E.B. (1983) *Existing Chemical Market Review: 1,3-Butadiene*, Washington DC, US Environmental Protection Agency, Regulatory Impacts Branch

Lonneman, W.A. (1977) *Ozone and hydrocarbon measurements in recent oxidant transport studies*. In: *Proceedings of an International Conference on Photochemical Oxidant Pollution and Its Control, 1976* (*EPA-600/3/77-001a; PB-264 232*), Research Triangle Park, NC, US Environmental Protection Agency, pp. 211-223

Lonneman, W.A., Kopczynski, S.L., Darley, P.E. & Sutterfield, F.D. (1974) Hydrocarbon composition of urban air pollution. *Environ. Sci. Technol.*, *8*, 229-236

Lonneman, W.A., Seila, R.L. & Bufalini, J.J. (1978) Ambient air hydrocarbon concentrations in Florida. *Environ. Sci. Technol.*, *12*, 459-463

Lwoff, A. (1953) Lysogeny. *Bacteriol. Rev.*, *17*, 269-337

Malvoisin, E. & Roberfroid, M. (1982) Hepatic microsomal metabolism of 1,3-butadiene. *Xenobiotica*, *12*, 137-144

Malvoisin, E., Lhoest, G., Poncelet, F., Roberfroid, M. & Mercier, M. (1979) Identification and quantitation of 1,2-epoxybutene-3 as the primary metabolite of 1,3-butadiene. *J. Chromatogr.*, *178*, 419-425

Mannsville Chemical Products Corp. (1983) *Butadiene (Chemical Products Synopsis)*, Cortland, NY

McCann, J., Choi, E., Yamasaki, E. & Ames, B.N. (1975) Detection of carcinogens as mutagens in the *Salmonella*/microsome test: Assay of 300 chemicals. *Proc. natl Acad. Sci. USA*, *72*, 5135-5139

McMichael, A.J., Spirtas, R., Gamble, J.F. & Tousey, P.M. (1976) Mortality among rubber workers: Relationship to specific jobs. *J. occup. Med.*, *18*, 178-185

de Meester, C., Poncelet, F., Robergroid, M. & Mercier, M. (1978) Mutagenicity of butadiene and butadiene monoxide. *Biochem. biophys. Res. Comm.*, *80*, 298-305

de Meester, C., Poncelet, F., Roberfroid, M. & Mercier, M. (1980) The mutagenicity of butadiene toward *Salmonella typhimurium*. *Toxicol. Lett.*, *6*, 125-130

Meinhardt, T.J., Young, R.J. & Hartle, R.W. (1978) Epidemiologic investigations of styrene-butadiene rubber production and reinforced plastics production. *Scand. J. Work Environ. Health*, *4* (Suppl. 2), 240-246

Meinhardt, T.J., Lemen, R.A., Crandall, M.S. & Young, R.J. (1982) Environmental epidemiologic investigation of the styrene-butadiene rubber industry. Mortality patterns with discussion of the hematopoietic and lymphatic malignancies. *Scand. J. Work Environ. Health*, *8*, 250-259

Miller, L.M. (1978) *Investigation of Selected Potential Environmental Contaminants: Butadiene and Its Oligomers (EPA-560/2-78-008; NTIS PB-291684)*, Washington, DC, US Environmental Protection Agency, Office of Toxic Substances

Monson, R.R. & Nakano, K.K. (1976) Mortality among rubber workers. I. White male union employees in Akron, Ohio. *Am. J. Epidemiol.*, *103*, 284-296

National Fire Protection Association (1984) *Fire Protection Guide on Hazardous Materials*, 8th ed., Quincy, MA, pp. 325M-19, 49-22

National Institute for Occupational Safety and Health (1980) *Health Hazard Evaluation Report HE-80-188-797, Metamora Products Corporation, Elkland, PA (NTIS PB82-188368)*, Cincinnati, OH

National Institute for Occupational Safety and Health (1984) *Current Intelligence Bulletin No. 41: 1,3-Butadiene (DHHS (NIOSH) Publ. No. 84-105)*, Cincinnati, OH

National Toxicology Program (1984) *Toxicology and Carcinogenesis Studies of 1,3-Butadiene (CAS No. 106-99-0) in B6C3F1 Mice (Inhalation Studies) (Technical Report Series No. 288)*, Research Triangle Park, NC

Natusch, D.F.S. (1978) Potentially carcinogenic species emitted to the atmosphere by fossil-fueled power plants. *Environ. Health Perspect.*, *22*, 79-90

Neligan, R.E. (1962) Hydrocarbons in the Los Angeles atmosphere. A comparison between the hydrocarbons in automobile exhaust and those found in the Los Angeles atmosphere. *Arch. environ. Health*, *5*, 581-591

NIH/EPA Chemical Information System (1983) *Carbon-13 NMR Spectral Search System, Mass Spectral Search System,* and *Infrared Spectral Search System*, Arlington, VA, Information Consultants, Inc.

Owen, P.E., Pullinger, D.H., Glaister, J.R. & Gaunt, I.F. (1985) *1,3-Butadiene: Two-year inhalation toxicity/carcinogenicity study in the rat* (Abstract No. P34). In: Hanhijärvi, H., ed., *26th Congress of the European Society of Toxicology, 16-19 June,* Kuopio, University of Kuopio, p. 69

Parsons, T.B. & Wilkins, G.E. (1976) *Biological Effects and Environmental Aspects of 1,3-Butadiene. Final Report (EPA-560/2-76-004; PB-253 982)*, Washington DC, US Environmental Protection Agency, Office of Toxic Substances

Perry, P. & Evans, H.J. (1975) Cytological detection of mutagen-carcinogen exposure by sister chromatid exchange. *Nature, 258,* 121-125

Perry, R.H. & Green, D.W., eds (1984) *Perry's Chemical Engineers' Handbook*, 6th ed., New York, McGraw-Hill, pp. 3-28

Polakowska, R. & Putrament, A. (1979) Mitochondrial mutagenesis in *Saccharomyces cerevisiae*. II. Methyl methanesulphonate and diepoxybutane. *Mutat. Res., 61,* 207-213

Poncelet, F., de Meester, C., Duverger-van Bogaert, M., Lambotte-Vanderpaer, M., Roberfroid, M. & Mercier, M. (1980) Influence of experimental factors on mutagenicity of vinylic monomers. *Arch. Toxicol., Suppl. 4,* 63-66

Pope, S., Baker, J.M. & Parish, J.H. (1984) Assay of cytotoxicity and mutagenicity of alkylating agents by using *Neurospora* spheroplasts. *Mutat. Res., 125,* 43-53

Porfirio, B., Dallapiccola, B., Mokini, V., Alimena, G. & Gandini, E. (1983) Failure of diepoxybutane to enhance sister chromatid exchange levels in Fanconi's anemia patients and heterozygotes. *Human Genet., 63,* 117-120

Rosenkranz, H.S. & Poirier, L.A. (1979) Evaluation of the mutagenicity and DNA-modifying activity of carcinogens and noncarcinogens in microbial systems. *J. natl Cancer Inst., 62,* 873-892

Rubber Manufacturers' Association (1984) *1,3-Butadiene (March 4; 5 PH 4:20)*, Washington DC

Sadtler Research Laboratories (1980) *The Sadtler Standard Spectra Collection, Cumulative Index*, Philadelphia, PA

Sandhu, S.S., Waters, M.D., Mortelmans, K.E., Evans, E.L., Jotz, M.M., Mitchell, A.D. & Kasica, V. (1984) Evaluation of diallate and triallate herbicides for genotoxic effects in a battery of in vitro and short-term in vivo tests. *Mutat. Res., 136,* 173-183

Sankaranarayanan, K., Ferro, W. & Zijlstra, J.A. (1983) Studies on mutagen-sensitive strains of *Drosophila melanogaster*. III. A comparison of the mutagenic sensitivities of the *ebony* (UV and X-ray sensitive) and *Canton-S* (wild-type) strains to MMS, ENU, DEB, DEN and 2,4,6-Cl_3-PDMT. *Mutat. Res., 110,* 59-70

Sax, N.I. (1984) *Dangerous Properties of Industrial Materials*, 6th ed., New York, Van Nostrand Reinhold, p. 545

Schneider, W., Frohne, J.C. & Bruderreck, H. (1978) Determination of hydrocarbons in the parts per 10^9 range using glass capillary columns coated with aluminium oxide. *J. Chromatogr., 155,* 311-327

Shugaev, B. (1969) Concentrations of hydrocarbons in tissues as a measure of toxicity. *Arch. environ. Health, 18*, 878-882

Siddiqi, A.A. & Worley, F.L., Jr (1977) Urban and industrial air pollution in Houston, Texas. I. Hydrocarbons. *Atmos. Environ., 11*, 131-143

Simmon, V.F. (1979) In vitro assays for recombinogenic activity of chemical carcinogens and related compounds with *Saccharomyces cerevisiae* D3. *J. natl Cancer Inst., 62*, 901-909

Simmon, V.F., Rosenkranz, H.S., Zeiger, E. & Poirier, L.A. (1979) Mutagenic activity of chemical carcinogens and related compounds in the intraperitoneal host-mediated assay. *J. natl Cancer Inst., 62*, 911-918

Startin, J.R. & Gilbert, J. (1984) Single ion monitoring of butadiene in plastics and foods by coupled mass spectrometry-automatic headspace gas chromatography. *J. Chromatogr., 294*, 427-430

Taylor, D.G. (1977) *NIOSH Manual of Analytical Methods*, 2nd Ed., Vol. 2 (*DHEW (NIOSH) Publication No. 77-157-B*), Washington DC, US Government Printing Office, pp. S91-1 — S91-9

Työsuojeluhallitus (National Finnish Board of Occupational Safety and Health) (1981) *Airborne Contaminants in the Workplace* (Safety Bulletin 3) (Finn.), Tampere, p. 9

US Environmental Protection Agency (1978) Interim primary drinking water regulations. *Fed. Regist., 43*, 29135-29150

US Food and Drug Administration (1984) Food and drugs. *US Code Fed. Regul., Title 21*, Parts 175.125, 175.300, 177.2600, pp. 138, 146, 284

US International Trade Commission (1979) *Synthetic Organic Chemicals, US Production and Sales, 1978 (USITC Publication 1001)*, Washington DC, US Government Printing Office, p. 223

US International Trade Commission (1984) *Synthetic Organic Chemicals, US Production and Sales, 1983 (USITC Publication 1588)*, Washington DC, US Government Printing Office, pp. 17, 20, 138, 161

US Occupational Safety and Health Administration (1983) *General Industry. OSHA Safety and Health Standards (29 CFR 1910) (OSHA 2206)* (revised), Washington DC, p. 599

Verschueren, K. (1983) *Handbook of Environmental Data on Organic Chemicals*, 2nd ed., New York, Van Nostrand Reinhold Co., pp. 295-297

Volkova, Z.A. & Bagdinov, Z.M. (1969) Problems of labor hygiene in rubber vulcanization. *Hyg. Sanit., 34*, 326-333

Voogd, C.E., van der Stel, J.J. & Jacobs, J.J.J.A.A. (1981) The mutagenic action of aliphatic epoxides. *Mutat. Res., 89*, 269-282

Watson, W.A.F. (1972) Studies on a recombination-deficient mutant of *Drosophila*. II. Response to X-rays and alkylating agents. *Mutat. Res., 14*, 299-307

Weast, R.C., ed. (1984) *CRC Handbook of Chemistry and Physics*, 65th ed., Boca Raton, FL, CRC Press, Inc., pp. C-184, D-202

Wiencke, J.K., Vosika, J., Johnson, P., Wang, N. & Garry, V.F. (1982) Differential induction of sister chromatid exchange by chemical carcinogens in lymphocytes cultured from patients with solid tumors. *Pharmacology*, *24*, 67-73

Wilson, R.H., Hough, G.V. & McCormick, W.E. (1948) Medical problems encountered in the manufacture of American-made rubber. *Ind. Med.*, *17*, 199-207

Windholz, M., ed. (1983) *The Merck Index*, 10th ed., Rahway, NJ, Merck & Co., p. 209

Zimmermann, F.K. (1971) Induction of mitotic gene conversion by mutagens. *Mutat. Res.*, *11*, 327-337

Zimmermann, F.K. & Vig, B.K. (1975) Mutagen specificity in the induction of mitotic crossing-over in *Saccharomyces cerevisiae*. *Mol. gen. Genet.*, *139*, 255-268

4-VINYLCYCLOHEXENE

This substance was considered by a previous Working Group, in February 1976 (IARC, 1976). Since that time, new data have become available, and these have been incorporated into the monograph and taken into consideration in the present evaluation.

1. Chemical and Physical Data

1.1 Synonyms and trade names

Chem. Abstr. Services Reg. No.: 100-40-3

Chem. Abstr. Name: Cyclohexene, 4-ethenyl-

IUPAC Systematic Name: 4-Vinylcyclohexene

Synonyms: Butadiene dimer; 1-cyclohexene, 4-vinyl; cyclohexenylethylene; 4-ethenyl-1-cyclohexene; 4-ethenylcyclohexene; NCI-C54999; 1,2,3,4-tetrahydrostyrene; vinylcyclohexene; 1-vinyl-3-cyclohexene; 1-vinylcyclohex-3-ene; 1-vinylcyclohexene-3; 4-vinyl-1-cyclohexene; 4-vinylcyclohexene-1

1.2 Structural and molecular formulae and molecular weight

$$CH = CH_2$$

C_8H_{12} Mol. wt: 108.18

1.3 Chemical and physical properties of the pure substance

(*a*) *Description*: Colourless liquid (Hawley, 1981; National Toxicology Program, 1985)

(b)   *Boiling-point*: 128.9°C (Weast, 1984)

(c)   *Melting-point*: -109°C (Sax, 1984)

(d)   *Density*: d_4^{20} 0.8299 (Weast, 1984)

(e)   *Spectroscopy data*: Ultraviolet (Perkampus et al., 1968), infrared (Sadtler Research Laboratories, 1980; prism [6321[a]], grating [10854]), nuclear magnetic resonance (Sadtler Research Laboratories, 1980; proton [9681], C-13 [987]) and mass spectral data (NIH/EPA Chemical Information System, 1983) have been reported.

(f)   *Solubility*: Soluble in diethyl ether, benzene and petroleum ether (Weast, 1984)

(g)   *Volatility*: Vapour pressure, 25.8 mm Hg at 38°C; relative vapour density (air = 1), 3.76 (Sax, 1984)

(h)   *Stability*: Flash-point, 15.6°C (open-cup) (Sax, 1984); temperatures above 26.6°C and prolonged exposure to oxygen lead to discolouration and gum formation (Hawley, 1981); highly inflammable (Buckingham, 1982); can react with oxidizing materials (Sax, 1984)

(i)   *Conversion factor:* mg/m³ = 4.42 × ppm[b]

1.4 Technical products and impurities

4-Vinylcyclohexene is available commercially in bulk quantities in 97% purity with about 3% 1,5-cyclooctadiene and traces of 1,5,9-cyclododecatriene and 1,2-divinylcyclobutane (Miller, 1978). *tert*-Butylcatechol (50-200 mg/kg) is added as a stabilizer to inhibit oxidation; water (200 mg/kg) is also usually present (E.I. duPont de Nemours & Co., 1984). The commercial product is not believed to contain significant quantities of 1,3-butadiene.

2. Production, Use, Occurrence and Analysis

2.1 Production and use

(a)   *Production*

4-Vinylcyclohexene is prepared commercially by catalytic dimerization of 1,3-butadiene, which is heated in the vapour phase at 425°C and under 13 atm pressure in the presence of a

---

[a]Spectrum number in Sadtler compilation

[b]Calculated from: mg/m³ = (molecular weight/24.45) × ppm, assuming standard temperature (25°C) and pressure (760 mm Hg)

silicon carbide catalyst. It has also been produced using copper or chromium naphthenate or resinate salts at 100-150°C and 40-1000 atm (Kirshenbaum, 1978). Other catalysts described in the literature include nickel dicarbonylphosphite, dicyclopentadienyl nickel, cobalt, rhodium and platinum. Dimerization of 1,3-butadiene to 4-vinylcyclohexene can occur spontaneously: when stored for 30 days at 46°C, approximately 1.6% of the butadiene dimerizes; after 30 days at 75°C, 16% dimerizes. 4-Vinylcyclohexene is also isolated as a by-product of 1,5-cyclooctadiene/cyclododecatriene manufacture (Miller, 1978).

Three companies manufacture 4-vinylcyclohexene in the USA (Anon., 1984), but recent production volumes have not been reported. One US firm imports 4-vinylcyclohexene from the Federal Republic of Germany.

(b)   Use

4-Vinylcyclohexene has been used in the manufacture of flame retardants and for the production of insecticidal compounds with ethylene chlorohydrin. These products result from typical addition and ring-opening reactions (E.I. duPont de Nemours & Co., 1984). The monomer has been used as a precursor for ethylcyclohexyl carbinol plasticizers, as an intermediate for thiocyanate insecticides and as an antioxidant

4-Vinylcyclohexene can be converted to 4-epoxyethyl-1,2-epoxycyclohexane (4-vinyl-cyclohexene diepoxide; see Fig. 1) *via* a two-step process of calcium hypochlorite treatment and subsequent dehydrohalogenation. The diepoxide is used in the manufacture of polyesters, coatings and plastics (Miller, 1978).

(c)   Regulatory status and guidelines

No data were available to the Working Group.

2.2 Occurrence

(a)   Natural occurrence

It is not known whether 4-vinylcyclohexene occurs as a natural product.

(b)   Occupational exposure

4-Vinylcyclohexene is formed as a dimer of 1,3-butadiene during its manufacture and use. In a survey of several Italian rubber goods manufacturing plants, workplace concentrations of 4-vinylcyclohexene in personal air samples were highest in the vulcanization area of a shoe-sole factory (30-210 $\mu g/m^3$). In a tyre-retreading factory, concentrations ranged from non-detectable in the vulcanization area to 0-3 $\mu g/m^3$ in the extrusion area. Levels in the extrusion area of an electrical cable insulation plant were 0-10 $\mu g/m^3$ (Cocheo *et al.*, 1983).

In another study of a rubber vulcanization area, air concentrations of 4-vinylcyclohexene in a tyre curing room ranged from 54.4-97.7 ppb (240-430 $\mu g/m^3$) (Rappaport & Fraser, 1977).

(c)   Miscellaneous

Commercial acrylonitrile-butadiene-styrene products, such as plastic sheets, ladles, graters and lunch trays were found to contain 14-210 mg/kg 4-vinylcyclohexene (Tan & Okada, 1981).

2.3 Analysis

4-Vinylcyclohexene can be monitored in workplace air by gas chromatography with flame ionization detection at levels down to 1 ppm (4.4 mg/m³) (Bianchi & Muccioli, 1981). Levels in the low μg/m³ range were detected by collecting large volumes of air (120 l) on multiple charcoal tubes, desorbing with trichlorofluoromethane and analysing by gas chromatography/mass spectrometry (GC/MS) (Cocheo *et al.*, 1983).

4-Vinylcyclohexene was determined in polybutadiene and acrylonitrile-butadiene-styrene polymers by dissolving the polymers in tetrahydrofuran and *N,N*-dimethylformamide, respectively, and analysing by GC/MS. Detection limits were in the range of 4-10 ppm (17.7-44.2 mg/m³). Migration of 4-vinylcyclohexene from acrylonitrile-butadiene-styrene sheet into four solvents simulating foods was evaluated by a similar method, with a detection limit of approximately 0.05 ppm (0.22 mg/m³) (Tan & Okada, 1981).

A purge-trap GC/MS method was used to detect 4-vinylcyclohexene in the gases released from styrene-butadiene rubber at 150°C (Khalil & Koski, 1982).

3. Biological Data Relevant to the Evaluation of Carcinogenic Risk to Humans

3.1 Carcinogenicity studies in animals

(a)   Oral administration

Mouse: Groups of 50 male and 50 female B6C3F₁ mice, eight weeks of age, were administered 200 or 400 mg/kg bw 4-vinylcyclohexene (purity, >98%, with at least seven impurities found by gas chromatography and containing 50 mg/kg *tert*-butylcatechol added as an inhibitor of peroxide formation) in corn oil by gavage on five days per week for 103 weeks. Survival among high-dose animals was poor; males: controls, 74%; low-dose, 78%; and high-dose, 14%; females: controls, 80%; low-dose, 78%; and high-dose, 34%. Groups of 50 males and 50 females received corn oil only and served as controls. The incidence of ovarian tumours was related statistically to treatment: granulosa-cell tumours or carcinomas — 1/49 controls, 10/48 ($p = 0.005$, life-table test) low-dose, and 13/47 ($p < 0.001$) high-dose; mixed-cell tumours (benign) — 0/49 controls, 25/48 ($p < 0.001$) low-dose, and 11/47 ($p < 0.001$) high-dose. In addition, adrenal cortical adenomas were observed in females: 0/50 controls, 3/49 low-dose and 4/48 high-dose (life-table, $p = 0.011$; trend, $p < 0.01$). In high-dose males, there was an increased incidence of lung tumours and lymphomas: broncho-alveolar adenomas or carcinomas — 4/49 controls, 11/50 low-dose and 4/50 [3/7 two-year survivors ($p = 0.03$)] high-dose ($p = 0.011$, life-table trend); malignant lymphomas — 4/50 controls, 7/50 low-dose and 5/50 [4/7 two-year survivors ($p = 0.002$)] high-dose ($p < 0.01$, life-table trend) (National Toxicology Program, 1985).

Rat: Groups of 50 male and 50 female Fischer 344/N rats, seven weeks of age, were administered 200 or 400 mg/kg bw 4-vinylcyclohexene (purity, >98%, with at least seven impurities found by gas chromatography and containing 50 mg/kg *tert*-butylcatechol added as an inhibitor of peroxide formation) in corn oil by gavage on five days per week for 103 weeks. Survival among high-dose animals was poor; males: controls, 64%; low-dose, 26%; and high-dose, 10%; females: controls, 80%; low-dose, 56%; and high-dose, 26%. Groups of 50 males and 50 females received corn oil only by gavage and served as controls. Skin papillomas or carcinomas were observed in males: 0/50 controls, 1/50 low-dose and 4/50 ($p = 0.001$, life-table test) high-dose animals; and clitoral-gland adenomas or squamous-cell carcinomas in females: 1/50 controls, 5/50 ($p = 0.04$) low-dose and 0/49 high-dose animals (National Toxicology Program, 1985). [The Working Group considered that the biological significance of these data could not be assessed because of the poor survival of the treated animals.]

(b) Skin application

Mouse: A group of 30 male Swiss ICR/HA mice, eight weeks old, received thrice-weekly topical applications of 45 mg 4-vinylcyclohexene (purified by removing autooxidation products with ferrous sulphate) in 0.1 ml of a 50% solution in benzene on the clipped dorsal skin for life. Median survival time was 375 days. Skin tumours were found in six males (one with a squamous-cell carcinoma and five with squamous papillomas) [$p = 0.04$]. In a vehicle-control group of 150 mice, ten developed skin papillomas and one a carcinoma (Van Duuren *et al.*, 1963).

Because the 4-vinylcyclohexene used in the study described above may have been contaminated with a minute amount of the hydrogen peroxide formed by autooxidation, a further study was carried out using 'oxygen-free material'. In this experiment, one-fifth of the dose used in the previous study (9 mg in 0.1 ml of a 10% solution in benzene) was applied thrice weekly for life to 30 male Swiss ICR/Ha mice. The median survival time was 565 days; no carcinogenic effect was observed (Van Duuren, 1965).

3.2 Other relevant biological data

(a) Experimental systems
Toxic effects

The oral LD_{50} for 4-vinylcyclohexene was 2.6 g/kg bw in Carworth-Wistar rats (Smyth *et al.*, 1969). LC_{50} values [exposure period not specified] of 27 000 mg/m³ (6095 ppm) in rats and 47 000 mg/m³ (10 610 ppm) in mice have been reported (Bykov, 1968). The percutaneous LD$_{50}$ in rabbits was 17 g/kg bw (Smyth *et al.*, 1969).

Exposure of rats and mice to 1000 mg/m³ (226 ppm) 4-vinylcyclohexene by inhalation for 6 h per day over four months was reported to inhibit weight gain and to cause leucocytosis, leucopenia and impairment of haemodynamics (Bykov, 1968).

In subchronic studies, groups of male and female mice received 0-1.2 g/kg bw 4-vinyl-cyclohexene by gavage on five days per week for 13 weeks; male and female rats received 0-800 mg/kg bw according to the same schedule. Hyaline droplet degeneration of the proximal convoluted tubules of the kidney, the severity of which was dose-related, was observed in male rats, and a reduction in the number of primary follicles and mature graafian follicles was seen in the ovaries of female mice given the highest dose (National Toxicology Program, 1985).

In rats and mice receiving 200 or 400 mg/kg bw 4-vinylcyclohexene by gavage for 103 weeks (see section 3.1), treatment-related, non-neoplastic lesions were induced in mice, including inflammation and epithelial hyperplasia of the forestomach, lung congestion and atrophy of the red pulp of the spleen; those seen in rats included hyperplasia of the forestomach (National Toxicology Program, 1985).

Effects on reproduction and prenatal toxicity

No data were available to the Working Group.

Absorption, distribution, excretion and metabolism

Wistar rat- and Swiss mouse-liver microsomal mixed-function oxidases metabolize 4-vinylcyclohexene (1) (see Fig. 1) to 4-vinyl-1,2-epoxycyclohexane (2), 4-epoxyethylcyclohexene (3) and traces of 4-epoxyethyl-1,2-epoxycyclohexane (4). These epoxides are further hydrolysed by epoxide hydrolase to the corresponding diols: 4-vinylcyclohexane-1,2-diol (5), 4-dihydroxyethylcyclohexene (6) and possibly 4-epoxyethylcyclohexane-1,2-diol (7). The last two metabolites may be further metabolized to 4-dihydroxyethyl-1,2-epoxycyclohexane (8) and the tetrol 4-dihydroxyethylcyclohexane-1,2-diol (9) (Gervasi *et al.*, 1981; Watabe *et al.*, 1981).

Mutagenicity and other short-term tests

4-Vinylcyclohexene (3.3-1000 µg/plate) was not mutagenic to *Salmonella typhimurium* TA1535, TA1537, TA98 or TA100 in the presence or absence of a metabolic system (S9) from the liver of Aroclor-induced rats or hamsters, when tested in the liquid preincubation assay (National Toxicology Program, 1985).

Several metabolites of 4-vinylcyclohexene (see Fig. 1) have been tested in short-term tests. *4-Epoxyethyl-1,2-epoxycyclohexane* (4) was mutagenic to *S. typhimurium* TA100 in the liquid preincubation assay (0.33-33 mM) (Turchi *et al.*, 1981), plate incorporation assay (1-10 µmol/plate) (Watabe *et al.*, 1980) and spot test (Wade *et al.*, 1979). *4-Vinyl-1,2-epoxycyclohexane* (2) was not mutagenic to strain TA100 in the liquid preincubation assay (0.33-1.0 mM) (however, due to its high toxicity, it could not be tested adequately) (Turchi *et al.*, 1981) or to strains TA1535, TA1537, TA1538, TA98 or TA100 in the plate incorporation assay (0.1-10 µmol/plate) (Watabe *et al.*, 1980). *4-Epoxyethylcyclohexene* (3) was not

Fig. 1. Possible pathways for metabolism of 4-vinylcyclohexene (1) by hepatic microsomes

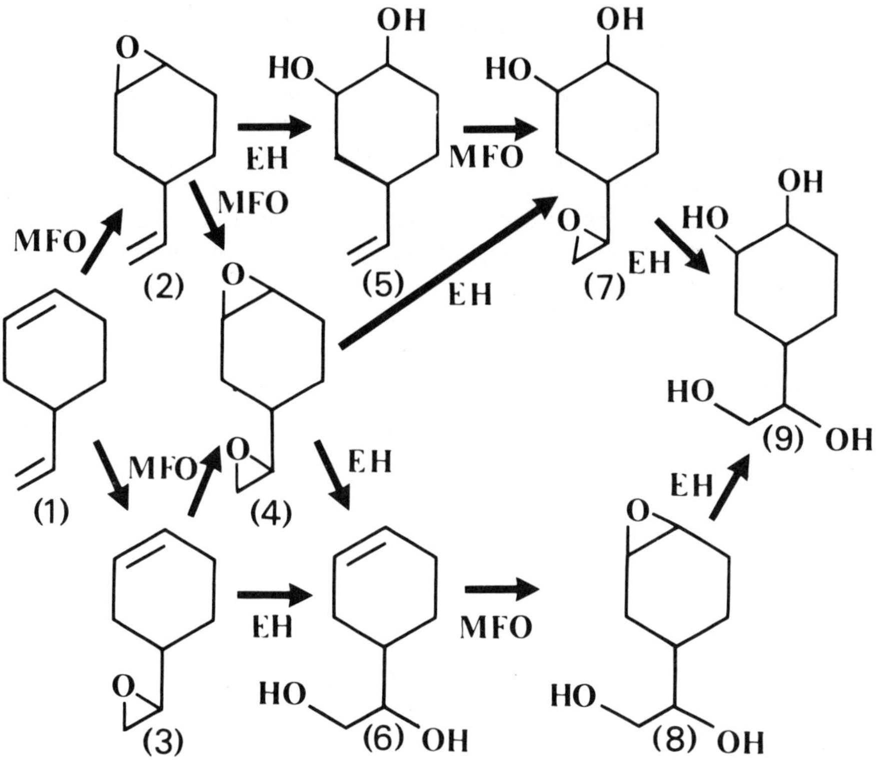

(1) 4-Vinylcyclohexene; (2) 4-vinyl-1,2-epoxycyclohexane; (3) 4-epoxyethylcyclohexene; (4) 4-epoxyethyl-1,2-epoxycyclohexane (4-vinylcyclohexene diepoxide); (5) 4-vinylcyclohexane-1,2-diol; (6) 4-dihydroxyethylcyclohexene; (7) 4-epoxyethylcyclohexane-1,2-diol; (8) 4-dihydroxyethyl-1,2-epoxycyclohexane; (9) 4-dihydroxyethylcyclohexane-1,2-diol; EH, epoxide hydrolase; MFO, mixed-function oxidases

mutagenic to strains TA1535, TA1537, TA1538, TA98 or TA100 in the plate incorporation assay (0.1-10 μmol/plate) (Watabe *et al.*, 1980). *4-Epoxyethylcyclohexane-1,2-diol* (7) was not mutagenic to strain TA100 in the liquid preincubation assay (0.33-10 mM) (Turchi *et al.*, 1981).

Intraperitoneal administration to Swiss mice of two doses of 500 mg/kg bw 4-vinyl-cyclohexene (1) in corn oil at 24-h intervals induced liver microsomal NADPH cytochrome c reductase and aminopyrine *N*-demethylase. The same treatment with 4-vinyl-1,2-epoxycyclohexane (2) induced the same enzymes plus epoxide hydrolase and increased the concentration of cytochrome P-450. Liver glutathione depletion was also observed following treatment with either compound or with 4-epoxyethyl-1,2-epoxycyclohexane, most probably as a result of conjugation of 4-vinylcyclohexene and/or its metabolites (Giannarini *et al.*, 1981).

Like other vinylalicyclic compounds, 4-vinylcyclohexene destroys hepatic cytochrome P-450 when incubated *in vitro* in the presence of liver microsomes from phenobarbital-treated mice (Testai *et al.*, 1982).

4-Epoxyethyl-1,2-epoxycyclohexane (4), but not *4-vinyl-1,2-epoxycyclohexane* (2) or *4-epoxyethylcyclohexane-1,2-diol* (7), induced 6-thioguanine-resistant mutants in cultured Chinese hamster V79 cells when tested at 0.3-20 mM (Gervasi *et al.*, 1981; Turchi *et al.*, 1981). 4-Vinyl-1,2-epoxycyclohexane and 4-epoxyethylcyclohexane-1,2-diol, tested at 2.0 mM, induced micronuclei, but 4-epoxyethyl-1,2-epoxycyclohexane did not; all three metabolites induced chromosomal damage (bridges and lagging chromosomes in anaphase) in V79 cells (Turchi *et al.*, 1981).

(b) Humans

Toxic effects

Keratitis, rhinitis, headache, hypotonia, leucopenia, neutrophilia, lymphocytosis and impairment of pigment and carbohydrate metabolism have been noted in workers exposed to 4-vinylcyclohexene (Bykov, 1968).

Effects on reproduction and prenatal toxicity
No data were available to the Working Group.

Absorption, distribution, excretion and metabolism
No data were available to the Working Group.

Mutagenicity and chromosomal effects
No data were available to the Working Group.

3.3 Case reports and epidemiological studies of carcinogenicity to humans

No data were available to the Working Group.

4. Summary of Data Reported and Evaluation

4.1 Exposure data

4-Vinylcyclohexene is formed as a dimer of 1,3-butadiene in the production and use of 1,3-butadiene. Occupational exposures to low levels have been measured in the rubber industry.

4.2 Experimental data

4-Vinylcyclohexene was tested for carcinogenicity in mice and rats by gastric intubation in corn oil. Treatment-related increases in the incidence of granulosa-cell and mixed-cell tumours of the ovary were observed in mice. High mortality was observed in male mice; increases in the incidence of lung tumours and lymphomas were statistically significant only by lifetable analysis. In rats, decreased survival, particularly in the high-dose group, compromised the study; however, there was no clear evidence of carcinogenicity in animals of either sex receiving the low dose. 4-Vinylcyclohexene, possibly contaminated with hydrogen peroxide, was tested in male mice by skin application; a marginal increase in the incidence of skin tumours was observed in one experiment.

No data were available to evaluate the reproductive effects or prenatal toxicity of 4-vinylcyclohexene to experimental animals.

4-Vinylcyclohexene was not mutagenic to *Salmonella typhimurium* in the presence or absence of an exogenous metabolic system.

Overall assessment of data from short-term tests: 4-Vinylcyclohexene[a]

	Genetic activity			Cell transformation
	DNA damage	Mutation	Chromosomal effects	
Prokaryotes		−		
Fungi/Green plants				
Insects				
Mammalian cells (*in vitro*)				
Mammals (*in vivo*)				
Humans (*in vivo*)				
Degree of evidence in short-term tests for genetic activity: **Inadequate**				Cell transformation: No data

[a]The groups into which the table is divided and the symbol '−' are defined on pp. 19-20 of the Preamble; the degrees of evidence are defined on pp. 20-21.

4.3 Human data

No data were available to evaluate the reproductive effects or prenatal toxicity of 4-vinylcyclohexene to humans.

No case report or epidemiological study was available to evaluate the carcinogenicity of 4-vinylcyclohexene to humans.

4.4 Evaluation[1]

There is *limited evidence* for the carcinogenicity of 4-vinylcyclohexene to experimental animals.

No data on humans were available.

In the absence of epidemiological data, no evaluation of the carcinogenicity of 4-vinyl-cyclohexene to humans could be made.

5. References

Anon. (1984) Buyers Guide, 1985. *Chem. Week*, October, p. 658

Bianchi, A. & Muccioli, G. (1981) Work environment and synthetic polymer production (Ital.). *Ind. Chim. Petrolifera*, 9, 77-80

Buckingham, J., ed. (1982) *Dictionary of Organic Compounds*, 5th ed., Vol. 5, New York, Chapman and Hall, p. 5711

Bykov, L.A. (1968) *Maximum permissible concentration of vinylcyclohexene in the air of industrial buildings* (Russ). In: *Proceedings of a Conference on the Toxicology and Hygiene of Petrochemical Industrial Products*, Moscow, pp. 32-34 [*Chem. Abstr., 75,* 40038y]

Cocheo, V., Bellomo, M.L. & Bombi, G.G. (1983) Rubber manufacture: Sampling and identification of volatile pollutants. *Am. ind. Hyg. Assoc. J., 44,* 521-527

E.I. duPont de Nemours & Co. (1984) *Vinylcyclohexene (Technical Bulletin)*, Wilmington, DE

Gervasi, P.G., Abbondandolo, A., Citti, L. & Turchi, G. (1981) *Microsomal 4-vinylcyclohexene mono-oxygenase and mutagenic activity of metabolic intermediates.* In: Gut, I., Cikrt, M. & Plaa, G.L., eds, *Xenobiotics: Biotransformation and Pharmacokinetics*, Berlin, Springer, pp. 205-210

Giannarini, C., Citti, L., Gervasi, P.G. & Turchi, G. (1981) Effects of 4-vinylcyclohexene and its main oxirane metabolite on mouse hepatic microsomal enzymes and glutathione levels. *Toxicol. Lett., 8,* 115-121

Hawley, G.G., ed. (1981) *The Condensed Chemical Dictionary*, 10th ed., New York, Van Nostrand Reinhold, p. 1085

---

[1]For definition of the italicized term, see Preamble, p. 18.

IARC (1976) *IARC Monographs on the Evaluation of Carcinogenic Risk of Chemicals to Man*, Vol. 11, *Cadmium, Nickel, Some Epoxides, Miscellaneous Industrial Chemicals and General Considerations on Volatile Anaesthetics*, Lyon, pp. 277-281

Khalil, H. & Koski, U. (1982) GC/MS and accessories: Characterization of residual trace organics in raw and vulcanized rubbers. *Elastomerics, 114*, 25-28

Kirshenbaum, I. (1978) *Butadiene*. In: Mark, H.F., Othmer, D.F., Overberger, C.G. & Seaborg, G.T., eds, *Kirk-Othmer Encyclopedia of Chemical Technology*, 3rd ed., Vol. 4, New York, John Wiley & Sons, p. 315

Miller, L.M. (1978) *Investigation of Selected Potential Environmental Contaminants: Butadiene and its Oligomers (EPA-560/2-78-008; NTIS PB-291 684)*, Philadelphia, PA, Franklin Research Center, pp. 10-11, 15-16

National Toxicology Program (1985) *NTP Technical Report on the Toxicology and Carcinogenicity Studies of 4-Vinylcyclohexene (CAS No. 100-40-3) in F344/N Rats and B6C3F$_1$ Mice (Gavage Studies) (Technical Report Series No. 303)*, Research Triangle Park, NC

NIH/EPA Chemical Information System (1983) *Carbon-13 NMR Spectral Search System, Mass Spectral Search System*, and *Infrared Spectral Search System*, Arlington, VA, Information Consultants, Inc.

Perkampus, H.H., Sandeman, I. & Timmons, C.J., eds (1968) *DMS UV Atlas of Organic Compounds*, Vol. IV, New York, Plenum Press, spectrum no. A1/17

Rappaport, S.M. & Fraser, D.A. (1977) Air sampling and analysis in a rubber vulcanization area. *Am. ind. Hyg. Assoc. J., 38*, 205-210

Sadtler Research Laboratories (1980) *The Sadtler Standard Spectra Collection, Cumulative Index*, Philadelphia, PA

Sax, N.I. (1984) *Dangerous Properties of Industrial Materials*, 6th ed., New York, Van Nostrand Reinhold, p. 833

Smyth, H.F., Jr, Carpenter, C.P., Weil, C.S., Pozzani, U.C., Striegel, J.A. & Nycum, J.S. (1969) Range-finding toxicity data: List VII. *Am. ind. Hyg. Assoc. J., 30*, 470-476

Tan, S. & Okada, T. (1981) Hygienic studies on plastic containers and packages. VII. Determination of 4-vinyl-1-cyclohexene in synthetic resins containing butadiene (Jpn.). *Shokuhin Eiseigaku Zasshi, 22*, 155-161

Testai, E., Citti, L., Gervasi, P.-G. & Turchi, G. (1982) Suicidal inactivation of hepatic cytochrome P-450 *in vitro* by some aliphatic olefins. *Biochem. biophys. Res. Comm., 107*, 633-641

Turchi, G., Bonatti, S., Citti, L., Gervasi, P.G., Abbondandolo, A. & Presciuttini, S. (1981) Alkylating properties and genetic activity of 4-vinylcyclohexene metabolites and structurally related epoxides. *Mutat. Res., 83*, 419-430

Van Duuren, B.L. (1965) *Carcinogenic epoxides, lactones and hydroperoxides*. In: Wogan, G.N., ed., *Mycotoxins in Foodstuffs*, Cambridge, MA, Massachusetts Institute of Technology Press, pp. 275-285

Van Duuren, B.L., Nelson, N., Orris, L., Palmes, E.D. & Schmitt, F.L. (1963) Carcinogenicity of epoxides, lactones and peroxy compounds. *J. natl Cancer Inst.*, *31*, 41-55

Wade, M.J., Moyer, J.W. & Hine, C.-H. (1979) Mutagenic action of a series of epoxides. *Mutat. Res.*, *66*, 367-371

Watabe, T., Hiratsuka, A., Isobe, M. & Ozawa, N. (1980) Metabolism of *d*-limonene by hepatic microsomes to non-mutagenic epoxides toward *Salmonella typhimurium*. *Biochem. Pharmacol.*, *29*, 1068-1071

Watabe, T., Hiratsuka, A., Ozawa, N. & Isobe, M. (1981) A comparative study on the metabolism of *d*-limonene and 4-vinylcyclohex-1-ene by hepatic microsomes. *Xenobiotica*, *11*, 333-344

Weast, R.C., ed. (1984) *CRC Handbook of Chemistry and Physics*, 65th ed., Boca Raton, FL, CRC Press, p. C-254

VINYLIDENE COMPOUNDS

VINYLIDENE CHLORIDE

This substance was considered by a previous Working Group, in February 1978 (IARC, 1979a). Since that time, new data have become available, and these have been incorporated into the monograph and taken into consideration in the present evaluation.

1. Chemical and Physical Data

1.1 Synonyms and trade names

Chem. Abstr. Services Reg. No.: 75-35-4

Chem. Abstr. Name: Ethene, 1,1-dichloro-

IUPAC Systematic Name: 1,1-Dichloroethylene

Synonyms: as-Dichloroethylene; 1,1-DCE; dichloroethene; VC; VDC; vinylidene chloride, monomer; vinylidene dichloride

1.2 Structural and molecular formulae and molecular weight

$$CH_2 = CCl_2$$

$C_2H_2Cl_2$ Mol. wt: 96.94

1.3 Chemical and physical properties of the pure substance

(*a*) *Description*: Colourless volatile liquid, with a mild, sweet odour resembling that of chloroform (Hawley, 1981; Verschueren, 1983; Windholz, 1983; Sax, 1984)

(*b*) *Boiling-point*: 37°C (Weast, 1984)

(*c*) *Melting-point*: -122.1°C (Weast, 1984)

(*d*) *Density*: d_4^{20} 1.218 (Weast, 1984)

—195—

(e) *Spectroscopy data*: Ultraviolet (National Toxicology Program, 1982), infrared (Sadtler Research Laboratories, 1980; prism [11632[a]], grating, [29675]), nuclear magnetic resonance (Sadtler Research Laboratories, 1980; proton [6385], C-13 [1090]) and mass spectral data (NIH/EPA Chemical Information System, 1983) have been reported.

(f) *Solubility*: Slightly soluble in water (0.25 g/100 g at 25°C (Dow Chemical Co., 1985)); soluble in ethanol, acetone and benzene; very soluble in diethyl ether and chloroform (Grasselli & Ritchey, 1975).

(g) *Volatility*: Vapour pressure, 591 mm Hg at 25°C; relative vapour density (air = 1), 3.25; saturation concentration, 2640 g/m³ at 20°C (Verschueren, 1983)

(h) *Stability*: Flash-point, -28°C (closed-cup) (Dow Chemical Co., 1985); polymerizes readily (Hawley, 1981); extremely inflammable; absorbs oxygen rapidly, forming explosive peroxides (Buckingham, 1982); can react vigorously with oxidizing materials (Sax, 1984)

(i) *Conversion factor*: mg/m³ = 3.96 × ppm[b]

1.4 Technical products and impurities

Vinylidene chloride is available commercially as a colourless liquid, free of suspended matter and sediment. Typical specifications are as follows: purity, 99.8 wt % min; acetylene, 25 mg/kg max; water, 50 mg/kg max; acidity (as HCl), 10 mg/kg max; polymer content, free and clear; individual halogenated impurities, 0.10 wt % max; total halogenated impurities, 0.20 wt % max; hydroquinone monomethyl ether (as a stabilizer), 180-220 mg/kg; peroxides (as H_2O_2), 10 mg/kg max (Dow Chemical Co., 1981). Dichloroacetylene (see p. 369 of this volume) has been reported to be an impurity in some commercial samples of vinylidene chloride (Reichert *et al.*, 1980).

2. Production, Use, Occurrence and Analysis

2.1 Production and use

(a) Production

Vinylidene chloride was first isolated by Regnault in 1838. A US company initiated research into vinylidene chloride polymerization techniques in the 1930s (Shelton *et al.*, 1971) and began commercial marketing of the first copolymers in 1939 (Wessling & Edwards, 1971).

---

[a]Spectrum number in Sadtler compilation

[b]Calculated from: mg/m³ = (molecular weight/24.45) × ppm, assuming standard temperature (25°C) and pressure (760 mm Hg)

Vinylidene chloride is produced commercially by the dehydrochlorination of 1,1,2-trichloroethane by lime or sodium hydroxide (Wessling & Edwards, 1971) and is extracted from the reactor by distillation, with the removal of oxygen to prevent polymerization. An azeotropic distillation column is used to dry the monomer (Shelton *et al.*, 1971). The monomethyl ether of hydroquinone is added to commercial grades of vinylidene chloride as an inhibitor (Gibbs & Wessling, 1983). The starting material, 1,1,2-trichloroethane, is often available as a by-product in the isolation of 1,2-dichloroethane (see IARC, 1979b) (Shelton *et al.*, 1971).

Seven manufacturers in western Europe reported a combined capacity for vinylidene chloride production of 352 000 tonnes in 1983: Belgium (160 000 tonnes), Federal Republic of Germany (100 000), France (50 000), The Netherlands (12 000) and the UK (30 000). In 1985, western European capacity had decreased to an estimated 130 000 tonnes.

Two firms in the USA are currently manufacturing vinylidene chloride. Another had previously produced vinylidene chloride, but ceased commercial sale of the product in 1967 (Shelton *et al.*, 1971). An estimated 90 700 tonnes per year of the monomer were produced in the USA during the early 1980s (Gibbs & Wessling, 1983).

Three companies in Japan accounted for the annual production of approximately 22 700 tonnes of vinylidene chloride monomer in the early 1980s (Gibbs & Wessling, 1983).

(b)   Use

Vinylidene chloride copolymerizes readily with other vinyl monomers, such as acrylonitrile, alkyl acrylates and methacrylates, vinyl acetate and vinyl chloride (Shelton *et al.*, 1971; Gibbs & Wessling, 1983). The US International Trade Commission (1984) reported the production of 45 800 tonnes of polyvinylidene chloride resins in 1983 (US International Trade Commission, 1984). The monomer is used in the USA almost exclusively as a comonomer, primarily with vinyl chloride.

Vinylidene chloride-vinyl chloride copolymers (Saran resins) have been used widely as films for food packaging. An oxygen barrier is created by adding a layer of vinylidene chloride copolymer to a multilayer film. These copolymers can also be used as extrusion resins for the production of piping, tubing and filaments. As moulded thermoplastic resins, they are resistant to chemicals and have a long life, making them appropriate for use in gasoline filters, valves, pipe fittings and chemical processing equipment (Gibbs & Wessling, 1983).

Vinylidene chloride polymers used as lacquer resins are resistant to gasoline, solvents and oils. They are used as interior coatings for ship tanks, railroad tank cars and fuel storage tanks and as exterior coatings for steel piles and structures. Copolymer latex formulated from vinylidene chloride is incorporated into cement to impart strength to the mortar or concrete. The latexes are used as barrier coatings on paper products and plastic films, and as binders for paints and nonwoven fabrics (Gibbs & Wessling, 1983).

Microspheres of vinylidene chloride copolymer can be added to reinforced polyesters, printing inks and composites for use in furniture, marble and marine applications (Gibbs & Wessling, 1983).

Halogenated polymers such as polyvinylidene chloride have been used as flame-retardant binders in carpet backing and for cotton batt (Gibbs & Wessling, 1983).

Vinylidene chloride copolymer fibres were widely used previously as monofilaments in automobile seat covers, outdoor furniture, venetian blind tape, brush bristles, insect screening, window awning fabric and agricultural shade cloth. As a multifilament yarn, it has been used for draperies, upholstery, dolls' hair, dust mops and industrial fabric (Wessling & Edwards, 1971).

(c)   Regulatory status and guidelines

Occupational exposure limits to vinylidene chloride have been set by 11 countries by regulation or recommended guideline (Table 1).

Table 1. National occupational exposure limits for vinylidene chloride[a]

Country	Year	Concentration (mg/m³)	Interpretation[b]
Belgium	1978	40	TWA
Finland	1981	40	TWA
		80 (15 min)	STEL
Germany, Federal Republic of	1984	40	TWA
The Netherlands	1978	40	TWA
Poland	1976	50	Ceiling
Romania	1975	500	TWA
		700	Ceiling
Sweden	1984	20	TWA
		40	STEL
Switzerland	1978	40	TWA
UK	1985	40	TWA
		80 (10 min)	STEL
USA			
ACGIH	1984	20	TWA
		80	STEL
NIOSH	1978	4	TWA
USSR	1977	50	Ceiling

[a]From National Institute for Occupational Safety and Health (NIOSH) (1978); International Labour Office (1980); Työsuojeluhallitus (1981); American Conference of Governmental Industrial Hygienists (ACGIH) (1984); Arbetarskyddsstyrelsens Författningssamling (1984); Deutsches Forschungsgemeinschaft (1984); Health and Safety Executive (1985)

[b]TWA, time-weighted average; STEL, short-term exposure limit

The US Food and Drug Administration (1984) permits the use of vinylidene chloride copolymers as components of articles intended for use in contact with food, including adhesives, resinous and polymeric coatings for polyolefin films, coating for nylon or polycarbonate films and paper or paperboard (providing the finished copolymers contain at least 50 wt % of polymer units derived from vinylidene chloride), cellophane, semirigid and rigid acrylic and modified acrylic plastics, polyethylene-phthalate polymers, packaging materials for use during the irradiation of prepackaged food (providing the film contains not less than 70 wt % of vinylidene chloride and has a viscosity of 0.5-1.5 cP), and polymer modifiers in semi-rigid and rigid vinyl chloride plastics.

Vinylidene chloride-methyl acrylate copolymers may be used in contact with food providing that (1) less than 15 wt % of polymer units are derived from methyl acrylate, (2) the average molecular weight of the copolymer is not less than 50 000, and (3) the residual vinylidene chloride will not exceed 10 mg/kg (US Food and Drug Administration, 1984).

The US Environmental Protection Agency (1984a) has identified vinylidene chloride as a hazardous waste under the Resource Conservation and Recovery Act of 1976.

2.2 Occurrence

(a) Natural occurrence

It is not known whether vinylidene chloride occurs as a natural product.

(b) Occupational exposure

On the basis of the US National Occupational Health Survey, it has been estimated that 6500 workers are potentially exposed to vinylidene chloride in the USA, primarily during production and polymerization (National Institute for Occupational Safety and Health, 1978). Air levels in monomer and polymer plants have been reported to be 90-100 $\mu g/m^3$ and 25-50 $\mu g/m^3$, respectively (US Environmental Protection Agency, 1984b). Ott et al. (1976) reported peak exposure levels in a vinylidene chloride-ethyl acrylate copolymer monofilament fibre production plant of as high as 7600 mg/m^3. Estimated 8-h time-weighted average concentrations in various industries are presented by job classifications in Table 2.

Workers in manufacturing facilities in which vinyl chloride is used in polymerization processes (e.g., polyvinyl chloride) have been reported to be exposed to vinylidene chloride (Jaeger, 1975; Ott et al., 1975) at concentrations of <20 mg/m^3 and usually at trace amounts (Kramer & Mutchler, 1972). Levels of 8 mg/m^3 vinylidene chloride have been reported in the atmosphere of submarines, and levels of 0-8 mg/m^3 have been found in spacecraft (Altman & Dittmer, 1966).

Oblas et al. (1980) found air levels of 2.6-256 $\mu g/m^3$ at several telephone offices across the USA.

(c) Air

Singh et al. (1981) have estimated that 2-5% of manufactured vinylidene chloride in the USA is emitted to the air. Air levels at a number of sites in the USA are listed in Table 3. The

Table 2. Occupational exposures to vinylidene chloride in various industries

Industry	Job classification	Concentration (mg/m³ air)	Reference
Monomer production (1975)	Production operators	~40	Thiess et al. (1979)
Polymerization	Production operators (1952-1955)	<100	Ott et al. (1976)
	Laboratory technicians (1952)	<40	
Polymerization (1976)	Production operators	<20-120	Thiess et al. (1979)
Polymerization (1976)	Production operators	0.004-5.7	Meyer (1978)
Fibre production (1960-1965)	Production operators	60-280	Ott et al. (1976)
	Foreman and utility men	40-100	

Table 3. Airborne vinylidene chloride concentrations in the USA

State	Concentration (µg/m³)	Reference
Arizona	0.120	Singh et al. (1981)
California	0.02-0.05	Singh et al. (1981); Hunt et al. (1984)
Colorado	0.06	Hunt et al. (1984)
Louisania	0.02-26	Hunt et al. (1984)
Michigan	24	Hunt et al. (1984)
North Carolina	11.2	Hunt et al. (1984)
Texas	0.07-46	Hunt et al. (1984)
Virginia	0.41	Hunt et al. (1984)

US Environmental Protection Agency (1984b, 1985) estimated the median ambient air level of vinylidene chloride in suburban/urban areas of the USA to be 20 ng/m³ but found ambient levels in industrial source areas to be much higher (median, 14 µg/m³).

(d) Water

Vinylidene chloride has been detected in effluent discharged from chemical manufacturing plants in The Netherlands at a concentration of 32 µg/l (Eurocop-Cost, 1976) and in effluent discharged by chemical and latex manufacturing plants in the USA. Levels of vinylidene chloride in industrial raw and treated waste-water from a number of industries are given in Table 4.

Table 4. Vinylidene chloride concentrations in industrial waste-water[a]

Industry	Mean concentration ($\mu g/l$)	
	Raw waste-water	Treated waste-water
Soap and detergent manufacture	18	not available
Paint and ink formulation	78	19
Organic chemicals and plastics production	200	6.8
Non-ferrous metals manufacturing	200	120
Metal finishing	760	not available

[a]From US Environmental Protection Agency (1984b)

Vinylidene chloride has been detected in approximately 3% of US drinking-water supplies. It has been estimated on the basis of several national drinking-water surveys that 52 000 persons in the USA are exposed to concentrations of 5-10 $\mu g/l$ vinylidene chloride (Cothern et al., 1984). The general US population is exposed to <0.6 μg from ingestion of drinking water; surface- and ground-water levels of 0.2-0.5 $\mu g/l$ were reported (US Environmental Protection Agency, 1984b). Pellizzari et al. (1979) reported mean levels in drinking-water in New Orleans and Baton Rouge, LA, of 0.2 $\mu g/l$. Vinylidene chloride has also been identified in well, river and other untreated water in other areas of the USA (Shackelford & Keith, 1976).

Vinylidene chloride was detected in no raw water sample and in only 1/90 treated water samples (<1 $\mu g/l$) from 30 Canadian potable water treatment facilities serving about 5.5 million consumers across Canada (Otson et al., 1982a,b).

As part of the Nationwide Urban Runoff Program, concentrations of 1.5-4 $\mu g/l$ were measured in water in Eugene, OR, USA (Cole et al., 1984). Vinylidene chloride levels in ground-water at a chemical-waste dump site in the Netherlands were 0.01-2.8 $\mu g/l$, while levels in the Rhine River were 0.3-80 $\mu g/l$ (Wegman et al., 1981).

(e)   Soil

DeLeon et al. (1980) analysed over 100 soil samples within and around chemical waste disposal sites for vinylidene chloride. One of three samples collected from a single midwestern US chemical disposal site contained 21.9 $\mu g/g$ (dry weight) vinylidene chloride.

(f)   Food

Vinylidene chloride monomer has been detected in liver pâté (< 0.005 mg/kg), biscuits (<0.005 mg/kg), potato crisps (<0.005 mg/kg) and cheese (<0.005 mg/kg) (Gilbert et al., 1980).

(g)   *Human samples*

Levels of vinylidene chloride in the breath of residents in North Carolina and New Jersey, USA, ranged from undetectable to 14 μg/m^3 (Wallace *et al.*, 1982, 1984).

(h)   *Other*

Residual, unpolymerized vinylidene chloride has been detected in US and UK Saran food packaging films at 0.02-58 mg/kg. Film manufactured in earlier years had higher amounts of residual monomer (Birkel *et al.*, 1977; Gilbert & Shepherd, 1981; US Environmental Protection Agency, 1984b).

Vinylidene chloride occurs as an impurity in trichloroethylene (Vlasov & Bodyagin, 1970), in vinyl chloride monomer (limit of detection, 5 mg/kg) (Sassu *et al.*, 1968; Kiezel *et al.*, 1975), in technical-grade 1,1,1-trichloroethane (30-900 mg/l) (Henschler *et al.*, 1980) and at a level of 0.011% in commercial chloroprene (Kurginyan & Shirinyan, 1969).

2.3 Analysis

Selected methods for the analysis of vinylidene chloride in various matrices are identified in Table 5.

The analytical method of the US National Institute for Occupational Safety and Health for vinylidene chloride in air (Taylor, 1978) is validated for the range of concentrations 2-12 mg/m^3 with 1 mg/m^3 the lower quantified limit. This method has been extended to higher concentrations, encompassing the limits for occupational exposures recommended by the American Conference of Governmental Industrial Hygienists (Foerst, 1979; Sidhu, 1980). Tenax sorbent, rather than charcoal, has been suggested for extraction of environmental samples (Pellizzari, 1979). Gas chromatographic analysis with a more sensitive and selective halide-specific detector (electrolytic conductivity, electrochemical), rather than a flame ionization detector, has been recommended for monitoring lower concentrations (Driscoll *et al.*, 1984).

The purge-and-trap methods recommended by the US Environmental Protection Agency (1984c,d,e) for the analysis of vinylidene chloride in water range from a fairly sensitive gas chromatographic method with an electrolytic conductivity detector to less sensitive gas chromatography/mass spectrometry methods for confirmation of the identity of components in the sample. Applications of these methods have been discussed (Ramstad *et al.*, 1981; McMahon, 1983). Improved separations have been reported using capillary, rather than packed, gas chromatography columns (Lao *et al.*, 1982; Dreisch & Munson, 1983). Static headspace analysis (Otson *et al.*, 1982b), vacuum transfer to a cryogenic trap (Comba & Kaiser, 1983), purge and on-column trapping (Otson & Williams, 1982) and purge closed-loop methods (Wang & Lenahan, 1984) have also been described for determination of vinylidene chloride in water. The purge-and-trap gas chromatography/mass spectrometry method has been adapted for the analysis of volatile organics, including vinylidene chloride, in fish (Easley *et al.*, 1981; limit of detection, 10 μg/kg) and in body tissue (Lin *et al.*, 1982; limit of detection, 10 μg/kg).

Table 5. Methods for the analysis of vinylidene chloride

Sample matrix	Sample preparation	Assay procedure[a]	Limit of detection	Reference
Air	Adsorb (charcoal); desorb (carbon disulphide)	GC/FID	1 mg/m^{3b}	Taylor (1978); Foerst (1979)
	Adsorb (Tenax); desorb (heat, purge with helium); trap (liquid nitrogen cold trap); desorb as vapour onto GC column	GC/MS	1 μg/l	Pellizzari (1979); Wallace et al. (1982, 1984)
Water	Purge (nitrogen or helium); trap (OV-1/Tenax/silica gel); desorb as vapour (heat, purging with nitrogen or helium) onto GC column	GC/ECD[c]	0.13 μg/l	US Environmental Protection Agency (1984c)
	Purge (nitrogen or helium); trap (OV-1/Tenax/silica gel); desorb as vapour (heat, purging with nitrogen or helium) onto GC column	GC/MS	2.8 μg/l	US Environmental Protection Agency (1984d)
	Add stable isotope-labelled vinylidene chloride to water sample as internal standard; purge, trap and desorb onto GC column as above	GC/MS	10 μg/l	US Environmental Protection Agency (1984e)
Soil	Extract (n-hexane); add internal standard	GC/EC	10 μg/g	DeLeon et al. (1980)
Body tissue	Mince tissue; add to isooctane/water; purge (60°C, helium); trap (Tenax); desorb (heat, helium) onto GC column	GC/ECD	~10 μg/kg (50 pg)	Lin et al. (1982)
Foods[d]	Withdraw vapour sample from headspace at 90°C	GC/EC	1 μg/kg (validated at 4-50 μg/kg)	Warner et al. (1983)
Polymer film[e]	Dissolve (tetrahydrofuran); inject solution	GC/EC	1 μg/g (validated at 1-3 μg/g)	Warner et al. (1983)
	Dissolve (tetrahydrofuran); inject solution	GC/MS	1 μg/g	Tan & Okada (1979)
	Dissolve (carbon tetrachloride/tetrahydrofuran); inject	GC/FID	1 μg/g	Motegi et al. (1976)

[a]Abbreviations: GC/FID, gas chromatography/flame ionization detection; GC/MS, gas chromatography/mass spectrometry; GC/ECD, gas chromatography/electrolytic conductivity detection; GC/EC, gas chromatography/electron capture detection

[b]7 μg vinylidene chloride collected by drawing 7 l of air sample through 100 mg charcoal

[c]Microcoulometric detector also acceptable

[d]Food-simulating solvents used to determine the migration of vinylidene chloride from polymer film (food packing material) into food

[e]Food packaging material

Headspace sampling with gas chromatography/electron capture detection has been recommended for the determination of vinylidene chloride residues in foods (e.g., from packaging materials) (Crosby, 1982; Warner *et al.*, 1983).

3. Biological Data Relevant to the Evaluation of Carcinogenic Risk to Humans

3.1 Carcinogenicity studies in animals[1]

(a) Oral administration

Mouse: Groups of 50 male and 50 female B6C3F1/N mice, nine weeks old, received 2 or 10 mg/kg bw vinylidene chloride (99% pure, with <0.1% of *cis*- or 0.1% *trans*-dichloroethylene and the stabilizer, hydroquinone monomethyl ether) in corn oil by gavage on five days per week for 104 weeks. Groups of 50 males and 50 females received corn oil only and served as vehicle controls. A reduction in body weight was observed in male and female mice receiving the lower dose. Survival rates at the end of the experiment were: 33/50 (66%) vehicle control, 35/50 (70%) low-dose and 36/50 (72%) high-dose males; and 40/50 (80%) vehicle control, 32/50 (64%) low-dose and 42/50 (84%) high-dose females. A statistically significant increase in the combined incidence of lymphomas and leukaemia was observed in low-dose females compared to vehicle controls: 7/48 (15%) control, 15/49 (31%) low-dose ($p = 0.05$, Fisher exact test) and 7/50 (14%) high-dose females. The increased incidence of lymphomas and leukaemias in low-dose females was not considered to be the result of treatment because no significantly increased incidence of these malignancies was observed in high-dose females or in low- or high-dose males (National Toxicology Program, 1982).

Rat: A group of 24 female BDIV rats [age unspecified] received a single dose of 150 mg/kg bw vinylidene chloride (99% pure, containing 0.03% 4-methoxyphenol) in olive oil by stomach tube on day 17 of gestation. Their progeny (89 males and 90 females) received weekly doses of 50 mg/kg bw vinylidene chloride in 0.3 ml olive oil for life, beginning at weaning. A vehicle-control group of 14 females received 0.3 ml olive oil on day 17 of gestation, and their progeny (53 males and 53 females) received 0.3 ml olive oil weekly for life, beginning at weaning. All survivors were killed at 120 weeks or when moribund. Litter sizes, preweaning mortality, survival rates and body-weight gain were similar in vinylidene chloride-treated and vehicle-control groups. No statistically significant increase in the incidence of tumours was noted in treated animals, although tumours that were not seen in controls appeared at a variety of sites in treated animals. Hyperplastic liver nodules were

---

[1]The Working Group was aware of a study in progress in which vinylidene chloride is being tested in a two-stage model in mice for initiating and promoting activity (IARC, 1984).

found in 2/23 dams treated with vinylidene chloride during pregnancy and in 2/81 male and 6/80 female progeny; no such effect was seen in controls ($p = 0.04$) (Ponomarkov & Tomatis, 1980).

Groups of 50 male and 50 female Fischer 344/N rats, nine weeks of age, received 1 or 5 mg/kg bw vinylidene chloride (99% pure, with <0.1% *cis*- or 0.1% *trans*-dichloroethylene and the stabilizer, hydroquinone monomethyl ether) in corn oil by gavage on five days per week for 104 weeks. A group of 50 males and 50 females received corn oil only and served as vehicle controls. Survival rates at the end of the study period were: 20/50 (40%) vehicle-control, 24/50 (48%) low-dose and 37/50 (74%) high-dose males; and 27/50 (54%) vehicle-control, 28/50 (56%) low-dose and 29/50 (58%) high-dose females. The large number of accidental deaths in control and low-dose males may have influenced the incidence of late-appearing tumours in these groups. The pattern of neoplasms in the treated animals resembled that in controls, and no significant increase in tumour incidence was observed (National Toxicology Program, 1982). [The Working Group noted the poor survival.]

Groups of 47-48 male and 48 female Sprague-Dawley rats, six to seven weeks of age, were administered 50, 100 or 200 mg/l vinylidene chloride (99.5% pure, with 1-5 mg/l hydroquinone monomethyl ether) in drinking-water *ad libitum* for two years (average time-weighted daily doses: males, 7, 10 or 20 mg/kg bw; females, 9, 14 or 30 mg/kg bw). A group of 80 males and 80 females received drinking-water only. Mortality and body-weight gain were similar in the treated and control groups; no statistically significant increase in tumour incidence was found (Quast *et al.*, 1983).

Groups of 50 male and 50 female Sprague-Dawley rats, nine weeks of age, were administered 0.5, 5, 10 or 20 mg/kg doses of vinylidene chloride (99.9% pure, with 0.04% 1,2-dichloroethylene and 0.002% mono- and dichloroacetylene in olive oil by gastric intubation on four to five days per week for 52 weeks, followed by observation for lifespan (147 weeks). A group of 100 animals of each sex served as vehicle controls for the lowest-dose group, and a separate group of 100 animals of each sex served as vehicle controls for the remaining groups. The pattern of different neoplasms and their incidences were comparable among treated and control animals (Maltoni *et al.*, 1984, 1985). [The Working Group noted that preliminary reports of the studies had been reviewed previously (IARC, 1979a).]

(b)   Inhalation exposure

Mouse: Groups of 36 male and 36 female CD-1 mice, two months of age, were exposed to 0 or 220 mg/m^3 (55 ppm) vinylidene chloride (99% pure) [impurities unspecified] in air for 6 h per day on five days per week for 12 months, at which time the experiment was terminated. An increase in the incidence of bronchioalveolar adenomas was observed in males (1/26 controls *versus* 6/35 treated), and increases in the incidence of angiosarcomas of the liver also occurred (0/26 control males *versus* 2/35 treated; 0/36 female controls *versus* 1/35 treated). Three hepatomas (in two males and one female) and two skin keratoacanthomas were also reported to occur in treated mice [sex unspecified] (Lee *et al.*, 1977, 1978). [The Working Group noted the short duration of the experiment.]

Groups of 8-12 male and 8-12 female CD-1 mice, two months of age, were exposed to 55 ppm (220 mg/m³) vinylidene chloride (99% pure; impurities unspecified) in air for 6 h per day on five days per week for one, three or six months and maintained without treatment for a further 12-month observation period. Untreated control groups of 16-28 mice of each sex were available. There was a dose-related decrease in survival in males and females. When treatment groups were pooled, the incidence of hepatocellular tumours was 10/60 (17%) in controls and 4/28 (14%) in treated males; bronchioalveolar tumours were seen in 16/120 (13%) controls, 4/28 (14%) treated males and 1/28 (3%) treated females; one treated male had a haemangiosarcoma of the mesentery (Hong *et al.*, 1981). [The Working Group noted the small number of animals, the short treatment period and the poor survival.]

Groups of 30 male and 30 female Swiss mice (60 males and 60 females received the highest dose), nine or 16 weeks of age, were exposed to 10, 25, 50, 100 or 200 ppm (40, 100, 200, 400 or 800 mg/m³) vinylidene chloride (99.9% pure, with 0.04% 1,2-dichloroethylene, 0.002% mono- and dichloroacetylene and the stabilizer paramethoxyphenol at the highest dose) in air for 4 h per day, on four to five days per week for 52 weeks (two days at 200 and 100 ppm, one week at 50 ppm) and observed for lifespan (126 weeks). A group of 100 animals of each sex, not kept in inhalation chambers, served as one group of controls (A). Groups exposed to 50, 100 and 200 ppm suffered high mortality within two to four days and were withdrawn from the study. In order to increase the power of the study, an additional group of 120 animals of each sex was then exposed to 25 ppm concurrently with a separate control group of 90 mice of each sex which were not kept in inhalation chambers (control B). Comparisons of tumour incidences between control B and the groups exposed concurrently to 25 ppm showed increases in the incidences of tumours at several sites: kidney adenocarcinomas in male mice (control B, 0/87; 25 ppm, 25/120); pulmonary adenomas in male mice (control B, 3/87; 25 ppm, 16/120) and female mice (control B, 3/89; 25 ppm, 11/119); and mammary tumours in female mice (control B, 1/89; 25 ppm, 12/119). Increased incidences were also seen in exposed groups containing smaller numbers of animals: kidney adenocarcinomas in male mice (control A, 0/99; 10 ppm, 0/30; 25 ppm, 3/30); pulmonary adenomas in male mice (control A, 3/99; 10 ppm, 11/30; 25 ppm, 7/30) and female mice (control A, 4/98; 10 ppm, 3/30; 25 ppm, 7/30); and mammary tumours in female mice (control A, 2/98; 10 ppm, 6/30; 25 ppm, 4/30) (Maltoni *et al.*, 1984, 1985). [The Working Group noted that preliminary reports of these studies had been reviewed previously (IARC, 1979a).]

Rat: A group of 36 male and 36 female CD rats, two months of age, were exposed to 0 or 220 mg/m³ (55 ppm) vinylidene chloride (>99% pure) [impurities unspecified] in air for 6 h per day on five days per week for up to 12 months, at which time the experiment was terminated and all survivors killed. Two rats developed angiosarcomas, one in a mesenteric lymph node and one in the subcutaneous tissue. No such tumour occurred in controls (Lee *et al.*, 1977, 1978). [The Working Group noted the short duration of the experiment and limited reporting.]

One group of four, two groups of eight and one group of 14 males; and one group of four, two groups of eight and one group of 16 female CD rats, two months of age, were exposed to 55 ppm (220 mg/m³) vinylidene chloride (99% pure) [impurities unspecified] in air for 6 h per day on five days per week for one, three, six or ten months, respectively. Following treatment, all groups were maintained without further exposure for 12 months, at which time the remaining animals were sacrificed. Corresponding male and female control groups of four to 16 rats were maintained on filtered air for the same treatment periods and then maintained for a further 12-month period. Survival rates were similar in treated and control groups: 21/34 vinylidene-treated male rats compared with 28/36 control males, and 27/36 vinylidene-treated females compared with 24/36 control females at the end of the study. No treatment-related tumour was reported, although a single hepatic haemangiosarcoma was observed in a male rat that had been exposed to vinylidene chloride for six months (Hong *et al.*, 1981). [The Working Group noted the small group sizes and the short exposure periods.]

Groups of 30 male and 30 female Sprague-Dawley rats, 16 weeks of age, were exposed to 10, 25, 50 or 100 ppm (40, 100, 200 or 400 mg/m^3) vinylidene chloride (99.9% pure, with 0.04% 1,2-dichloroethylene and 0.002% mono- and dichloroacetylene) for 4 h per day on four to five days per week for 52 weeks, followed by observation for lifetime (137 weeks). One additional group of 60 animals of each sex was initially exposed to 200 ppm (800 mg/m^3) for two days, then 150 ppm (600 mg/m^3) for 4 h per day four to five times per week for 52 weeks; frequency of dosing was reduced periodically to four times per week due to toxicity. Groups of 100 animals of each sex were used as controls. The pattern of neoplasms and their incidences were comparable among treated and control animals (Maltoni *et al.*, 1984). [The Working Group noted that preliminary reports of these studies had been reviewed previously (IARC, 1979a).]

Groups of 103-104 male and 103-104 female Sprague-Dawley rats, six to seven weeks of age, were exposed by inhalation to 10 or 40 ppm (40 or 160 mg/m^3) vinylidene chloride (purity, 99% [impurities unspecified]; stabilized with hydroquinone monomethyl ether) for 6 h per day on five days per week for one month. Exposure was then increased to 25 or 75 ppm (100 or 300 mg/m^3) vinylidene chloride for 17 months because of the lack of treatment-related effects. Surviving animals were held for an additional six months. Groups of 86 male and 86 female rats served as controls. Groups of four to five rats of each sex were removed from each exposure group for interim evaluations. There was no treatment-related effect on body-weight gain or survival, except for an increase in mortality among females exposed to 75 ppm at months 15, 17 and 21. No treatment-related neoplasm was observed (Quast *et al.*, 1986). [The Working Group noted that exposure was stopped after 18 months.]

Hamster: A group of 30 male and 30 female Chinese hamsters, 29 weeks of age, were exposed to 25 ppm (100 mg/m^3) vinylidene chloride (99.9% pure, with 0.04% 1,2-dichloroethylene and 0.002% mono- and dichloroacetylene) in air for 4 h per day on four to five days per week for 52 weeks and observed for lifetime (164 weeks). A group of 18 males and 17 females, not housed in chambers, were used as controls. The pattern of neoplasms and their incidences were comparable among treated and control animals (Maltoni *et al.*, 1984). [The Working Group noted that preliminary reports of this study had been reviewed previously (IARC, 1979a).]

(c)   Subcutaneous administration

Mouse: In one of several experiments designed to investigate the potential carcinogenicity of a number of halogenated hydrocarbons, a group of 30 female Ha:ICR Swiss mice, six to eight weeks of age, received weekly subcutaneous injections of 2 mg vinylidene chloride [purity unspecified] in 0.05 ml trioctanoin into the left flank for 78 weeks. Groups of 30 animals each received treatment with either trioctanoin only or β-propiolactone (0.30 mg in 0.05 ml trioctanoin), the latter serving as positive controls. An additional group of 100 mice served as untreated controls. No vinylidene chloride-treated animal developed a local sarcoma, compared with 24 mice in the positive-control group (Van Duuren *et al.*, 1979). [The Working Group noted that only tissues from the injection site and the liver were examined histologically.]

(d)   Skin application

Mouse: Vinylidene chloride was tested for initiating activity in a two-stage mouse-skin assay. A group of 30 female Ha:ICR Swiss mice, six to eight weeks of age, received a single topical application of 121 mg vinylidene chloride [purity unspecified] in 0.2 ml acetone on the dorsal skin, followed 14 days later by thrice-weekly applications of 5 μg 12-0-tetra-decanoylphorbol 13-acetate (TPA) in 0.2 ml acetone for 428-576 days. Groups of 30 animals received no treatment, treatment with acetone only, treatment with TPA only, or treatment with 7,12-dimethylbenz[*a*]anthracene and TPA, and served as untreated, vehicle, TPA-treated or positive controls, respectively. All animals were examined daily and weighed monthly. Complete autopsies were performed at termination of the study or at death, and all abnormal-appearing tissues and organs were examined histopathologically; routine sections of skin, liver, stomach and kidney were examined. In 90 TPA-control mice, a total of seven skin papillomas was observed in six mice, and two had squamous-cell carcinomas. In the vinylidene chloride/TPA group of 30 mice, a total of nine skin papillomas was observed in eight mice, and one had a squamous-cell carcinoma ($p < 0.005$). In 100 control mice receiving no treatment and in 30 mice receiving acetone alone, no papilloma or carcinoma was observed. In the positive control group, 317 papillomas developed in 29 mice, and 18 had carcinomas ($p < 0.0005$) (Van Duuren *et al.*, 1979).

Vinylidene chloride was also tested as a complete carcinogen on mouse skin. A group of 30 female Ha:ICR Swiss mice, six to eight weeks of age, received thrice-weekly topical applications of 40 or 121 mg vinylidene chloride in 0.2 ml acetone on the dorsal skin for 440-594 days. Controls received no treatment or treatment with acetone only. No skin papilloma was observed in the vinylidene chloride-treated animals; two papillomas of the forestomach were observed in the group treated with the high dose (Van Duuren *et al.*, 1979).

3.2 Other relevant biological data

The biological effects of vinylidene chloride have been reviewed (Haley, 1975; US Environmental Protection Agency, 1976; Warren & Ricci, 1978; Henschler, 1979).

(a) *Experimental systems*

Toxic effects

The results of acute toxicity studies on vinylidene chloride have been highly variable; the lethal concentrations are dependent on dietary parameters (fed or fasted animals) and on the hepatic glutathione content, which exhibits significant diurnal variations (Jaeger *et al.*, 1973a, 1974). The LC_{50} by inhalation for a 4-h exposure was 40 000-60 000 mg/ m^3 (10 000-15 000 ppm) in fed rats and 2000-10 000 mg/ m^3 (500-2500 ppm) in fasted rats; death was due to vascular collapse and shock (Jaeger *et al.*, 1973b). The LC_{50} of vinylidene chloride in rats, following exposure for 4 h and observation for two weeks, was 25 400 mg/ m^3 (6350 ppm) (Siegel *et al.*, 1971).

The oral LD_{50} in mice is approximately 200 mg/kg bw (Jones & Hathway, 1978a); that in normal rats is 1500 mg/kg bw, and that in adrenalectomized rats, 80 mg/kg bw (Jenkins *et al.*, 1972).

In a two-year study of male and female Sprague-Dawley rats receiving 60-70, 100-120 or 200-230 mg/l vinylidene chloride in their drinking-water (calculated equivalent doses of 5-12, 8-20 or 16-40 mg/kg bw per day), no toxicological effect was noted except for a non-dose-related decrease in survival of male rats at 18 and 24 months (Norris, 1977).

Injury to liver parenchymal cells was observed in fasted rats exposed to 800 mg/ m^3 (200 ppm) vinylidene chloride for 4 h (Reynolds *et al.*, 1975, 1980). Inhalation of 2000 mg/ m^3 (500 ppm) during 20 exposures of 6 h caused nasal irritation, reduced weight gain and histopathological changes in the liver in rats (Gage, 1970). In inhalation studies in which rats, guinea-pigs, dogs, rabbits and monkeys were exposed to a mean level of 190 mg/ m^3 (48 ppm) for 90 days, there was significant mortality among guinea-pigs and monkeys and liver damage but no change in haematological parameters in all species (Prendergast *et al.*, 1967).

Rats exposed for 90 days to 100 or 300 mg/ m^3 (25 or 75 ppm) in air showed minimal toxicological effects in the liver (fatty liver changes and hepatocellular hypertrophy in the portal area) (Norris, 1977; Quast *et al.*, 1983). Following exposure to up to 320 mg/ m^3 (80 ppm) vinylidene chloride for 22-23 h per day for seven days, mice were more susceptible than rats to its hepatotoxicity (Short *et al.* 1977a,b).

Minimal changes in the liver, characterized by an increase in cytoplasmic vacuolization of occasional individual hepatocytes, were noted in Sprague-Dawley rats given 200 mg/l vinylidene chloride in their drinking-water for 90 days (calculated dose of 6-8 mg/kg bw per day) (Norris, 1977).

Vinylidene chloride increases the levels of serum alanine α-ketoglutarate transaminase and hepatic triglycerides and decreases those of hepatic glucose-6-phosphatase and glutathione in rats. The lethality and hepatotoxicity of vinylidene chloride are increased by fasting (which leads to decreased hepatic glutathione concentrations) (Jaeger *et al*, 1973a,c) and by phenobarbital and 3-methylcholanthrene (which induce microsomal enzymes) (Carlson & Fuller, 1972).

Various epoxides (1,1,1-trichloropropane-2,3-oxide, 2,3-epoxypropan-1-ol, styrene oxide and cyclohexene oxide) enhanced the hepatotoxicity of vinylidene chloride in male rats and decreased the acute oral LD_{50} (Andersen *et al.*, 1977). Pretreatment with acetone was reported to potentiate vinylidene chloride-induced hepatotoxicity (Hewitt & Plaa, 1983). The hepatotoxicity of orally administered vinylidene chloride was greater when administered in oil than in aqueous Tween-80 (Chieco *et al.*, 1981).

Simultaneous administration of vinyl chloride (see IARC, 1979c) with vinylidene chloride prevented the hepatoxicity associated with vinylidene chloride inhalation in fasted rats (Jaeger, 1975).

Pretreatment of rodents with diethyldithiocarbamate, carbon disulphide, pyrazole, 3-aminotriazole, carbon tetrachloride, thiram or disulfiram resulted in different degrees of protection against the acute toxicity of vinylidene chloride (Short *et al.*, 1977a,b; Andersen *et al.*, 1978; Masuda & Nakayama, 1983).

Oral doses of 100-200 mg/kg bw vinylidene chloride were reported to cause selective damage of pulmonary Clara cells in mice (Forkert & Reynolds, 1982).

Effects on reproduction and prenatal toxicity

In an experiment reported in an abstract, CD rats and CD-1 mice were exposed to vinylidine chloride for 23 h per day for up to ten days during gestation. LC_{50} values were 80 ppm (317 mg/m³) in mice and >460 ppm (1820 mg/m³) in rats. When exposure was begun on day 7, no litter was produced by mice exposed to 30 ppm (119 mg/m³) or 55 ppm (218 mg/m³) vinylidene chloride; in rats, no effect on litters was reported with concentrations of up to 460 ppm (1820 mg/m³). The authors concluded that malformations could not be attributed to exposure of mice to 15 ppm (60 mg/m³) and of rats to 460 ppm (1820 mg/m³) vinylidine chloride (Short *et al.*, 1976).

Sprague-Dawley rats were exposed to 80, 316 or 630 mg/m³ (20, 80 or 160 ppm) vinylidene chloride for 7 h per day on gestation days 6-15, and New Zealand rabbits were exposed to 316 or 630 mg/m³ on gestation days 6-18. Maternal toxicity was apparent with 316 mg/m³ in rats and with 630 mg/m³ in rabbits. In rabbits, resorptions were increased in the group receiving 630 mg/m³. Skeletal variations occurred significantly more often in rats given both 316 and 630 mg/m³ and in rabbits given 630 mg/m³ (Murray *et al.*, 1979).

In Sprague Dawley rats given 200 mg/ml vinylidene chloride in the drinking-water on gestation days 6-15, no adverse effect was observed (Murray *et al.*, 1979). In a three-generation study in which Sprague-Dawley rats received 50, 100 or 200 mg/l vinylidene chloride in drinking-water, survival was comparable in six sets of litters over three generations in control and exposed groups. There was no evidence of adverse effects on the reproductive capacity of animals of either sex (Nitschke *et al.*, 1983).

Absorption, distribution, excretion and metabolism

As the dose of radioactive vinylidene chloride to rats is increased from 1 to 50 mg/kg bw orally or from 40 to 800 mg/m³ (10 to 200 ppm) by inhalation, the metabolic pathways become saturated, so that a smaller percentage of the dose administered is metabolized and more is eliminated *via* the lungs as vinylidene chloride. With 1 mg/kg bw orally or 40 mg/m³ by inhalation, there was no difference in elimination by fed *versus* fasted rats; with 50 mg/kg bw orally or 800 mg/m³ by inhalation, there was a significant increase in the excretion of vinylidene chloride *via* the lungs and a decrease in urinary excretion of radioactivity in fed *versus* fasted rats (Norris, 1977). This pattern is explained by a saturable, dose-dependent metabolism of vinylidene chloride, which has been well established in pharmacokinetic studies (Andersen *et al.*, 1979a,b; Filser & Bolt, 1979, 1981; Dallas *et al.*, 1983). Comparative studies in mice and rats have revealed that mice, which are more susceptible to vinylidene chloride than rats, biotransform the chemical to a greater extent than rats (Jones & Hathway, 1978a; McKenna *et al.*, 1980). In addition, the alkylation of proteins by metabolites of [1,2-^{14}C]-vinylidene chloride was greater in mice than in rats (McKenna *et al.*, 1980).

The main excretory route for ^{14}C-vinylidene chloride in rats after intragastric, intravenous or intraperitoneal administration is pulmonary: both unchanged vinylidene chloride and related CO_2 are excreted by that route; other vinylidene chloride metabolites are eliminated *via* the kidneys. Biotransformation of vinylidene chloride gives thiodihydroxy-acetic (thiodiglycolic) acid and an *N*-acetyl-*S*-cysteinylacetyl derivative as major urinary metabolites, together with substantial amounts of chloroacetic, dithiohydroxyacetic (dithioglycolic) and thiohydroxyacetic (thioglycolic) acids (Jones & Hathway, 1978b). Methylthioacetylamino-ethanol has also been isolated as a urinary metabolite of vinylidene chloride in rats (Reichert *et al.*, 1979). Pretreatment of rats with compounds that deplete hepatic glutathione leads to a decrease in the rate of metabolism of vinylidene chloride, which is consistent with the observation of an increase in toxicity (Andersen *et al.*, 1980). Mice but not rats excrete a small amount of *N*-acetyl-*S*-(2-carboxymethyl)cysteine, and mice excrete more *N*-acetyl-*S*-derivative than rats (Jones & Hathway, 1978a).

Treatment of mice with disulfiram reduced levels of covalently bound radioactivity in the liver and kidney after intraperitoneal administration of 3 mg/kg bw ^{14}C-vinylidene chloride (Short *et al.*, 1977b).

Experiments in which a mixture of vinylidene chloride and air was passed through a mouse-liver microsomal system and subsequently through a trap with 4-(4-nitrobenzyl)-pyridine failed to demonstrate the presence of an alkylating intermediate (Bartsch *et al.*, 1979).

Metabolic conversion of vinylidene chloride into an epoxide which can rearrange to the corresponding acyl chloride has been proposed (Henschler, 1977; Jones & Hathway, 1978a,b). Studies on the biotransformation of vinylidene chloride in hepatic microsomes *in vitro* support this view (Costa & Ivanetich, 1982).

Mutagenicity and other short-term tests

Vinylidene chloride is mutagenic to *Salmonella typhimurium his*G46, TA1530, TA1535, TA1537, TA92, TA98 and TA100 and to *Escherichia coli* WP2 uvrA at concentrations in the range of 0.02-50%, only in the presence of an exogenous metabolic system. Positive results have been obtained with metabolic systems prepared from the liver, lung and kidneys of several rodent species, as well as from human liver (Bartsch *et al.*, 1975a, 1976, 1979; Jones & Hathway, 1978c; Oesch *et al.*, 1983). Reverse mutations were induced in *E. coli* K12 by vinylidene chloride (2.5 mM) in the presence of liver microsomes from phenobarbital-induced mice (Greim *et al.*, 1975).

Doses of vinylidene chloride greater than 20 mM induced mitotic gene conversions and point mutations in *Saccharomyces cerevisiae* D7 in the presence, but not in the absence of a metabolic system (S9) from the liver of Aroclor-induced mice. In an intrasanguinous host-mediated assay using *S. cerevisiae* D7 as the indicator organism, male Swiss CD mice received multiple doses of vinylidene chloride by gavage (total dose, 2500 mg/kg bw); gene conversions and point mutations were induced in yeast recovered from liver and kidney but not from lung (Bronzetti *et al.*, 1981).

Vinylidene chloride (tested at up to 10% v/v) did not induce 8-azaguanine- or ouabain-resistant mutants in cultured Chinese hamster V79 cells in the presence of a phenobarbital-induced mouse- or rat-liver metabolic system (S15) (Drevon & Kuroki, 1979).

Vinylidene chloride (2.1 mM) induced unscheduled DNA synthesis in isolated hepatocytes from phenobarbital-induced rats (Costa & Ivanetich, 1984).

At concentrations of 3 and 30 mM (0.3 and 3 mg/ml), vinylidine chloride did not induce chromosomal aberrations in Chinese hamster Don-6 cells (Sasaki *et al.*, 1980). Chromosomal aberrations were not induced by vinylidine chloride (0.5-2 mg/ml) in cultured Chinese hamster lung cells in the absence of an exogenous metabolic system (Ishidate *et al.*, 1983).

Groups of male CD-1 mice were exposed for 6 h to 40 or 200 mg/m³ (10 or 50 ppm) ^{14}C-vinylidine chloride. DNA purified from kidneys and livers of animals exposed to 50 ppm contained 30 and six alkylations per 10^6 nucleotides, respectively; and with 10 ppm, kidney DNA contained 11 and liver 0.94 alkylations/10^6 nucleotides. DNA binding decreased (with biphasic kinetics) with increasing time after exposure. Unscheduled DNA synthesis, measured by ^{3}H-thymidime incorporation, was increased by 38% (statistically significant) in the kidneys of mice treated with 50 ppm vinylidene chloride. No treatment-related unscheduled DNA synthesis was seen in the livers of mice treated with 50 ppm, or in the kidneys or livers of mice treated with 10 ppm (Reitz *et al.*, 1980).

Vinylidene chloride was inactive in the dominant lethal mutation test in male CD-1 mice exposed by inhalation to 40, 120 or 200 mg/m³ (10, 30 or 50 ppm) for 6 h per day for five days (Anderson *et al.*, 1977) and in male CD rats exposed for 6 h per day on five days per week to 220 mg/m³ (55 ppm) vinylidene chloride (Short *et al.*, 1977c).

Mutagenicity of metabolites

Chloroacetic acid was not mutagenic to *Salmonella typhimurium* TA100 in the absence of an exogenous metabolic system (McCann *et al.*, 1975) or to TA1530 in the presence or absence of liver S9 from phenobarbital-induced mice (Bartsch *et al.*, 1975b; Malaveille *et al.*, 1975). The compound was not mutagenic to *Escherichia coli* strains WP2, WP100 *uvrA⁻ recA⁻*, GY5027 *envA⁻ uvrB⁻* or GY4015 *amp* (Mamber *et al.*, 1983, 1984).

Chloroacetic acid (2.1 mM) did not induce 8-azaguanine- or ouabain-resistant mutants in cultured Chinese hamster V79 cells (Huberman *et al.*, 1975).

(b) Humans

Toxic effects

Vinylidene chloride is a central nervous system depressant. Repeated exposures to low concentrations may cause liver and renal dysfunction (Torkelson & Rowe, 1981). Skin contact with vinylidene chloride causes irritation, which may be due partly to the presence of hydroquinone monomethyl ether inhibitor (Chivers, 1972). Contact with the eye causes conjunctivitis and transient corneal injury (Gibbs & Wessling, 1983). In one study, spirometry, blood chemistry (including liver and renal tests), haematological parameters and blood pressure measurements did not differ in vinylidene chloride workers and controls. Measured past time-weighted average concentrations ranged from <5 to 70 ppm (20-280 mg/m³) (Ott *et al.*, 1976).

Effects on reproduction and prenatal toxicity
No data were available to the Working Group.

Absorption, distribution, excretion and metabolism
No data were available to the Working Group.

Mutagenicity and chromosomal effects
No data were available to the Working Group.

3.3 Case reports and epidemiological studies of carcinogenicity to humans

Ott *et al.* (1976) investigated the cancer risk among a cohort of 138 US workers exposed to vinylidene chloride, where vinyl chloride was not used as a copolymer. Twenty-seven workers were lost to follow-up but considered to be alive in the analyses; 55 people had less than 15 years since first exposure, and only five deaths were observed. The authors reported that no finding was 'statistically attributable' to vinylidene chloride exposure.

Thiess *et al.* (1979) reported preliminary results of a study of the mortality experience of a cohort of 629 male (447 German and 182 foreign workers) employed at two plants in the Federal Republic of Germany that had produced vinylidene chloride and polyvinylidene chloride since 1955. Vital status was ascertained for 97% of the 447 German workers. Of the 182 foreign workers, 65 had worked for less than one year, and only 24% (44) were traced. The observed deaths were compared with local and regional rates, without making allowance for latent period. Within the study period (approximately 20 years), 39 deaths were observed, whereas 57 and 36 would have been expected, respectively. Five cases of lung carcinoma were observed, whereas 3.9 and 2.2 were expected; this result was not statistically significant. Workers in the factory were also potentially exposed to vinyl chloride (see IARC, 1979c) and acrylonitrile (see IARC, 1979d).

[The Working Group noted that both of these studies suffered from the limited size of the cohorts, the short observation period and the small numbers of deaths from specific causes. The fact that no allowance was made for latent period may have resulted in an overestimation of the expected numbers and an underestimation of risk.]

In an attempt to identify the specific exposure associated with an excess lung cancer risk noted previously in a US synthetic chemicals plant, Waxweiler *et al.* (1981) considered 19 chemicals, one of which was vinylidene chloride. Company personnel assigned a rank of exposure to vinylidene chloride (from 0 to 5) to each job in the plant for each year since its start in 1942. These exposure data were then linked with detailed, individual work histories so as to obtain for each of the 4806 male workers ever employed in the plant an estimate of his exposure to vinylidene chloride; 'doses' were calculated by multiplying the exposure rank of a job by the number of days worked at that job. Cumulative 'doses' for 45 workers who died from lung cancer during the study period (1942-1973) were then compared with expected 'doses' based on the cumulative exposure of subcohorts of fellow workers matched individually to the cases by year of birth and age of hire into the plant. This comparison failed to suggest any specific association between exposure to vinylidene chloride in the plant and excess lung cancer risk.

4. Summary of Data Reported and Evaluation

4.1 Exposure data

Vinylidene chloride has been available commercially since 1939. Polyvinylidene and copolymers of vinylidene chloride are used extensively in food packaging films, in lacquer resins, in textiles and in chemical processing equipment. Exposure to vinylidene chloride occurs during its production and conversion to the polymer. It has been detected at low levels in ambient air and drinking-water.

4.2 Experimental data

Vinylidene chloride was tested for carcinogenicity in mice and rats by oral administration and inhalation exposure, in mice by subcutaneous administration and topical application and in hamsters by inhalation. Studies in mice and rats by oral administration gave negative results. In inhalation studies, no treatment-related neoplasm was observed in rats or hamsters. In mice, treatment-related increases in the incidence of kidney adenocarcinomas were observed in male mice, as were increases in mammary carcinomas in females and pulmonary adenomas in male and female mice. In skin-painting studies in female mice, vinylidene chloride showed activity as an initiator, but in a study of repeated skin application, no skin tumour occurred. No tumour at the injection site was seen in mice given repeated subcutaneous administrations.

Inhalation exposure of pregnant rats and rabbits to vinylidene chloride induced embryotoxicity or malformations; no adverse effect occurred in the absence of signs of maternal toxicity. Fertility was not affected in animals of either sex.

Vinylidene chloride was mutagenic to bacteria in the presence of an exogenous metabolic system. It induced mutation and mitotic gene conversion in yeast in the presence of an exogenous metabolic system and in a host-mediated assay in mice. It induced unscheduled DNA synthesis in rat hepatocytes, but was not mutagenic to and did not induce chromosomal aberrations or sister chromatid exchanges in cultured mammalian cells. It alkylated DNA and induced DNA repair in the liver and kidney of mice exposed by inhalation. It did not induce dominant lethal mutations in male mice exposed by inhalation.

Overall assessment of data from short-term tests: Vinylidene chloride[a]

	Genetic activity			Cell transformation
	DNA damage	Mutation	Chromosomal effects	
Prokaryotes		+		
Fungi/Green plants		+		
Insects				
Mammalian cells (*in vitro*)	+	−	−	
Mammals (*in vivo*)	+		−	
Humans (*in vivo*)				
Degree of evidence in short-term tests for genetic activity: **Sufficient**				Cell transformation: No data

[a]The groups into which the table is divided and the symbols '+' and '−' are defined on pp. 19-20 of the Preamble; the degrees of evidence are defined on pp. 20-21.

4.3 Human data

No data were available to evaluate the reproductive effects or prenatal toxicity of vinylidene chloride to humans.

The limitations of the two available cohort studies did not permit an assessment of the carcinogenicity of vinylidene chloride to humans, and the increased risk of lung cancer observed in the third study could not be linked specifically to exposure to vinylidene chloride.

4.4 Evaluation[1]

There is *limited evidence* for the carcinogenicity of vinylidene chloride to experimental animals.

There is *inadequate evidence* for the carcinogenicity of vinylidene chloride to humans.

In the absence of adequate epidemiological data, no evaluation of the carcinogenicity of vinylidene chloride to humans could be made.

[1]For definition of the italicized terms, see Preamble, pp. 18 and 22.

5. References

Altman, P.L. & Dittmer, D.S. (1966) *Environmental Biology*, Bethesda, MD, Federation of American Societies for Experimental Biology, pp. 326, 328

American Conference of Governmental Industrial Hygienists (1984) *Threshold Limit Values for Chemical Substances and Physical Agents in the Work Environment and Biological Exposure Indices with Intended Changes for 1984-85*, Cincinnati, OH, p. 33

Andersen, M.E., Jones, R.A. & Jenkins, L.J., Jr (1977) Enhancement of 1,1-dichloroethylene toxicity by pretreatment of fasted male rats with 2,3-epoxypropan-1-ol. *Drug chem. Toxicol.*, *1*, 63-74

Andersen, M.E., Jones, R.A. & Jenkins, L.J., Jr (1978) The acute toxicity of single, oral doses of 1,1-dichloroethylene in the fasted, male rat: Effect of induction and inhibition of microsomal enzyme activities on mortality. *Toxicol. appl. Pharmacol.*, *46*, 227-234

Andersen, M.E., French, J.E., Gargas, M.L., Jones, R.A. & Jenkins, L.J., Jr (1979a) Saturable metabolism and acute toxicity of 1,1-dichloroethylene. *Toxicol. appl. Pharmacol.*, *47*, 385-393

Andersen, M.E., Gargas, M.L., Jones, R.A. & Jenkins, L.J., Jr (1979b) The use of inhalation techniques to assess the kinetic constants of 1,1-dichloroethylene metabolism. *Toxicol. appl. Pharmacol.*, *47*, 395-409

Andersen, M.E., Thomas, O.E., Gargas, M.L., Jones, R.A. & Jenkins, L.J., Jr (1980) The significance of multiple detoxification pathways for reactive metabolites in the toxicity of 1,1-dichloroethylene. *Toxicol. appl. Pharmacol.*, *52*, 422-432

Anderson, D., Hodge, M.C.E. & Purchase, I.F.H. (1977) Dominant lethal studies with the halogenated olefins vinyl chloride and vinylidene dichloride in male CD-1 mice. *Environ. Health Perspect.*, *21*, 71-78

Arbetarskyddsstyrelsens Författningssamling (National Swedish Board of Occupational Safety and Health) (1984) *Hygienic Limit Values (AFS 1984:5)* (Swed.), Stockholm, p. 34

Bartsch, H., Malaveille, C., Montesano, R. & Tomatis, L. (1975a) Tissue-mediated mutagenicity of vinylidene chloride and 2-chlorobutadiene in *Salmonella typhimurium*. *Nature*, *255*, 641-643

Bartsch, H., Malaveille, C. & Montesano, R. (1975b) Human, rat and mouse liver-mediated mutagenicity of vinyl chloride in *S. typhimurium* strains. *Int. J. Cancer*, 15, 429-437

Bartsch, H., Malaveille, C. & Montesano, R. (1976) *The predictive value of tissue-mediated mutagenicity assays to assess the carcinogenic risk of the chemicals.* In: Montesano, R., Bartsch, H. & Tomatis, L., eds, *Screening Tests in Chemicals Carcinogenesis (IARC Scientific Publications No. 12)*, Lyon, International Agency for Research on Cancer, pp. 467-491

Bartsch, H., Malaveille, C., Barbin, A. & Planche, G. (1979) Mutagenic and alkylating metabolites of halo-ethylenes, chlorobutadienes and dichlorobutenes produced by rodent or human liver tissues. Evidence for oxirane formation by P450-linked microsomal mono-oxygenases. *Arch. Toxicol.*, *41*, 249-277

Birkel, T.J., Roach, J.A.G. & Sphon, J.A. (1977) Determination of vinylidene chloride in Saran films by electron capture gas-solid chromatography and confirmation by mass spectrometry. *J. Assoc. off. anal. Chem.*, *60*, 1210-1213

Bronzetti, G., Bauer, C., Corsi, C., Leporini, C., Nieri, R. & del Carratore, R. (1981) Genetic activity of vinylidene chloride in yeast. *Mutat. Res.*, *89*, 179-185

Buckingham, J., ed. (1982) *Dictionary of Organic Compounds*, 5th ed., Vol. 2, New York, Chapman and Hall, p. 1733 [D-02638]

Carlson, G.P. & Fuller, G.C. (1972) Interaction of modifiers of hepatic microsomal drug metabolism and the inhalation of toxicity of 1,1-dichloroethylene. *Res. Commun. chem. Pathol. Pharmacol.*, *4*, 553-559

Chieco, P., Moslen, M.T. & Reynolds, E.S. (1981) Effect of administrative vehicle on oral 1,1-dichloroethylene toxicity. *Toxicol. appl. Pharmacol.*, *57*, 146-155

Chivers, C.P. (1972) Two cases of occupational leucoderma following contact with hydroquinone monomethyl ether. *Br. J. ind. Med.*, *29*, 105-107

Cole, R.H., Frederick, R.E., Healy, R.P. & Rolan, R.G. (1984) Preliminary findings of the priority pollutant monitoring project of the Nationwide Urban Runoff Program. *J. Water Pollut. Control Fed.*, *56*, 898-908

Comba, M.E. & Kaiser, K.L.E. (1983) Determination of volatile contaminants at the ng.l^{-1}-level in water by capillary gas chromatographic with electron capture detection. *Int. J. environ. anal. Chem.*, *16*, 17-31

Costa, A.K. & Ivanetich, K.M. (1982) Vinylidene chloride: Its metabolism by hepatic microsomal cytochrome P-450 in vitro. *Biochem. Pharmacol.*, *31*, 2083-2092

Costa, A.K. & Ivanetich, K.M. (1984) Chlorinated ethylenes: Their metabolism and effect of DNA repair in rat hepatocytes. *Carcinogenesis*, *5*, 1629-1636

Cothern, C.R., Coniglio, W.A. & Marcus, W.L. (1984) *Techniques for the Assessment of the Carcinogenic Risk to the US Population due to the Exposure from Selected Volatile Organic Compounds from Drinking Water Via the Ingestion, Inhalation and Dermal Routes* (*US NTIS PB84-213941*), Washington DC, US Environmental Protection Agency, Office of Drinking Water

Crosby, N.T. (1982) Analysis for residual monomer levels in plastics and in foods. *Anal. Proc.*, *19*, 428-430

Dallas, C.E., Weir, F.W., Feldman, S., Putcha, L. & Bruckner, J.V. (1983) The uptake and disposition of 1,1-dichloroethylene in rats during inhalation exposure. *Toxicol. appl. Pharmacol.*, *68*, 140-151

DeLeon, I.R., Maberry, M.A., Overton, E.B., Raschke, C.K., Remele, P.C., Steele, C.F., Warren, V.L. & Laseter, J.L. (1980) Rapid gas chromatographic method for the determination of volatile and semivolatile organochlorine compounds in soil and chemical waste disposal site samples. *J. chromatogr. Sci.*, *18*, 85-88

Deutsche Forschungsgemeinschaft (1984) *Maximal Concentrations in the Workplace and Biological Occupational Limit Value* (Ger.), Part XX, Weinheim, Verlag Chemie GmbH, p. 28

Dow Chemical Co. (1981) *Vinylidene Chloride, MEHQ Inhibited (Sales Specification)*, Midland, MI

Dow Chemical Co. (1985) *Material Safety Data Sheet: Vinylidene Chloride, MEHQ Inhibited (Product Code: 91637)*, Midland, MI

Dreisch, F.A. & Munson, T.O. (1983) Purge-and-trap analysis using fused silica capillary column GC/MS. *J. chromatogr. Sci.*, *21*, 111-118

Drevon, C. & Kuroki, T. (1979) Mutagenicity of vinyl chloride, vinylidene chloride and chloroprene in V79 Chinese hamster cells. *Mutat. Res.*, *67*, 173-182

Driscoll, J.N., Conron, D.W. & Ferioli, P. (1984) Comparison of a new electrochemical detector for gas chromatographic analysis with the electrolytic conductivity detector. *J. Chromatogr.*, *302*, 269-276

Easley, D.M., Kleopfer, R.D. & Carasea, A.M. (1981) Gas chromatographic-mass spectrometric determination of volatile organic compounds in fish. *J. Assoc. off. anal. Chem.*, *64*, 653-656

Eurocop-Cost (1976) *Analysis of Organic Micropollutants in Water, A Comprehensive List of Polluting Substances which have been Identified in Various Fresh Waters, Effluent Discharges, Aquatic Animals and Plants, and Bottom Sediments (Cost-Project 64b)*, 2nd ed., Luxemburg, Commission of the European Communities, European Cooperation and Coordination in the Field of Scientific and Technical Research, p. 41

Filser, J.G. & Bolt, H.M. (1979) Pharmacokinetics of halogenated ethylenes in rats. *Arch. Toxicol.*, *42*, 123-136

Filser, J.G. & Bolt, H.M. (1981) Inhalation pharmacokinetics based on gas uptake studies. I. Improvement of kinetic models. *Arch. Toxicol.*, *47*, 279-292

Foerst, D. (1979) A sampling and analytical method for vinylidene chloride in air. *Am. ind. Hyg. Assoc. J.*, *40*, 888-893

Forkert, P.-G. & Reynolds, E.S. (1982) 1,1-Dichloroethylene-induced pulmonary injury. *Exp. Lung Res.*, *3*, 57-68

Gage, J.C. (1970) The subacute inhalation toxicity of 109 industrial chemicals. *Br. J. ind. Med.*, *27*, 1-18

Gibbs, D.S. & Wessling, R.A. (1983) *Vinylidene chloride and polyvinylidene chloride*. In: Mark, H.F., Othmer, D.F., Overberger, C.G. & Seaborg, G.T., eds, *Kirk-Othmer Encyclopedia of Chemical Technology*, 3rd ed., Vol. 23, New York, John Wiley & Sons, pp. 764-798

Gilbert, J. & Shepherd, M.J. (1981) Headspace gas chromatography for the analysis of vinyl chloride and other monomers in plastic packaging and in foods. *J. Assoc. publ. Anal.*, *19*, 39-49

Gilbert, J., Shepherd, M.J., Startin, J.R. & McWeeny, D.J. (1980) Gas chromatographic determination of vinylidene chloride monomer in packaging films and in foods. *J. Chromatogr.*, *197*, 71-78

Grasselli, J.G. & Ritchey, W.M., eds (1975) *CRC Atlas of Spectral Data and Physical Constants for Organic Compounds*, Vol. 3, Cleveland, OH, CRC Press, Inc., p. 281

Greim, H., Bonse, G., Radwan, Z., Reichert, D. & Henschler, D. (1975) Mutagenicity *in vitro* and potential carcinogenicity of chlorinated ethylenes as a function of metabolic oxirane formation. *Biochem. Pharmacol.*, *24*, 2013-2017

Haley, T.J. (1975) Vinylidene chloride: A review of the literature. *Clin. Toxicol.*, *8*, 633-643

Hawley, G.G., ed. (1981) *The Condensed Chemical Dictionary*, 10th ed., New York, Van Nostrand Reinhold Co., p. 1086

Health and Safety Executive (1985) *Occupational Exposure Limits 1985 (Guidance Note EH40/85)*, London, Her Majesty's Stationery Office, p. 11

Henschler, D. (1977) Metabolism and mutagenicity of halogenated olefins — A comparison of structure and activity. *Environ. Health Perspec.*, *21*, 61-64

Henschler, D. (1979) *Toxicologic-occupational establishment of MAC-values. Vinylidene chloride* (Ger.). In: *Gesundheitsschädliche Arbeitsstoffe*, 7th ed., Weinheim, Verlag Chemie GmbH, pp.

Henschler, D., Reichert, D. & Metzler, M. (1980) Identification of potential carcinogens in technical grade 1,1,1-trichloroethane. *Int. Arch. occup. environ. Health*, *47*, 263-268

Hewitt, W.R. & Plaa, G.L. (1983) Dose-dependent modification of 1,1-dichloroethylene toxicity by acetone. *Toxicol. Lett.*, *16*, 145-152

Hong, C.B., Winston, J.M., Thornburg, L.P., Lee, C.C. & Woods, J.S. (1981) Follow-up study on the carcinogenicity of vinyl chloride and vinylidene chloride in rats and mice: Tumor incidence and mortality subsequent to exposure. *J. Toxicol. environ. Health*, *7*, 909-924

Huberman, E., Bartsch, H. & Sachs, L. (1975) Mutation induction in Chinese hamster V79 cells by two vinyl chloride metabolites, chloroethylene oxide and 2-chloroacetaldehyde. *Int. J. Cancer*, *16*, 639-644

Hunt, W.F., Jr, Faoro, R.B. & Duggan, G.M. (1984) *Compilation of Air Toxic and Trace Metal Summary Statistics (EPA-450/4-84-015)*, Research Triangle Park, NC, US Environmental Protection Agency, Office of Air and Radiation, Office of Air Quality, Planning and Standards, pp. 4, 41

IARC (1979a) *IARC Monographs on the Evaluation of the Carcinogenic Risk of Chemicals to Humans*, Vol. 19, *Some Monomers, Plastics and Synthetic Elastomers, and Acrolein*, Lyon, pp. 439-459

IARC (1979b) *IARC Monographs on the Evaluation of the Carcinogenic Risk of Chemicals to Humans*, Vol. 20, *Some Halogenated Hydrocarbons*, Lyon, pp. 429-448

IARC (1979c) *IARC Monographs on the Evaluation of the Carcinogenic Risk of Chemicals to Humans*, Vol. 19, *Some Monomers, Plastics and Synthetic Elastomers and Acrolein*, Lyon, pp. 377-438

IARC (1979d) *IARC Monographs on the Evaluation of the Carcinogenic Risk of Chemicals to Humans*, Vol. 19, *Some Monomers, Plastics and Synthetic Elastomers and Acrolein*, Lyon, pp. 47-113

IARC (1984) *Information Bulletin on the Survey of Chemicals Being Tested for Carcinogenicity*, No. 11, Lyon, p. 162

International Labour Office (1980) *Occupational Exposure Limits for Airborne Toxic Substances, A Tabular Compilation of Values from Selected Countries*, 2nd (rev.) ed. (*Occupational Safety and Health Series No. 37*), Geneva, pp. 216-217

Ishidate, M., Jr *et al.* (1983) *The Data Book of Chromosomal Aberration Tests* in vitro *on 587 Chemical Substances Using a Chinese Hamster Fibroblast Cell Line (CHL cells)*, Tokyo, The Realize Inc., p. 582

Jaeger, R.J. (1975) Vinyl chloride monomer: Comments on its hepatotoxicity and interaction with 1,1-dichloroethylene. *Ann. N.Y. Acad. Sci.*, *246*, 150-151

Jaeger, R.J., Conolly, R.B. & Murphy, S.D. (1973a) Diurnal variation of hepatic glutathione concentration and its correlation with 1,1-dichloroethylene inhalation toxicity in rats. *Res. Commun. chem. Pathol. Pharmacol.*, *6*, 465-471

Jaeger, R.J., Trabulus, M.J. & Murphy, S.D. (1973b) The interaction of adrenalectomy, partial adrenal replacement therapy, and starvation with hepatotoxicity and lethality of 1,1-dichloroethylene intoxication (Abstract no. 133). *Toxicol. appl. Pharmacol.*, *25*, 491

Jaeger, R.J., Trabulus, M.J. & Murphy, S.D. (1973c) Biochemical effects of 1,1-dichloroethylene in rats: Dissociation of its hepatotoxicity from a lipoperoxidative mechanism. *Toxicol. appl. Pharmacol.*, *24*, 457-467

Jaeger, R.J., Conolly, R.B. & Murphy, S.D. (1974) Effect of 18 hr fast and glutathione depletion on 1,1-dichloroethylene-induced hepatotoxicity and lethality in rats. *Exp. mol. Pathol.*, *20*, 187-198

Jenkins, L.J., Jr, Trabulus, M.J. & Murphy, S.D. (1972) Biochemical effects of 1,1-dichloroethylene in rats: Comparison with carbon tetrachloride and 1,2-dichloroethyene. *Toxicol. appl. Pharmacol.*, *23*, 501-510

Jones, B.K. & Hathway, D.E. (1978a) Differences in metabolism of vinylidene chloride between mice and rats. *Br. J. Cancer*, *37*, 411-417

Jones, B.K. & Hathway, D.E. (1978b) The biological fate of vinylidene chloride in rats. *Chem.-biol. Interactions*, *20*, 27-41

Jones, B.K. & Hathway, D.E. (1978c) Tissue-mediated mutagenicity of vinylidene chloride in *Salmonella typhimurium* TA1535. *Cancer Lett.*, *5*, 1-6

Kiezel, L., Liszka, M. & Rutkowski, M. (1975) Gas chromatographic determination of trace impurities in distillates of vinyl chloride monomer (Pol.). *Chem. Anal. (Warsaw)*, *20*, 555-562 [*Chem. Abstr.*, *83*, 212233s]

Kramer, C.G. & Mutchler, J.E. (1972) The correlation of clinical and environmental measurements for workers exposed to vinyl chloride. *Am. ind. Hyg. Assoc. J., 33*, 19-30

Kurginyan, K.A. & Shirinyan, V.T. (1969) Identification and quantitative determination of some impurities in chloroprene (Russ.). *Arm. Khim. Zh., 22*, 61-65 [*Chem. Abstr., 71*, 29974x]

Lao, R.C., Thomas, R.S., Bastien, P., Halman, R.A. & Lockwood, J.A. (1982) Analysis of organic priority and non-priority pollutants in environmental samples by GC/MS/computer systems. *Pergamon Ser. environ. Sci., 7*, 107-118

Lee, C.C., Bhandari, J.C., Winston, J.M., House, W.B., Peters, P.J., Dixon, R.L. & Woods, J.S. (1977) Inhalation toxicity of vinyl chloride and vinylidene chloride. *Environ. Health Perspect., 21*, 25-32

Lee, C.C., Bhandari, J.C., Winston, J.M., House, W.B., Dixon, R.L. & Woods, J.S. (1978) Carcinogenicity of vinyl chloride and vinylidene chloride. *J. Toxicol. environ. Health, 4*, 15-30

Lin, S.-N., Fu, F.W.-Y., Bruckner, J.V. & Feldman, S. (1982) Quantitation of 1,1- and 1,2-dichloroethylene in body tissues by purge-and-trap gas chromatography. *J. Chromatogr., 244*, 311-320

Malaveille, C., Bartsch, H., Barbin, A., Camus, A.M., Montesano, R., Croisy, A. & Jacquignon, P. (1975) Mutagenicity of vinyl chloride, chloroethyleneoxide, chloroacetaldehyde and chloroethanol. *Biochem. biophys. Res. Commun., 63*, 363-370

Maltoni, C., Cotti, G. & Chieco, P. (1984) Chronic toxicity and carcinogenicity bioassays of vinylidene chloride. *Acta oncol., 5*, 91-145

Maltoni, C., Lefemine, G., Cotti, G., Chieco, P. & Patella, V. (1985) *Archives of Research on Industrial Carcinogenesis*, Vol. III, *Experimental Research on Vinylidene Chloride Carcinogenesis*, Princeton, NJ, Princeton Scientific Publishers

Mamber, S.W., Bryson, V. & Katz, S.E. (1983) The *Escherichia coli* WP2/WP100 rec assay for detection of potential chemical carcinogens. *Mutat. Res., 119*, 135-144

Mamber, S.W., Bryson, V. & Katz, S.E. (1984) Evaluation of the *Escherichia coli* K12 inductest for detection of potential chemical carcinogens. *Mutat. Res., 130*, 141-151

Masuda, Y. & Nakayama, N. (1983) Protective action of diethyldithiocarbamate and carbon disulphide against acute toxicities induced by 1,1-dichloroethylene in mice. *Toxicol. appl. Pharmacol., 71*, 42-53

McCann, J., Simmon, V., Streitwieser, D. & Ames, B.N. (1975) Mutagenicity of chloroacetaldehyde, a possible metabolic product of 1,2-dichloroethane (ethylene dichloride), chloroethanol (ethylene chlorohydrin), vinyl chloride, and cyclophosphamide. *Proc. natl Acad. Sci USA, 72*, 3190-3193

McKenna, M.J., Zempel, J.A. & Gehring, P.J. (1980) *A Comparison of the Pharmacokinetics of Inhaled Vinylidene Chloride in Rats and Mice*, Midland, MI, Dow Chemical USA, Toxicology Research Laboratory

McMahon, L.W. (1983) *Organic priority pollutants in wastewater.* In: Oakes, T.W., ed., *1982 UCC-ND/GAT Environmental Protection Seminar*, Oak Ridge, TN, Oak Ridge National Laboratory, pp. 220-249

Meyer, C. (1978) *Health Hazard Evaluation Determination Report No. HE 76-63-487, BASF Wyandotte, Corporation, South Kearny, NJ*, Cincinnati, OH, National Institute for Occupational Safety and Health

Motegi, S., Ueda, K., Tanaka, H. & Ohta, M. (1976) Determination of residual vinylidene chloride monomer in polyvinylidene chloride films used for fish jelly products. *Bull. Jpn. Soc. Sci. Fish., 42*, 1387-1394

Murray, F.J., Nitschke, K.D., Rampy, L.W. & Schwetz, B.A. (1979) Embryotoxicity and fetotoxicity of inhaled or ingested vinylidene chloride in rats and rabbits. *Toxicol. appl. Pharmacol., 49*, 189-202

National Institute for Occupational Safety and Health (1978) *Vinyl Halides Carcinogenicity (Current Intelligence Bulletin No. 28; DHEW (NIOSH) Pub. No. 79-102)*, Washington DC

National Toxicology Program (1982) *Carcinogenesis Bioassay of Vinylidene Chloride (CAS No. 75-35-4) in F344 Rats and B6C3F1 Mice (Gavage Study) (Technical Report Series No. 228)*, Research Triangle Park, NC

NIH/EPA Chemical Information System (1983) *Carbon-13 NMR Spectral Search System, Mass Spectral Search System*, and *Infrared Spectral Search System*, Arlington, VA, Information Consultants, Inc.

Nitschke, K.D., Smith, F.A., Jr, Quast, J.F., Norris, J.M. & Schwetz, B.A. (1983) A three-generation rat reproductive toxicity study of vinylidene chloride in the drinking water. *Fundam. appl. Toxicol., 3*, 75-79

Norris, J.M. (1977) *Toxicological and pharmacokinetic studies on inhaled and ingested vinylidene chloride in laboratory animals.* In: *Proceedings of the Technical Association of the Paper Industry (TAPPI) Paper Synthetics Conference, Chicago, IL, 1977*, Atlanta, GA, TAPPI

Oblas, D.W., Dugger, D.L. & Lieberman, S.I. (1980) The determination of organic species in the telephone central office ambient. *IEEE Trans. Components, Hybrids, Manuf. Technol., CHMT-3*, 17-20

Oesch, F., Protic-Sabljic, Friedberg, T., Klimisch, H.-J. & Glatt, H.R. (1983) Vinylidene chloride: Changes in drug-metabolizing enzymes, mutagenicity and relation to its targets for carcinogenesis. *Carcinogenesis, 4*, 1031-1038

Otson, R. & Williams, D.T. (1982) Headspace chromatographic determination of water pollutants. *Anal. Chem., 54*, 942-946

Otson, R., Williams, D.T. & Biggs, D.C. (1982a) Relationships between raw water quality, treatment, and occurrence of organics in Canadian potable water. *Bull. environ. Contam. Toxicol., 28*, 396-403

Otson, R., Williams, D.T. & Bothwell, P.D. (1982b) Volatile organic compounds in water at thirty Canadian potable water treatment facilities. *J. Assoc. off. anal. Chem.*, *65*, 1370-1374

Ott, M.G., Langner, R.R. & Holder, B.B. (1975) Vinyl chloride exposure in a controlled industrial environment. A long-term mortality experience in 594 employees. *Arch. environ. Health*, *30*, 333-339

Ott, M.G., Fishbeck, W.A., Townsend, J.C. & Schneider, E.J. (1976) A health study of employees exposed to vinylidene chloride. *J. occup. Med.*, *18*, 735-738

Pellizzari, E. (1979) *Analysis of Organic Air Pollutants by Gas Chromatography and Mass Spectroscopy (EPA-600/2-79-057)*, Research Triangle Park, NC, US Environmental Protection Agency

Pellizzari, E.D., Erickson, M.D. & Zweidinger, R.A. (1979) *Formulation of a Preliminary Assessment of Halogenated Organic Compounds in Man and Environmental Media (EPA-560/13-79/006; US NTIS PB80-112 170)*, Research Triangle Park, NC, p. 76

Ponomarkov, V. & Tomatis, L. (1980) Long-term testing of vinylidene chloride and chloroprene for carcinogenicity in rats. *Oncology*, *37*, 136-141

Prendergast, J.A., Jones, R.A., Jenkins, L.J., Jr & Siegel, J. (1967) Effects on experimental animals of long-term inhalatoin of trichloroethylene, carbon tetrachloride, 1,1,1-trichloroethane, dichlorodifluoromethane, and 1,1-dichloroethylene. *Toxicol. appl. Pharmacol.*, *10*, 270-289

Quast, J.F., Humiston, C.G., Wade, C.E., Ballard, J., Beyer, J.E., Schwetz, R.W. & Norris, J.M. (1983) A chronic toxicity and oncogenicity study in rats and subchronic toxicity study in dogs on ingested vinylidene chloride. *Fundam. appl. Toxicol.*, *3*, 55-62

Quast, J.F., McKenna, M.J., Rampy, L.W. & Norris, J.M. (1986) Chronic toxicity and oncogenicity study on inhaled vinylidene chloride in rats. *Fundam. appl. Toxicol.*, *6*, 105-144

Ramstad, T., Nestrick, T.J. & Peters, T.L. (1981) Applications of the purge-and-trap technique. *Am. Lab.*, *13*, 65-73

Reichert, D., Werner, H.W., Metzler, M. & Henschler, D. (1979) Molecular mechanism of 1,1-dichloroethylene toxicity: Excreted metabolites reveal different pathways of reactive metabolites. *Arch. Toxicol.*, *42*, 159-169

Reichert, D., Metzler, M. & Henschler, D. (1980) Decomposition of the neuro- and nephrotoxic compound dichloroacetylene in the presence of oxygen: Separation and identification of novel products. *J. environ. Pathol. Toxicol.*, *4*, 525-532

Reitz, R.H., Watanabe, P.G., McKenna, M.J., Quast, J.F. & Gehring, P.J. (1980) Effects of vinylidene chloride on DNA synthesis and DNA repair in the rat and mouse: A comparative study with dimethylnitrosamine. *Toxicol. appl. Pharmacol.*, *52*, 357-370

Reynolds, E.S., Moslen, M.T., Szabo, S., Jaeger, R.J. & Murphy, S.D. (1975) Hepatotoxicity of vinyl chloride and 1,1-dichloroethylene. Role of mixed function oxidase system. *Am. J. Pathol.*, *81*, 219-236

Reynolds, E.S., Moslen, M.T., Boor, P.J. & Jaeger, R.J. (1980) 1,1-Dichloroethylene hepatotoxicity. Time course of GSH changes and biochemical aberrations. *Am. J. Pathol.*, *101*, 331-342

Sadtler Research Laboratories (1980) *The Sadtler Standard Spectra Collection, Cumulative Index*, Philadelphia, PA

Sasaki, M., Sugimura, K., Yoshida, M.A. & Abe, S. (1980) Cytogenetic effects of 60 chemicals on cultured human and Chinese hamster cells. *Kromosomo II, 20*, 574-584

Sassu, G.M., Zilio-Grandi, F. & Conte, A. (1968) Gas chromatographic determination of impurities in vinyl chloride. *J. Chromatogr., 34*, 394-398

Sax, N.I. (1984) *Dangerous Properties of Industrial Materials*, 6th ed., New York, Van Nostrand Reinhold Co., p. 2730

Shackelford, W.M. & Keith, L.H. (1976) *Frequency of Organic Compounds Identified in Water (EPA-600/4-76-062)*, Athens, GA, US Environmental Protection Agency, Office of Research and Development, Environmental Research Laboratory

Shelton, L.G., Hamilton, D.E. & Fisackerly, R.H. (1971) *Vinyl and vinylidene chloride*. In: Leonard, E.C., ed., *Vinyl and Diene Monomers*, Part 3, New York, Wiley Interscience, pp. 1205-1289

Short, R.D., Minor, J.L., House, W.B., Marcus, W. & Lee, C.C. (1976) Continuous inhalation of 1,1-dichloroethylene (DCE) by rats and mice during gestation (Abstract No. 719). *Pharmacologist, 18*, 245

Short, R.D., Winston, J.M., Minor, J.L., Hong, C.-B., Seifter, J. & Lee, C.-C. (1977a) Toxicity of vinylidene chloride in mice and rats and its alteration by various treatments. *J. Toxicol. environ. Health, 3*, 913-921

Short, R.D., Winston, J.M., Minor, J.L., Seifter, J. & Lee, C.-C. (1977b) Effect of various treatments on toxicity of inhaled vinylidene chloride. *Environ. Health Perspect., 21*, 125-129

Short, R.D., Minor, J.L., Winston, J.M. & Lee, C.-C. (1977c) A dominant lethal study in male rats after repeated exposures to vinyl chloride or vinylidene chloride. *J. Toxicol. environ. Health, 3*, 965-968

Sidhu, K.S. (1980) A gas-chromatographic method for the determination of vinylidene chloride in air. *J. anal. Toxicol., 4*, 266-268

Siegel, J., Jones, R.A., Coon, R.A. & Lyon, J.P. (1971) Effects on experimental animals of acute, repeated and continuous inhalation exposures to dichloroethylene mixtures. *Toxicol. appl. Pharmacol., 18*, 168-174

Singh, H.B., Salas, L.J., Smith, A.J. & Shigeishi, H. (1981) Measurements of some potentially hazardous organic chemicals in urban environments. *Atmos. Environ., 15*, 601-612

Tan, S. & Okada, T. (1979) Determination of residual vinylidene chloride monomer in polyvinylidene chloride. Hygienic studies on plastic containers and packages. III. (Jpn). *J. Food hyg. Soc. Jpn, 20*, 223-227

Taylor, D.G. (1978) *NIOSH Manual of Analytical Methods*, 2nd Ed., Vol. 4 (*DHEW (NIOSH) Publ. No. 78-175*), Washington DC, US Government Printing Office, pp. 266-1 - 266-9

Thiess, A.M., Frentzel-Beyme, R. & Penning, E. (1979) *Mortality study of vinylidene chloride exposed persons*. In: Hien, C. & Kilian, D.J., eds, *Proceedings of the 5th Medichem Congress, San Francisco, CA, September 1977*, San Francisco, CA, University of California at San Francisco, pp. 270-278

Torkelson, T.R. & Rowe, V.K. (1981) *Halogenated aliphatic hydrocarbons*. In: Clayton, G.D. & Clayton, F.E., eds, *Patty's Industrial Hygiene and Toxicology*, Vol. 2B, 3rd rev. ed., New York, Wiley Interscience, pp. 3545-3550

Työsuojeluhallitus (National Finnish Board of Occupational Safety and Health) (1981) *Airborne Contaminants in the Workplace* (*Safety Bulletin 3*) (Finn.), Tampere, p. 27

US Environmental Protection Agency (1976) *Health and Environmental Impacts, Task 1, Vinylidene Chloride* (*EPA-560/6-76-023*), Washington DC, Office of Toxic Substances

US Environmental Protection Agency (1984a) Protection of environment. *US Code Fed. Regul., Title 40*, Part 261.33, p. 363

US Environmental Protection Agency (1984b) *Health Assessment Document; Vinylidene Chloride* (*EPA-600/8-83-031A; US NTIS PB84-126762*), Washington DC, Office of Health and Environmental Assessment

US Environmental Protection Agency (1984c) Method 601. Guidelines establishing test procedures for the analysis of pollutants under the Clean Water Act (40 CFR 136). Purgeable halocarbons. *Fed. Regist., 49*, 43261-43271

US Environmental Protection Agency (1984d) Method 624. Guidelines establishing test procedures for the analysis of pollutants under the Clean Water Act (40 CFR 136). Purgeables. *Fed. Regist., 49*, 43373-43383

US Environmental Protection Agency (1984e) Method 1624, Revision B. Guidelines establishing test procedures for the analysis of pollutants under the Clean Water Act (40 CFR 136). Volatile organic compounds by isotope dilution GC/MS. *Fed. Regist., 49*, 43407-43415

US Environmental Protection Agency (1985) *Health Assessment Document for Vinylidene Chloride,* (*EPA-600/8-83-031F*), Washington DC, Office of Health and Environmental Assessment

US Food and Drug Administration (1984) Food and drugs. *US Code Fed. Regul., Title 21*, Parts 175.105, 175.300, 175.360, 175.365, 176.170, 177.1010, 177.1200, 177.1630, 177.1990, 178.3790, 179.45, pp. 133, 145, 160-161, 176, 198, 211, 250, 268-269, 342, 356-357

US International Trade Commission (1984) *Synthetic Organic Chemicals, US Production and Sales, 1983* (*USITC Publication 1588*), Washington DC, US Government Printing Office, p. 138

Van Duuren, B.L., Goldschmidt, B.M., Loewengart, G., Smith, A.C., Melchionne, S., Seldman, I. & Roth, D. (1979) Carcinogenicity of halogenated olefinic and aliphatic hydrocarbons in mice. *J. natl Cancer Inst.*, *63*, 1433-1439

Verschueren, K. (1983) *Handbook of Environmental Data on Organic Chemicals*, 2nd ed., New York, Van Nostrand Reinhold Co., pp. 487-488

Vlasov, S.M. & Bodyagin, G.N. (1970) Gas chromatographic analysis of trichloroethylene (Russ.). *Tr. Khim. Khim. Tekhnol.*, *1*, 161-162 [*Chem. Abstr.*, *75*, 71124c]

Wallace, L., Zweidinger, R., Erickson, M., Cooper, S., Whitaker, D. & Pellizzari, E. (1982) Monitoring individual exposure. Measurements of volatile organic compounds in breathing-zone air, drinking water, and exhaled breath. *Environ. int.*, *8*, 269-282

Wallace, L.A., Pellizzari, E., Hartwell, T., Rosenzweig, M., Erickson, M., Sparacino, C. & Zelon, H. (1984) Personal exposure to volatile organic compounds. I. Direct measurements in breathing-zone air, drinking water, food, and exhaled breath. *Environ. Res.*, *35*, 293-319

Wang, T. & Lenahan, R. (1984) Determination of volatile halocarbons in water by purge-closed loop gas chromatography. *Bull. environ. Contam. Toxicol.*, *32*, 429-438

Warner, C., Modderman, J., Fazio, T., Beroza, M., Schwartzman, G., Fominaya, K. & Sherma, J., eds (1983) *Food Additives Analytical Manual*, Vol. 1, Arlington, VA, Asssociation of Official Analytical Chemists, pp. 348-357

Warren, H.S. & Ricci, B.E. (1978) *Vinylidene Chloride, I. An Overview. II. A Literature Collection 1947 to 1977 (ORNL/TIRC-77/3)*, Oak Ridge, TN, Oak Ridge National Laboratory

Waxweiler, R.J. Smith, A.H., Falk, H. & Tyroler, H.A. (1981) Excess lung cancer risk in a synthetic chemicals plant. *Environ. Health Perspect.*, *41*, 159-165

Weast, R.C., ed. (1984) *CRC Handbook of Chemistry and Physics*, 65th ed., Boca Raton, FL, CRC Press, p. C-295

Wegman, T.C.C., Bank, C.A. & Greve, P.A. (1981) Environmental pollution by a chemical waste dump. *Stud. environ. Sci.*, *17*, 349-357

Wessling, R.A. & Edwards, F.G. (1971) *Vinylidene chloride polymers*. In: Bikales, N.M., ed., *Encyclopedia of Polymer Science and Technology*, Vol. 14, New York, Wiley Interscience, pp. 540-579

Windholz, M., ed. (1983) *The Merck Index*, 10th ed., Rahway, NJ, Merck & Co., p. 143

VINYLIDENE FLUORIDE

1. Chemical and Physical Data

1.1 Synonyms and trade names

Chem. Abstr. Services Reg. No.: 75-38-7
Chem. Abstr. Name: Ethene, 1,1-difluoro-
IUPAC Systematic Name: 1,1-Difluoroethylene
Synonyms: VDF; vinylidene difluoride

1.2 Structural and molecular formulae and molecular weight

$$CH_2 = CF_2$$

$C_2H_2F_2$ Mol. wt: 64.04

1.3 Chemical and physical properties of the pure substance

(a) *Description*: Colourless gas with a faint ethereal odour (Hawley, 1981; Sax, 1984)

(b) *Boiling-point*: -83°C at 760 mm Hg (Hawley, 1981)

(c) *Melting-point*: -144°C at 760 mm Hg (Hawley, 1981)

(d) *Density*: d^{24} 0.617 g/cm³ (liquid) (Hawley, 1981); d^{21} 0.585 g/cm³ (liquid) (E.I. duPont de Nemours & Co., 1969)

(e) *Spectroscopy data*: Infrared (Sadtler Research Laboratories, 1980; prism [30862[a]], grating [3857p]) and mass spectral data (NIH/EPA Chemical Information System, 1983) have been reported.

---

[a]Spectrum number in Sadtler compilation

(f)   *Solubility*: Slightly soluble in water (0.018 g/ 100 g at 25°C and 760 mm Hg (E.I. duPont de Nemours & Co., 1969; National Fire Protection Association, 1984); soluble in ethanol and diethyl ether (Weast, 1984)

(g)   *Stability*: Inflammable (Hawley, 1981); emits toxic fluoride fumes when heated to decomposition; sensitive to heat or oxidizers (Sax, 1984)

(h)   *Reactivity*: Alkyl boron and alkyl hyponitrite compounds, among others, initiate polymerization (Dohany & Robb, 1980).

(i)   *Conversion factor:* mg/ m³ = 2.62 × ppm[a]

1.4 Technical products and impurities

Vinylidene fluoride is available in the USA in bulk quantities as a liquefied gas under pressure. The commercial product typically is 99.75 mol% min pure with noncondensible gases as oxygen, 0.05 mol% max, other impurities, 0.2 mol% max and moisture, 0.01 wt% max; it does not require an inhibitor. Other impurities present are vinyl fluoride (see p. 147 of this volume), difluoromethane, 1,1-difluoroethane, 1,1-difluoro-1-chloroethane and 1,1,1-trifluoroethane (Pennwalt Corp., 1984).

2. Production, Use, Occurrence and Analysis

2.1 Production and use

(a)   *Production*

Vinylidene fluoride was first produced in the early 1900s by the dehydrobromination of 1,1-difluoro-2-bromoethane. An industrial synthetic process was developed in the 1940s. Several methods for vinylidene fluoride production are based on pyrolysis, including the dechlorination of 1,2-dichloro-1,1-difluoroethane in the presence of a nickel catalyst and the dehydrofluorination of 1,1,1-trifluoroethane, which has been patented for the commercial production of vinylidene fluoride monomers. 1-Chloro-1,1-difluoroethane can be converted to vinylidene fluoride by a dehydrochlorination reaction in the presence of various catalysts (Wolinski, 1971).

---

[a]Calculated from: mg/ m³ = (molecular weight/ 24.45) × ppm, assuming standard temperature (25°C) and pressure (760 mm Hg)

Two companies in the USA are the major producers of vinylidene fluoride. Other manufacturers may produce the monomer as a specialty chemical. There are currently two producers in France, and two firms in the UK produced the monomer in the past (Chemical Sources Europe, 1980).

(b)   Use

Vinylidene fluoride monomer is used to manufacture polyvinylidene fluoride (PVDF) and elastomeric copolymers with chlorotrifluoroethylene or hexafluoropropylene.

Polyvinylidene fluoride

PVDF, developed in the 1960s, is thermally, chemically and ultraviolet-light-resistant. PVDF fluoroplastics are used for tank linings, pumps, valves, and solid or lined pipes in chemical processing equipment. Due to their resistance to corrosion, they are used to protect mechanical parts and pipes in the production of organic insecticides and bromine processing, in displacement bleaching units in pulp mills, in water-treatment in many nuclear power plants and for transporting corrosive chemicals used in metal etching operations for electronics manufacture. The monofilament form of PVDF is used as filter cloth in the pulp and paper industry (Dohany & Robb, 1980; Pennwalt Corp., 1983).

Because of the high melting-point of PVDF polymers, they are used as insulation for high-temperature wire and in aircraft missiles (US Environmental Protection Agency, 1980).

Protective paints and coatings formulated with PVDF resins, used as an exterior finish for metal siding and building parts, resist weathering and ultraviolet radiation for up to 30 years (US Environmental Protection Agency, 1980).

No data were available on the quantities of polyvinylidene fluoride produced in 1983. There is one manufacturer of PVDF in the USA, one in France, one in Belgium and one in Japan.

Elastomeric copolymers

Vinylidene fluoride can be copolymerized with chlorotrifluoroethylene or hexafluoropropylene to form fluoroelastomers *via* a free-radical mechanism using peroxide catalysts or irradiation techniques. A terpolymer also exists containing vinylidene fluoride, hexafluoropropylene and tetrafluoroethylene. The copolymers (primarily vinylidene fluoride-hexafluoropropylene) are used for their heat- and moisture-resistant properties, primarily in industrial, aerospace and automotive applications as gaskets, O-rings and seals and in hose linings, tubing, industrial gloves and autoclave and oven seals (Thompson & Barney, 1971).

Vinylidene fluoride-chlorotrifluoroethylene copolymers, available in powder form and as a film, are used as fluoroelastomers and as plastics for packaging materials, medical tubing and electrical components.

(c)   Regulatory status and guidelines

The National Institute for Occupational Safety and Health (1978) recommended that the time-weighted average exposure level be established at 3 mg/m^3. Polyvinylidene fluoride resins may be used as articles or components of articles intended for repeated use in contact with food (US Food and Drug Administration, 1984).

2.2 Occurrence

(*a*) *Natural occurrence*

It is not known whether vinylidene fluoride occurs as a natural product.

(*b*) *Occupational exposure*

No data were available to the Working Group

2.3 Analysis

Gas chromatography with thermal conduction detection has been used to detect vinylidene fluoride in the reaction product of the hydrofluorination of acetylene (Gil'burd *et al.*, 1967), and gas chromatography with flame ionization detection has been used to detect vinylidene fluoride in a prepared mixture of dichlorofluoromethane and its possible impurities (Ratcliffe & Targett, 1969).

3. Biological Data Relevant to the Evaluation of Carcinogenic Risk to Humans

3.1 Carcinogenicity studies in animals[1]

Oral administration

Rat: Groups of 30 and 35 male and 30 and 35 female Sprague-Dawley rats, 13 weeks of age, received daily doses of 4.12 and 8.25 mg/kg bw, respectively, vinylidene fluoride [purity unspecified] in olive oil by gastric intubation on four or five days per week for 52 weeks and were observed until 141 weeks. A group of 30 male and 30 female controls were given olive oil only. Liposarcomas were observed in the subcutaneous tissue and abdominal cavity in 0 control, 1 low-dose and 2 high-dose males, and in 0 control, 0 low-dose and 1 high-dose female. Among several thousand historical controls, the incidence of liposarcomas was reported to be 0.1%. A small number of lipomas was also observed. The incidences of mammary tumours were comparable in all groups, and one Zymbal-gland carcinoma was seen in a high-dose female (Maltoni & Tovoli, 1979). [The Working Group noted the limited duration of treatment].

---

[1]The Working Group was aware that a study of exposure of mice and rats by inhalation has been started (IARC, 1984).

3.2 Other relevant biological data

(a) Experimental systems

Toxic effects

The available data are inadequate to determine the acute inhalation toxicity of vinylidene fluoride (Carpenter *et al.*, 1949; Lester & Greenberg, 1950; Clayton, 1967).

Exposure of rats to 215 000 mg/m³ (82 000 ppm) vinylidene fluoride for 3.5 h produced no sign of hepatotoxicity (Jaeger *et al.*, 1975). However, rats pretreated with Aroclor 1254 on three consecutive days and then exposed for 6 h to 65 500 mg/m³ (25 000 ppm) had elevated serum levels of sorbitol dehydrogenase and histological signs of liver damage (Conolly *et al.*, 1979).

Newborn Wistar rats exposed to 5200 mg/m³ (2000 ppm) vinylidene fluoride for 8 h per day on five days per week for 10-14 weeks did not develop a significant number of ATPase-deficient foci in the liver (Stöckle *et al.*, 1979; Bolt *et al.*, 1982).

Effects on reproduction and prenatal toxicity

No data were available to the Working Group.

Absorption, distribution, excretion and metabolism

The inhalation pharmacokinetics of vinylidene fluoride have been studied in Wistar rats (Filser & Bolt, 1979, 1981). Vinylidene fluoride was taken up rapidly *via* the pulmonary route, but was less concentrated in the organism than other structurally-related halogenated olefins. In the state of equilibrium between gas phase and organism, the mean concentration (by volume) in the organism was only 23% of that in the gas phase. Metabolism proceeded very slowly and was saturable at exposure concentrations of about 260 mg/m³ (100 ppm). The maximal metabolic rate was 1% that of vinyl chloride and less than 20% that of vinyl fluoride (Filser & Bolt, 1979). Exposure of rats to vinylidene fluoride has been reported to result in some increase in the urinary excretion of fluoride (Dilley *et al.*, 1974).

Experiments in which a mixture of vinylidene fluoride and air was passed through a mouse-liver microsomal system and subsequently through a trap with 4-(4-nitrobenzyl)pyridine failed to demonstrate the presence of an alkylating intermediate (Bartsch *et al.*, 1979).

Vinylidene fluoride inhibits microsomal mixed-function oxidases *in vitro* (Bolt *et al.*, 1979).

Like other halogenated C_1 and C_2 compounds that are biotransformed to reactive metabolites, vinylidene fluoride causes changes in rat intermediary metabolism which lead to increased exhalation of acetone (Filser & Bolt, 1980; Filser *et al.*, 1982).

Mutagenicity and other short-term tests

Vinylidene fluoride vapours (50% v/v in air for 24 h) induced a marginal increase in the number of revertants in *Salmonella typhimurium* TA100 in the presence of a metabolic system from the liver of phenobarbital-induced mice (Bartsch *et al.*, 1979).

(b) Humans

No data were available to the Working Group.

3.3 Case reports and epidemiological studies of carcinogenicity to humans

No data were available to the Working Group.

4. Summary of Data Reported and Evaluation

4.1 Exposure data

Vinylidene fluoride has been produced commercially since the 1940s. It is used in the manufacture of polyvinylidene fluoride and elastomeric copolymers. Exposure is limited to the manufacture of the monomer and its use in the production of polyvinylidene fluoride and elastomeric copolymers.

4.2 Experimental data

In a limited study in one strain of rats by oral administration, a small number of liposarcomas was observed in treated animals.

No data were available to evaluate the reproductive effects or prenatal toxicity of vinylidine fluoride to experimental animals.

Vinylidene fluoride gave equivocal results for mutagenicity to *Salmonella typhimurium* when tested in the presence of an exogenous metabolic system.

4.3 Human data

No data were available to evaluate the reproductive effects or prenatal toxicity of vinylidine fluoride to humans.

No case report or epidemiological study was available to evaluate the carcinogenicity of vinylidene fluoride to humans.

4.4 Evaluation[1]

There is *inadequate evidence* for the carcinogenicity of vinylidene fluoride in experimental animals.

No data on humans were available.

In the absence of epidemiological data, no evaluation of the carcinogenicity of vinylidene fluoride to humans could be made.

---

[1]For definition of the italicized term, see Preamble, p. 18.

Overall assessment of data from short-term tests: Vinylidene fluoride[a]

	Genetic activity			Cell transformation
	DNA damage	Mutation	Chromosomal effects	
Prokaryotes		?		
Fungi/Green plants				
Insects				
Mammalian cells (*in vitro*)				
Mammals (*in vivo*)				
Humans (*in vivo*)				
Degree of evidence in short-term tests for genetic activity: **Inadequate**				Cell transformation: No data

[a]The groups into which the table is divided and the symbol ? are defined on pp. 19-20 of the Preamble; the degrees of evidence are defined on pp. 20-21.

5. References

Bartsch, H., Malaveille, C., Barbin, A. & Planche, G. (1979) Mutagenic and alkylating metabolites of halo-ethylenes, chlorobutadienes and dichlorobutenes produced by rodent or human liver tissues. Evidence for oxirane formation by P450-linked microsomal mono-oxygenases. *Arch. Toxicol., 41*, 249-277

Bolt, H.M., Filser, J.G., Wiegand, M., Buchter, A. & Bolt, W. (1979) Studies on liver microsomal metabolism and interaction of vinyl chloride and related compounds in relation to possible carcinogenicity. *Arh. hig. Rada Toksikol., 30 (suppl.)*, 369-377

Bolt, H.M., Laib, R.J. & Filser, J.G. (1982) Reactive metabolites and carcinogenicity of halogenated ethylenes. *Biochem. Pharmacol., 31*, 1-4

Carpenter, C.P., Smyth, H.F., Jr & Pozzani, U.C. (1949) The assay of acute vapor toxicity, and the grading and interpretation of results on 96 chemical compounds. *J. ind. Hyg. Toxicol., 31*, 343-346

Chemical Sources Europe (1980) *Chemical Sources Europe*, Mountain Lakes, NJ, p. 514

Clayton, J.W., Jr (1967) Fluorocarbon toxicity and biological action. *Fluorine Chem. Rev., 1*, 197-252

Conolly, R.B., Szabo, S. & Jaeger, R.J. (1979) Vinylidene fluoride: Acute hepatotoxicity in rats pretreated with PCB or phenobarbital. *Proc. Soc. exp. Biol. Med.*, 162, 163-169

Dilley, J.V., Carter, V.L., Jr & Harris, E.S. (1974) Fluoride ion excretion by male rats after inhalation of one of several fluoroethylenes or hexafluoropropene. *Toxicol. appl. Pharmacol.*, 27, 582-590

Dohany, J.E. & Robb, L.E. (1980) *Polyvinylidene fluoride.* In: Mark, H.F., Othmer, D.F., Overberger, C.G. & Seaborg, G.T., eds, *Kirk-Othmer Encyclopedia of Chemical Technology*, 3rd ed., Vol. 11, New York, John Wiley & Sons, pp. 64-74

E.I. DuPont de Nemours & Co. (1969) *Technical Report DP-6: Vinyl Fluoride, Vinylidene Fluoride*, Wilmington, DE

Filser, J.G. & Bolt, H.M. (1979) Pharmacokinetics of halogenated ethylenes in rats. *Arch. Toxicol.*, 42, 123-136

Filser, J.G. & Bolt, H.M. (1980) Characteristics of haloethylene-induced acetonemia in rats. *Arch. Toxicol.*, 45, 109-116

Filser, J.G. & Bolt, H.M. (1981) Inhalation pharmacokinetics based on gas uptake studies. I. Improvement of kinetic models. *Arch. Toxicol.*, 47, 279-292

Filser, J.G., Jung, P. & Bolt, H.M. (1982) Increased acetone exhalation induced by metabolites of halogenated C_1 and C_2 compounds. *Arch. Toxicol.*, 49, 107-116

Gil'burd, M.M., Mikityuk, L.P., Pazderskii, Y.A. & Syrvatka, B.G. (1967) Analysis of the reaction products of the hydrofluorination of acetylene (Russ.). *Sovrem. Metody Khim. Spektral. Anal. Mater.*, 246-252 [Chem. Abstr., 68, 46036y]

Hawley, G.G., ed. (1981) *The Condensed Chemical Dictionary*, 10th ed., New York, Van Nostrand Reinhold Co., p. 1086

IARC (1984) *Information Bulletin on the Survey of Chemicals Being Tested for Carcinogenicity*, No. 11, Lyon, p. 262

Jaeger, R.J., Connolly, R.B. & Murphy, S.D. (1975) Short-term inhalation toxicity of halogenated hydrocarbons. Effects on fasting rats. *Arch. environ. Health*, 30, 26-31

Lester, D. & Greenberg, L.A. (1950) Acute and chronic toxicity of some halogenated derivatives of methane and ethane. *Arch. ind. Hyg. occup. Med.*, 2, 335-344

Maltoni, C. & Tovoli, D. (1979) First experimental evidence of the carcinogenic effects of vinylidene fluoride. Long-term bioassays on Sprague-Dawley rats by oral administration. *Med. Lav.*, 5, 363-368

National Fire Protection Association (1984) *Fire Protection Guide on Hazardous Materials*, 8th ed., Quincy, MA, p. 325M-94

National Institute for Occupational Safety and Health (1978) *Vinyl Halides Carcinogenicity (Current Intelligence Bulletin No. 28; DHEW (NIOSH) Pub. No. 79-102)*, Cincinnati, OH

NIH/EPA Chemical Information System (1983) *Carbon-13 NMR Spectral Search System, Mass Spectral Search System*, and *Infrared Spectral Search System*, Arlington, VA, Information Consultants, Inc.

Pennwalt Corp. (1983) *Kynar® for CPI Systems* (*Technical Bulletin PL 70510-M-6-83-TR*), Philadelphia, PA

Pennwalt Corp. (1984) *Isotron 1132a, Vinylidene Fluoride Monomer* (*Technical Data, 04097*), Philadelphia, PA

Ratcliffe, D.B. & Targett, B.H. (1969) A gas-chromatographic determination of organo-halogen impurities in dichlorofluoromethane. *Analyst*, *94*, 1028-1032

Sadtler Research Laboratories (1980) *The Sadtler Standard Spectra Collection, Cumulative Index*, Philadelphia, PA

Sax, N.I. (1984) *Dangerous Properties of Industrial Materials*, 6th ed., New York, Van Nostrand Reinhold Co., p. 2730

Stöckle, G., Laib, R.J., Filser, J.G. & Bolt, H.M. (1979) Vinylidene fluoride: Metabolism and induction of preneoplastic hepatic foci in relation to vinyl chloride. *Toxicol. Lett.*, *3*, 337-342

Thompson, D.C. & Barney, A.L. (1971) *Vinylidene fluoride polymers (elastomers)*. In: Bikales, N.M., ed., *Encyclopedia of Polymer Science and Technology*, Vol. 14, New York, Wiley Interscience, pp. 610-617

US Environmental Protection Agency (1980) *TSCA Chemical Assessment Series, Chemical Hazard Information Profiles (CHIPs), August 1976 — August 1978* (*EPA-560/11-80-011*), Washington DC, pp. 277-289

US Food and Drug Administration (1984) Food and drugs. *US Code Fed. Regul.*, *Title 21*, Part 177.2510, p. 283

Weast, R.C., ed. (1984) *CRC Handbook of Chemistry and Physics*, 65th ed., Boca Raton, FL, CRC Press, p. C-295

Wolinski, L.E. (1971) *Fluorovinyl monomers*. In: Leonard, E.C., ed., *Vinyl and Diene Monomers*, Part 3, New York, Wiley-Interscience, pp. 1291-135

NYLON MONOMERS

11-AMINOUNDECANOIC ACID

1. Chemical and Physical Data

1.1 Synonyms and trade names

Chem. Abstr. Services Reg. No.: 2432-99-7
Chem. Abstr. Name: Undecanoic acid, 11-amino-
IUPAC Systematic Name: 11-Aminoundecanoic acid
Synonyms: Aminoundecanoic acid; ω-aminoundecanoic acid; 11-aminoundecylic acid

1.2 Structural and molecular formulae and molecular weight

$$H_2N - CH_2 - (CH_2)_9 - \overset{\overset{\displaystyle O}{\|}}{C} - OH$$

$C_{11}H_{23}NO_2$ Mol. wt: 201.35

1.3 Chemical and physical properties of the pure substance

(*a*)   *Description*: White crystalline solid (National Toxicology Program, 1982)

(*b*)   *Melting-point*: 188-191°C (National Toxicology Program, 1982); 190-192° C (Buckingham, 1982)

(*c*)   *Spectroscopy data*: Ultraviolet (National Toxicology Program 1982); infrared (Sadtler Research Laboratories, 1980; prism [15268[a]], grating [25137]; Pouchert, 1981 [345H[b]]), nuclear magnetic resonance (Pouchert, 1983 [491A]; National Toxicology Program, 1982) and mass spectral data (NIH/EPA Chemical Information System, 1983) have been reported.

---

[a]Spectrum number in Sadtler compilation

[b]Spectrum number in Pouchert compilation

(d) *Conversion factor:* mg/m^3 = 8.24 x ppm^a

1.4 Technical products and impurities

11-Aminoundecanoic acid is not available in commercial quantities but is manufactured for internal ('captive') use by a single company. No information was available on the technical product.

2. Production, Use, Occurrence and Analysis

2.1 Production and use

(a) *Production*

In the production of 11-aminoundecanoic acid, castor oil is transesterified with methanol to produce glycerol and methyl ricinoleate. A pyrolytic process converts methyl ricinoleate to methyl 10-undecylenate and heptaldehyde. Methyl 10-undecylenate is hydrolysed, and the resultant acid is treated with hydrogen bromide in the presence of peroxides to yield 11-bromoundecanoic acid. This compound is then converted to 11-aminoundecanoic acid (Naughton *et al.*, 1979).

There is currently one major industrial producer of 11-aminoundecanoic acid, based in France, which both processes the monomer and exports it to a US subsidiary for polymer production.

(b) *Use*

Nylon 11 polymers are the principal use of 11-aminoundecanoic acid. Nylon 11 is prepared by a melt condensation of the monomer for approximately 3 h at 215°C in a nitrogen atmosphere (Putscher, 1982). This catalytic process usually leaves no residual monomer (Welgos, 1982).

Nylon 11 polymers are resistant to chemicals, fuels, shock and vibration and are thus used in the automotive industry. Rollers and bearings for conveyors can also be constructed from Nylon 11. When fabricated into monofilament, Nylon 11 is used as a covering for braided cable, in fabrics such as filter cloth and netting and for flexible fishing line and brush bristles (Naughton *et al.*, 1979). Thermoplastic Nylon 11 is also used for dry or powder coatings that require no solvent, which are resistant to wear and impact. Nylon 11 polymers can be machined into flat or tubular film, which is used as packaging material (Naughton *et al.*, 1979).

---

^{a}Calculated from: mg/m^3 = (molecular weight/24.45) × ppm, assuming standard temperature (25°C) and pressure (760 mm Hg)

(*c*)   *Regulatory status and guidelines*

The US Food and Drug Administration (1984) permits the use of Nylon 11 resins in articles intended for use in contact with food. They are also approved for use as components of sideseam cements intended for single use in contact with food.

2.2 Occurrence

(*a*)   *Natural occurrence*

It is not known whether 11-aminoundecanoic acid occurs as a natural product.

(*b*)   *Occupational exposure*

No data were available to the Working Group.

2.3 Analysis

A method for the analysis of 11-aminoundecanoic acid in rodent feed, developed for the carcinogenesis study of the US National Toxicology Program (1982), involves extraction with dilute nitric acid, neutralization, reaction with dansyl chloride in acetonitrile and analysis by high-performance liquid chromatography with ultraviolet detection.

A method for identification of this chemical by field desorption mass spectrometry has been described (McEwen & Bolinski, 1975).

3. Biological Data Relevant to the Evaluation of Carcinogenic Risk to Humans

3.1 Carcinogenicity studies in animals

Oral administration

Mouse: Groups of 50 male and 50 female B6C3F$_1$ mice, six weeks of age, were fed a diet containing 7500 or 15 000 mg/kg (ppm) 11-aminoundecanoic acid (purity, $99.13 \pm 0.03\%$) for 103 weeks. An equal number of untreated mice served as controls. Survival was 74% of control, 68% of low-dose and 36% of high-dose males, and 85% of control, 76% of low-dose and 51% of high-dose females. All surviving animals were killed at 108-109 weeks. Increases in the incidence of malignant lymphomas occurred in male mice only: in 2/50 control, 9/50 ($p < 0.05$) low-dose, and 4/50 high-dose animals (National Toxicology Program, 1982; Dunnick *et al.*, 1983). [The Working Group noted the poor dose-related survival, which might have affected the incidence of late-developing tumours.]

Rat: Groups of 50 male and 50 female Fischer 344/N rats, six weeks of age, were fed a diet containing 7500 or 15 000 mg/kg (ppm) 11-aminoundecanoic acid (purity, 99.13 ± 0.03%) for 104 weeks. An equal number of untreated rats served as controls. Survival was 78% of control, 74% of low-dose and 60% of high-dose males and 76% of control, 64% of low-dose and 84% of high-dose females. All surviving animals were killed at 109 weeks. A treatment-related increase in the incidence of transitional-cell carcinoma of the urinary bladder was observed in males only: in 0/48 control, 0/48 low-dose and 7/49 ($p < 0.01$) high-dose animals; there were also 1/49 transitional-cell papilloma of the urinary bladder and 1/50 transitional-cell carcinoma of the kidney in the high-dose group. Dose-related transitional-cell hyperplasia of the urinary bladder and renal pelvis was observed in males and females. An increased incidence of calculi of the urinary bladder was seen in males in the high-dose group (1/48 (2%) control, 1/48 (2%) low-dose and 5/49 (10%) high-dose animals) only in animals that did not develop a transitional-cell carcinoma. Two of 50 high-dose females had transitional-cell carcinomas of the kidney, and no calculi were observed in these animals. Treatment-related neoplastic nodules of the liver were also observed in males: in 1/50 controls; 9/50 ($p < 0.01$) low-dose and 8/50 ($p < 0.01$) high-dose animals; in addition, 1/50 low-dose and 2/50 high-dose animals had hepatocellular carcinomas (National Toxicology Program, 1982; Dunnick *et al.*, 1983).

3.2 Other relevant biological data

(a) *Experimental systems*

Toxic effects

No mortality was observed after 14 days among male rats that received a single oral dose of 21.5 g/kg bw 11-aminoundecanoic acid; deaths occurred in 0/5, 1/5 and 5/5 female rats that received 10, 14.7 and 21 g/kg bw, respectively (National Toxicology Program, 1982).

In rats and mice given diets containing 7500 or 15 000 mg/kg 11-aminoundecanoic acid for 103-104 weeks (see section 3.1), dose-related effects included hyperplasia of the transitional epithelium of the renal pelvis and urinary bladder of rats of both sexes, calcification of the renal cortex and medulla in female rats and mineralization of the kidney and vacuolization of hepatocytes in male and female mice (National Toxicology Program, 1982; Dunnick *et al.*, 1983).

Effects on reproduction and prenatal toxicity

No data were available to the Working Group.

Absorption, distribution, excretion and metabolism

No data were available to the Working Group.

Mutagenicity and other short-term tests

No sex-linked recessive mutation was induced in *Drosophila melanogaster* that received an injection of 1000 µg 11-aminoundecanoic acid (Yoon *et al.*, 1985).

It was reported in an abstract [details not given] that 11-aminoundecanoic acid does not induce unscheduled DNA synthesis in hepatocytes of rats treated *in vivo* (Mirsalis *et al.*, 1983).

(*b*) *Humans*

No data were available to the Working Group.

3.3 Case reports and epidemiological studies of carcinogenicity to humans

No data were available to the Working Group.

4. Summary of Data Reported and Evaluation

4.1 Exposure data

11-Aminoundecanoic acid is synthesized by one company for the production of Nylon 11.

4.2 Experimental data

11-Aminoundecanoic acid was tested for carcinogenicity in mice and rats by administration in the diet. Increased incidences of transitional-cell carcinomas of the urinary bladder and neoplastic nodules of the liver were observed in male rats. Transitional-cell carcinomas of the kidney and epithelial hyperplasia of the urinary bladder and renal pelvis were observed in male and female rats. No clear evidence for an increased incidence of treatment-related tumours was seen in mice.

No data were available to evaluate the reproductive effects or prenatal toxicity of 11-aminoundecanoic acid to experimental animals.

11-Aminodecanoic acid was not mutagenic to *Drosophila melanogaster*.

4.3 Human data

No data were available to evaluate the reproductive effects or prenatal toxicity of 11-aminoundecanoic acid to humans.

No case report or epidemiological study was available to evaluate the carcinogenicity of 11-aminoundecanoic acid to humans.

Overall assessment of data from short-term tests: 11-Aminoundecanoic acid[a]

	Genetic activity			Cell transformation
	DNA damage	Mutation	Chromosomal effects	
Prokaryotes				
Fungi/Green plants				
Insects		−		
Mammalian cells (*in vitro*)				
Mammals (*in vivo*)				
Humans (*in vivo*)				
Degree of evidence in short-term tests for genetic activity: **Inadequate**				Cell transformation: No data

[a]The groups into which the table is divided and the symbol − are defined on pp. 19-20 of the Preamble; the degrees of evidence are defined on pp. 20-21.

4.4 Evaluation[1]

There is *limited evidence* for the carcinogenicity of 11-aminoundecanoic acid in experimental animals.

No data on humans were available.

In the absence of epidemiological data, no evaluation of the carcinogenicity of 11-aminoundecanoic acid to humans could be made.

5. References

Buckingham, J., ed. (1982) *Dictionary of Organic Compounds*, 5th ed., Vol. 1, New York, Chapman and Hall, pp. 338-339

Dunnick, J.K., Huff, J.E., Haseman, J.K. & Boorman, G.A (1983) Lesions of the urinary tract produced in Fischer 344 rats and B6C3F1 mice after chronic administration of 11-aminoundecanoic acid. *Fundam. appl. Toxicol.*, *3*, 614-618

[1]For definition of the italicized term, see Preamble, p. 18.

McEwen, C.N. & Bolinski, A.G. (1975) High resolution field desorption mass spectrometry by peak matching. *Biomed. mass Spectrom.*, *2*, 112-114

Mirsalis, J., Tyson, K., Beck, J., Loh, E., Steinmetz, K., Contreras, C., Austere, L., Martin, S. & Spalding, J. (1983) Induction of unscheduled DNA synthesis (UDS) in hepatocytes following *in vitro* and *in vivo* treatment (Abstract No. Ef-5). *Environ. Mutagenesis, 5*, 482

National Toxicology Program (1982) *NTP Technical Report on the Carcinogenesis Bioassay of 11-Aminoundecanoic Acid (CAS No. 2432-99-7) in F344 Rats and B6C3F1 Mice (Feed Study) (Technical Report Series No. 216)*, Research Triangle Park, NC

Naughton, F.C., Duneczky, F., Swenson, C.R., Kroplinksi, T. & Cooperman, M.C. (1979) *Castor oil.* In: Mark, H.F., Othmer, D.F., Overberger, C.G. & Seaborg, G.T., eds, *Kirk-Othmer Encyclopedia of Chemical Technology*, 3rd ed., Vol. 5, New York, John Wiley & Sons, pp. 1-15

NIH/EPA Chemical Information System (1983) *Carbon-13 NMR Spectral Search System, Mass Spectral Search System*, and *Infrared Spectral Search System*, Arlington, VA, Information Consultants

Pouchert, C.J., ed. (1981) *The Aldrich Library of Infrared Spectra*, 2nd ed., Milwaukee, WI, Aldrich Chemical Co., p. 345

Pouchert, C.J., ed. (1983) *The Aldrich Library of NMR Spectra*, 3rd ed., Vol. 1, Milwaukee, WI, Aldrich Chemical Co., p. 491

Putscher, R.E. (1982) *Polyamides (general).* In: Mark, H.F., Othmer, D.F., Overberger, C.G. & Seaborg, G.T., eds, *Kirk-Othmer Encyclopedia of Chemical Technology*, 3rd ed., Vol. 18, New York, John Wiley & Sons, pp. 328-371

Sadtler Research Laboratories (1980) *The Sadtler Standard Spectra Collection, Cumulative Index*, Philadelphia, PA

US Food and Drug Administration (1984) Food and drugs. *US Code Fed. Regul., Title 21*, Part 177.1500, p. 234

Welgos, R.J. (1982) *Polyamides (plastics).* In: Mark, H.F., Othmer, D.F., Overberger, C.G. & Seaborg, G.T., eds, *Kirk-Othmer Encyclopedia of Chemical Technology*, 3rd ed., Vol. 18, New York, John Wiley & Sons, pp. 406-425

Yoon, J.S., Mason, J.M., Valencia, R., Woodruff, R.C. & Simmering, S. (1985) Chemical mutagenesis testing in *Drosophila*. IV. Results of 45 coded compounds tested for the National Toxicology Program. *Environ. Mutagenesis, 7*, 349-367

CAPROLACTAM

This substance was considered by a previous Working Group, in February 1978 (IARC, 1979). Since that time, new data have become available, and these have been incoporated into the monograph and taken into consideration in the present evaluation.

1. Chemical and Physical Data

1.1 Synonyms and trade names

Chem. Abstr. Services Reg. No.: 105-60-2

Chem. Abstr. Name: 2*H*-Azepin-2-one, hexahydro-

IUPAC Systematic Name: Hexahydro-2*H*-azepin-2-one

Synonyms: 6-Aminocaproic acid lactam; aminocaproic lactam; 1-aza-2-cycloheptanone; 2-azacycloheptanone; 2*H*-azepin-7-one, hexahydro-; 6-caprolactam; ε-caprolactam; ω-caprolactam; caprolactam monomer; cyclohexanone iso-oxime; 2-A epinone, hexahydro-; hexahydro-2-azepinone; hexamethylenimine, 2-oxo-; 6-hexanelactam; hexanoic acid, 6-amino-, lactam; hexanoic acid, 6-amino-, cyclic lactam; hexanolactam; hexanone isoxime; 1,6-hexolactam; 2-ketohexamethyleneimine; 2-ketohexamethylenimine; NCI-C50646; 2-oxohexamethyleneimine; 2-oxohexamethylenimine; 2-perhydroazepinone

Trade names: A1030; A1030N0; Akulon; Akulon M 2W; Alkamid; Amilan CM 1001; Amilan CM 1011; Amilan CM 1001C; Amilan CM 1001G; ATM 2 (nylon); Bonamid; Capran 80; Capran 77C; Caprolon B; Caprolon V; Capron; Capron 8250; Capron 8252; Capron 8253; Capron 8256; Capron B; Capron GR 8256; Capron 8257; Capron GR 8258; Capron PK 4; Chemlon; CM 1001; CM 1011; CM 1031; CM 1041; Danamid; Dull 704; Durethan BK; Durethan BK 30S; Durethan BKV 30H; Durethan BKV 55H; Ertalon 6Sa; Extrom 6N; Grilon; Itamid; Itamid 250; Itamide 25; Itamide 35; Itamide 250; Itamide 350; Itamide 250G; Itamide S; Kaprolit; Kaprolit B; Kaprolon; Kaprolon B; Kapromin; Kapron; Kapron A; Kapron B; KS 30P; Maranyl F 114; Maranyl F 124; Maranyl F 500; Metamid; Miramid H 2; Miramid WM 55; Nylon A1035SF; Nylon CM 1031; Nylon X 1051; Orgamide; Orgamid RMNOCD; P 6 (polyamide); PA 6; PA 6 (polymer); PK 4; PKA; Plaskin 8200; Plaskon 201; Plaskon 8201; Plaskon 8205;

Plaskon 8207; Plaskon 8252; Plaskon 8202C; Plaskon 8201HS; Plaskon XP 607; Polyamide PK 4; Relon P; Renyl MV; SIPAS 60; Spencer 401; Spencer 601; Steelon; Stilon; Stylon; Tarlon X-A; Tarlon XB; Tarnamid T; Tarnamid T 2; Tarnamid T 27; TNK 2G5; Torayca N 6; UBE 1022B; Ultramid B 3; Ultramid B 4; Ultramid B 5; Ultramid BMK; Vidlon; Widlon; Zytel 211.

1.2 Structural and molecular formulae and molecular weight

$C_6H_{11}NO$ Mol. wt: 113.16

1.3 Chemical and physical properties of the pure substance

(a) *Description*: White, hygroscopic, crystalline solid (Hawley, 1981; Fisher & Crescentini, 1982; Sax, 1984)

(b) *Boiling-point*: 139°C at 12 mm Hg (Weast, 1984); 266.9°C at 760 mm Hg (Fisher & Crescentini, 1982)

(c) *Melting-point*: 69-71°C (Weast, 1984)

(d) *Density*: d_4^{75} 1.02 (Windholz, 1983)

(e) *Spectroscopy data*: Ultraviolet (Grasselli & Ritchey, 1975; National Toxicology Program, 1982), infrared (Sadtler Research Laboratories, 1980; prism [208[a]], grating [15262]), nuclear magnetic resonance (Sadtler Research Laboratories, 1980; proton [6492], C-13 [1620]) and mass spectral data (NIH/EPA Chemical Information System, 1983) have been reported.

(f) *Solubility*: Soluble in water (525 g/100 g at 25°C) and benzene; very soluble in ethanol and chloroform (Fisher & Crescentini, 1982; Weast, 1984); soluble in chlorinated solvents, petroleum distillates, cyclohexene and dimethyl formamide (Hawley, 1981; Windholz, 1983)

---

[a]Spectrum number in Sadtler compilation

(g) *Volatility*: Vapour pressure, 0.001 mm Hg at 20°C; relative vapour density (air = 1), 3.91; saturation concentration, 6 mg/m³ at 20°C (Verschueren, 1983)

(h) *Stability*: Flash-point, 125°C (open- or closed-cup); stabilized with alkalis (Fisher & Crescentini, 1982; Windholz, 1983); emits toxic fumes of nitric oxide when heated to decomposition (Sax, 1984)

(i) *Reactivity*: Hygroscopic (Windholz, 1983); can be hydrolysed, *N*-alkylated, *O*-alkylated, nitrosated, halogenated and subjected to many other reactions (Fisher & Crescentini, 1982)

(j) *Conversion factor*: mg/m³ = 4.63 × ppm[a]

1.4 Technical products and impurities

Caprolactam is available commercially in both molten and flake forms. The chemical is normally shipped in the molten form. Typical product specifications are as follows: appearance, white crystalline solid; solidification point (dry basis), 69°C min; water, 0.1% max; iron, 0.5 mg/kg max; cyclohexanone oxime, 10 mg/kg max; water insolubles, 10 mg/kg max (Allied Corp., 1982).

2. Production, Use, Occurrence and Analysis

2.1 Production and use

(a) Production

Caprolactam was first prepared by Gabriel and Maas in 1899 (Sweeny, 1968), but its potential economic importance was not realized until 1938 when it was polymerized by I.G. Farben in Germany. New and improved processes have been developed in several countries for the polymerization of caprolactam and for the commercial preparation of the monomer for use in the production of Nylon 6 (see IARC, 1979) fibres and plastics (Fisher & Crescentini, 1982).

Caprolactam is commonly prepared *via* the Beckmann rearrangement of cyclohexanone oxime. Selection of a particular process depends largely on the availability and cost of the feedstocks and the efficiency of their conversion to caprolactam. One US firm produces caprolactam by conversion of phenol to cyclohexanone by liquid-phase catalytic hydrogenation, reaction of cyclohexanone with hydroxylamine sulphate (produced in aqueous

---

[a]Calculated from: mg/m³ = (molecular weight/24.45) × ppm, assuming standard temperature (25°C) and pressure (760 mm Hg)

solution by the conventional Raschig process) to produce cyclohexanone oxime, and quantitative conversion of the oxime to caprolactam by the Beckmann rearrangement (Fisher & Crescentini, 1982).

In a process used in the Federal Republic of Germany, cyclohexane is oxidized to cyclohexanone by catalytic air oxidation. Hydroxylamine sulphate, used to prepare the cyclohexanone oxime, is produced by direct hydrogenation of nitric oxide over palladium catalyst. Cyclohexane can be converted directly to cyclohexanone oxime by the reaction of cyclohexane with nitrosyl chloride in the presence of ultraviolet light. In an alternative process, toluene is oxidized to benzoic acid, which is then hydrogenated over palladium catalyst to cyclohexanecarboxylic acid, followed by direct conversion to caprolactam by nitrosation with nitrosylsulphuric acid (Fisher & Crescentini, 1982).

Caprolactam has been produced commercially in the USA since 1955 (Saunders, 1982). Total annual world production capacity in 1985 was estimated to be more than 3 million tonnes. US capacity is about 560 000 tonnes (Anon., 1985), and production in 1983 was 445 000 tonnes, up from 298 000 tonnes in 1973. Two US firms produce caprolactam for internal consumption in the manufacture of Nylon 6 resins and fibres, while the third US producer sells all of its caprolactam externally (Fisher & Crescentini, 1982).

Europe has major production facilities for caprolactam (in thousand tonnes in 1980): total (1460), Belgium (230), Federal Republic of Germany (200), The Netherlands (200), Italy (170), Poland (115), the UK (65), the German Democratic Republic (60), Czechoslovakia (45). Spain and Switzerland had a combined capacity of 35 000 tonnes and Romania, Bulgaria, Hungary and Yugoslavia a total production capacity of 130 000 tonnes. The USSR had a total capacity of 260 000 tonnes (Fisher & Crescentini, 1982).

Japan had a total annual production capacity of 430 000 tonnes in 1980, which was divided between four major companies. Other Asian countries had the capacity to produce 280 000 tonnes a year, the Republic of Korea (40 000) and Taiwan (45 000) being the two major producers. India, Turkey and China also produce caprolactam (Fisher & Crescentini, 1982).

Latin America was expected to increase its production to 250 000 tonnes in 1985 with the construction of new facilities in Mexico (145 000). Brazil (35 000) and Argentina (70 000) are now the major South American producers (Fisher & Crescentini, 1982).

(b) Use

The major use of caprolactam is in the production of polycaprolactam, commonly known as Nylon 6. In the USA, 89% of the polymer is produced as fibres, 10% as resins and 1% for miscellaneous uses. Of the Nylon 6 fibres produced in the USA, 70% are used in rugs and carpets, 15% for textiles and clothing and 15% for tyre cords. Of the resins produced, 65% are used in automobile parts and 35% for wire and cable insulation. Nylon 6 is also used in additives to floor polishes, plasticizers for concrete patching cement, and dye stabilizers, and to manufacture brush bristles.

In western Europe, 70% of the caprolactam produced is used in Nylon 6 fibres and 30% for Nylon 6 resins. In Japan, about 80% is used to produce Nylon 6 fibres.

(c) Regulatory status and guidelines

Occupational exposure limits to caprolactam have been set by 16 countries by regulation or recommended guideline (Table 1).

The US Food and Drug Administration (1984) permits the use of caprolactam-(ethylene-ethyl acrylate) graft polymers as a component of side-seam cements intended for use in contact with food. Nylon 6 may be used for processing, handling and packaging food.

Table 1. National occupational exposure limits for caprolactam [dust (vapour)][a]

Country	Year	Concentration (mg/m³) dust (vapour)	Interpretation[b]
Australia	1978	1 (20)	TWA
Belgium	1978	1 (20)	TWA
Bulgaria	1971	10 (--)	Ceiling
Finland	1981	1 (20)	TWA
		3 (40)	Ceiling
German Democratic Republic	1979	10 (10)	TWA
		30 (30)	Ceiling
Germany, Federal Republic of	1984	25 (25)	TWA
Hungary	1974	10 (--)	Ceiling
Italy	1978	1 (20)	TWA
The Netherlands	1978	1 (20)	TWA
Poland	1976	10 (--)	Ceiling
Romania	1975	5 (--)	TWA
		10 (--)	Ceiling
Switzerland	1978	1 (25)	TWA
UK	1985	1 (20)	TWA
		3 (40)	STEL
USA (ACGIH)	1984	1 (20)	TWA
		3 (40)	STEL
USSR	1980	10 (--)	Ceiling
Yugoslavia	1971	200 (--)	Ceiling

[a]From International Labour Office (1980); Työsuojeluhallitus (1981); American Conference of Governmental Industrial Hygienists (ACGIH) (1984); Deutsche Forschungsgemeinschaft (1984); Health and Safety Executive (1985)

[b]TWA, time-weighted average; STEL, short-term exposure limit

2.2 Occurrence

(a) Natural occurrence

It is not known whether caprolactam occurs as a natural product.

(b) Occupational exposure

Concentrations of 20-40 mg/ m³ caprolactam were detected in a polymerization plant and in a weaving workshop (Lefaux, 1968). Workers were exposed to vapour condensation and dust containing an atmospheric concentration of 61 mg/ m³ caprolactam during fibre spinning (Hohensee, 1951). Air concentrations of up to 65 mg/ m³ caprolactam were reported in a monomer plant and up to 460 mg/ m³ in a polymerization plant (Ferguson & Wheeler, 1973). Levels of <0.6-18.2 mg/ m³ were reported in a plant manufacturing rayon filament (Fajen et al., 1982).

(c) Water

In a study of the suitability of using drinking-water supply pipes made of Nylon 6, the concentration of caprolactam in water after 1.5 days at 40°C was 1.06 mg/ l (Sheftel & Sova, 1974).

Caprolactam has been reported to be present in trace amounts in waste-waters from Nylon 6 plants in Japan (15 mg/ l) (Otsubo et al., 1974) and the USSR (Pevzner & Melent'eva, 1975). The monomer has been detected in (1) finished drinking-water in the USA (Safe Drinking Water Committee, 1977); (2) effluent water from landfill leachate in Delaware (Shackelford & Keith, 1976); (3) groundwater run-off from a shallow radioactive waste burial site, at a concentration of 0.3 μg/ l (Toste et al., 1984); and (4) the final effluent waste-water from a dye manufacturing plant, at levels of 36-150 μg/ l (Games & Hites, 1977). Due to its high solubility in water, caprolactam reportedly leaches out of polyamide fibre clothing placed in an aqueous solution containing components simulating perspiration (Statsek & Ivanova, 1978).

2.3 Analysis

Particulate caprolactam in air has been collected on glass fibre filters, extracted with dichloromethane and analysed by gas chromatography with flame ionization detection, in a detection range of 0.5-50 mg/ sample (Nelson, 1980).

Gutiérrez Jodra et al. (1980) have suggested using an impinger with dichloromethane for sample collection in air and using gas chromatography/ flame ionization detection, and have reported a linear response to concentrations of caprolactam in dichloromethane from 1-150 ppm (0-15 mg/ m³ air).

A method for the analysis of caprolactam in powdered rodent feed developed for the carcinogenesis study of the US National Toxicology Program (1982) involves extraction with methanol and gas chromatography with flame ionization detection and was used for concentrations in the range of 0.3-1.6% in feed.

3. Biological Data Relevant to the Evaluation of Carcinogenic Risk to Humans

3.1 Carcinogenicity studies in animals

Oral administration

Mouse: Groups of 50 male and 50 female B6C3F$_1$ mice, six weeks of age, were fed a diet containing 7500 or 15 000 mg/kg (ppm) caprolactam (minimum purity, >99.5%) for 103 weeks. An equal number of untreated mice of each sex served as controls. All surviving animals (>76%) were killed at 105 weeks. Slight decreases in body-weight gains were noted in animals of each sex. No treatment-related tumour was observed (National Toxicology Program, 1982).

Rat: Groups of 50 male and 50 female Fischer 344/N rats, six weeks of age, were fed a diet containing 3750 or 7500 mg/kg (ppm) caprolactam (minimum purity, >99.5%) for 103 weeks. An equal number of untreated rats of each sex served as untreated controls. All surviving animals (>64%) were killed at 105 weeks. Slight decreases in body-weight gains were observed in animals of each sex. No treatment-related tumour was observed (National Toxicology Program, 1982).

3.2 Other relevant biological data

(*a*)   *Experimental systems*

Toxic effects

The USSR literature on this topic has been summarized (Izmerov, 1983).

The oral LD$_{50}$ of caprolactam in male and female B6C3F$_1$ mice was 2.1 and 2.5 g/kg bw, respectively, and that in male and female Fischer 344/N rats was 1.6 and 1.2 g/kg bw, respectively (National Toxicology Program, 1982). The oral LD$_{50}$ in mice has also been reported to be 1 g/kg bw (Lomonova, 1966). The LC$_{50}$ for caprolactam dust in mice and rats exposed for 2 h was 450 mg/m^3 (100 ppm) and 300 mg/m^3 (65 ppm), respectively (Izmerov, 1983). In mice, the LD$_{50}$ by subcutaneous injection was 0.75 g/kg bw, by intraperitoneal injection, 0.57 g/kg bw, and by intravenous injection, 0.48 g/kg bw (Hohensee, 1951).

When male rats were exposed for 4 h per day to 125 mg/m^3 (27 ppm) caprolactam dust for 2.5 months, disturbances in nervous system function (increasing excitability), gonads (changes in spermatogenesis), respiratory system (decreased respiratory rate) and urinary function (decreased excretion of chloride) were observed. No adverse effect was noted in rats exposed to 11 mg/m^3 (Gabrielyan *et al.*, 1975).

Effects on reproduction and prenatal toxicity

Exposure of female rats to concentrations of 140 and 475 mg/m³ (30 or 100 ppm) caprolactam dust disrupted the oestrous cycle and reduced the proportion of inseminated rats that became pregnant (Khadzhieva, 1969a). [The Working Group noted that it was unclear whether these effects were seen in both groups.] Khadzhieva (1969b) also exposed rats to these concentrations for 4 h daily on gestation days 1-5, 6-12 or on day 13 after parturition; both concentrations increased pre- and post-implantation intrauterine deaths and reduced foetal body weight.

When pregnant Swiss-Webster mice were treated by oral intubation with 6.5-6.7 mg/kg bw ¹⁴C-caprolactam, rapid transfer of the radioactivity across the placenta was demonstrated by whole-body autoradiography, with near-complete elimination from the foetal and maternal compartments 24 h after treatment (Waddell *et al.*, 1984).

In male rats exposed for 4 h per day to 125 mg/m³ (27 ppm) caprolactam dust, spermatogenesis was reduced after 2.5 months. No effect was seen in animals exposed to 11 mg/m³ (2.4 ppm) (Gabrielyan *et al.*, 1975).

Absorption, distribution, excretion and metabolism

After its intraperitoneal injection to rats, caprolactam is excreted partly unchanged and partly as ε-aminocaproic acid. Three rabbits that received a single intraperitoneal injection of 400 mg/kg bw caprolactam excreted 9, 10 and 22% of the dose as unchanged lactam in the urine and faeces, but no additional amino acid could be detected in the urine (Goldblatt *et al.*, 1954).

The distribution of ¹⁴C-caprolactam was studied by whole-body autoradiography in male and female mice 3 h after oral administration of 6.4-6.9 mg/kg bw. Radioactivity was rapidly absorbed from the stomach and distributed throughout the entire animal; there was efficient elimination by the kidneys and liver. Material secreted by the liver into bile and intestinal contents did not appear to be reabsorbed *via* the enterohepatic circulation (Waddell *et al.*, 1984).

Mutagenicity and other short-term tests

Caprolactam (purity, >99%) was not mutagenic to *Salmonella typhimurium* TA1535, TA1537, TA1538, TA98 or TA100 when tested at up to 50 000 μg/plate in the presence or absence of a metabolic system (S9) from the liver of Aroclor-induced rats. Concentrations of up to 11 250 μg/ml failed to induce 6-thioguanine-resistant mutants in Chinese hamster ovary cells in the presence or absence of S9. In secondary cultures of Syrian hamster embryo cells, negative results were obtained in a focus assay for cell transformation (up to 6687 μg/ml) and for enhancement of viral cell transformation (SA7) (up to 10 000 μg/ml) (Greene *et al.*, 1979).

Recently, caprolactam was tested in a large number and variety of in-vitro short-term tests conducted at 59 laboratories engaged in the Collaborative Study on Short-term Tests for Genotoxicity and Carcinogenicity of the International Programme on Chemical Safety (Ashby *et al.*, 1985) (Table 2).

Table 2. Results of short-term tests on caprolactam

Test system	Organism/assay[a]	Reported results		Comments	Reference
		Without exogenous metabolic system	With exogenous metabolic system		
PROKARYOTES					
Mutation	*Salmonella typhimurium* TM 677 (forward mutation)	Negative	Negative	Tested at up to 500 μg/ml	Liber (1985)
	Salmonella typhimurium (reverse mutation)	Negative	Negative	Tested at up to 10 000 μg/plate	Baker & Bonin (1985); Matsushima *et al.* (1985); Rexroat & Probst (1985); Zeiger & Haworth (1985)
FUNGI					
Mutation	*Saccharomyces cerevisiae* XVI85-14C (reverse mutation)	Negative	Positive	At 100-2000 μg/ml	Harrington & Nestmann (1985)
	Saccharomyces cerevisiae XVI85-14C (reverse mutation; his$^-$/his$^+$; trp$^-$/trp$^+$)	Positive	Negative	At 100-800 μg/ml, at pH 4.1 and pH 6.3	Mehta & von Borstel (1985)
	Saccharomyces cerevisiae XVI85-14C (reverse mutation; arg$^-$/arg$^+$)	Positive	Positive	At 200-800 μg/ml, at pH 6.3	Mehta & von Borstel (1985)
	Saccharomyces cerevisiae D6, DG1-M, D7, PV-2, PV-3, RM52 (reverse mutation)	Negative	Negative	Tested at up to 5000 μg/ml	Arni (1985); Inge-Vechtomov *et al.* (1985); Mehta & von Borstel (1985); Parry & Eckardt (1985a,b)
	Saccharomyces cerevisiae PV-1 (forward mutation)	Negative	Negative	Tested at up to 1000 μg/ml	Inge-Vechtomov *et al.* (1985)

Table 2 (contd)

Test system	Organism/assay[a]	Reported results Without exogenous metabolic system	With exogenous metabolic system	Comments	Reference
	Saccharomyces cerevisiae D5 (petite mutation)	Negative	Not tested	Tested at up to 2000 μg/ml	Ferguson (1985)
	Schizosaccharomyces pombe P1 (forward mutation)	Negative	Negative	Tested at up to 1900 μg/ml	Loprieno et al. (1985)
	Aspergillus nidulans B5 (forward mutation)	Negative	Not tested	Tested at up to 1000 μg/ml	Carere et al. (1985)
	Saccharomyces cerevisiae D7, JD1, PV-2, PV-3 (gene conversion)	Negative	Negative	Tested at up to 5000 μg/ml	Arni (1985); Brooks et al. (1985); Inge-Vechtomov et al. (1985); Parry & Eckardt (1985a)
	Saccharomyces cerevisiae D7-144 (gene conversion)	Negative	Negative	Tested at pH 4.1 at up to 100 μg/ml	Mehta & von Borstel (1985)
	Sacchromyces cerevisiae D7-144 (gene conversion)	Positive	Positive	At 400-800 μg/ml, at pH 6.3	Mehta & von Borstel (1985)
	Saccharomyces cerevisiae D6, D61-M, D7, PV-2, PV-3 (mitotic crossing-over)	Negative	Negative	Tested at up to 15 000 μg/ml	Arni (1985); Inge-Vechtomov et al. (1985); Parry & Eckardt (1985a,b); Zimmermann et al. (1985)
	Aspergillus nidulans P1 (mitotic crossing-over)	Negative	Not tested	Tested at up to 500 μg/ml	Carere et al. (1985)
Chromosomal effects	*Saccharomyces cerevisiae* D61M (aneuploidy)	Equivocal	Not tested	Tested at up to 15 000 μg/ml	Zimmermann et al. (1985)
	Saccharomyces cerevisiae D61M, D6 (aneuploidy)	Negative	Negative	Tested at up to 5000 μg/ml	Parry & Eckardt (1985b)

Table 2 (contd)

Test system	Organism/assay[a]	Reported results		Comments	Reference
		Without exogenous metabolic system	With exogenous metabolic system		
	Aspergillus nidulans P1 (aneuploidy)	Negative	Not tested	Tested at up to 500 μg/ml	Carere *et al.* (1985)
INSECTS					
Mutation	*Drosophila melanogaster* (wing spots)	Positive	Not tested	Tested at 442-1768 mM (6 h) and 8.8-44.2 mM (96 h)	Würgler *et al.* (1985)
	Drosophila melanogaster (eye spots)	Positive	Not tested	At 400 mM	Fujikawa *et al.* (1985)
	Drosophila melanogaster (eye spots)	Positive	Not tested	At 5 mM	Vogel (1985)
MAMMALIAN CELLS IN VITRO					
DNA damage	Chinese hamster ovary cells (single-strand breaks)	Negative	Negative	Tested at up to 100 mM	Douglas *et al.* (1985); Lakhanisky & Hendrickx (1985)
	Primary rat hepatocytes (single-strand breaks)	Negative	Not tested	Tested at up to 3390 μg/ml	Bradley (1985)
	Primary rat hepatocytes (unscheduled DNA synthesis)	Negative	Not tested	Tested at up to 10 mM	Glauert *et al.* (1985); Probst & Hill (1985); Williams *et al.* (1985)
	HeLa S3 cells (unscheduled DNA synthesis)	Negative	Negative	Tested at up to 1 mM	Barrett, R.H. (1985); Martin & Campbell (1985)

Table 2 (contd)

Test system	Organism/assay[a]	Reported results		Comments	Reference
		Without exogenous metabolic system	With exogenous metabolic system		
Mutation	Chinese hamster V79 cells (6TG^s/6TG^r)	Negative	Negative	Tested at up to 4000 μg/ml	Fox & Delow (1985); Kuroda et al. (1985)
	Chinese hamster V79 cells (8AG^s/8AG^r)	Negative	Negative	No dose indicated	Lee & Webber (1985)
	Chinese hamster V79 cells (Oua^s/Oua^r)	Not tested	Negative	Tested at up to 1mM	Kuroki & Munakata (1985)
	Chinese hamster ovary cells (6TG^s/6TG^r; Oua^s/Oua^r)	Negative	Negative	Tested at up to 2000 μg/ml	Zdzienicka & Simons (1985)
	Mouse lymphoma L5178Y cells (TFT^s/TFT^r)	Negative	Negative	Tested at up to 11 320 μg/ml	Amacher & Turner (1985); Lee & Webber (1985); Myhr et al. (1985); Oberly et al. (1985)
	Mouse lymphoma L5178Y cells (BrdUrd^s/BrdUrd^r; 6TG^s/6TG^r)	Negative	Negative	Tested at up to 15 000 μg/ml	Knaap & Langebroek (1985)
	Mouse lymphoma L5178Y cells (TFT^s/TFT^r; Oua^s/Oua^r)	Uncertain	Not tested	Tested at up to 1000 μg/ml	Styles et al. (1985)
	Mouse lymphoma L5178Y cells (6TG^s/6TG^r)	Negative	Negative	Tested at up to 200 μg/ml (fluctuation test)	Garner & Campbell (1985)
	Mouse BALB/c 3T3 cells (Oua^s/Oua^r)	Not tested	Uncertain	Tested at up to 15 000 μg/ml	Matthews et al. (1985)
	Human lymphoblastoid TK6 cells (TFT^s/TFT^r)	Negative	Negative	Tested at up to 8000 μg/ml	Crespi et al. (1985)

Table 2 (contd)

Test system	Organism/assay[a]	Reported results		Comments	Reference
		Without exogenous metabolic system	With exogenous metabolic system		
	Human lymphoblastoid AHH-1 cells (6TG^s/6TG^r)	Negative	Not tested	Tested at up to 5000 µg/ml	Crespi et al. (1985)
Chromosomal effects	Chinese hamster ovary cells (aberrations)	Negative	Negative	Tested at up to 150 mM	Gulati et al. (1985); Natarajan et al. (1985); Palitti et al. (1985)
	Chinese hamster liver cells (aberrations)	Negative	Not tested	Tested at up to 2000 µg/ml	Danford (1985)
	Chinese hamster lung cells (aberrations)	Negative	Positive	Tested at up to 12 000 µg/ml; positive only at highest dose	Ishidate & Sofuni (1985)
	Rat liver RL4 cells (aberrations)	Negative	Not tested	Tested at up to 1000 µg/ml	Priston & Dean (1985)
	Human lymphocytes (aberrations)	Positive	Positive	At 270–2750 µg/ml	Howard et al. (1985)
	Chinese hamster ovary cells (sister chromatid exchange)	Negative	Negative	Tested at up to 150 mM	Douglas et al. (1985); Gulati et al. (1985); Lane et al. (1985); Natarajan et al. (1985)
	Chinese hamster V79 cells (sister chromatid exchange)	Negative	Negative	Tested at up to 50 mM	van Went (1985)
	Rat liver RL4 cells (sister chromatid exchange)	Negative	Not tested	Tested at up to 1000 µg/ml	Priston & Dean (1985)

Table 2 (contd)

Test system	Organism/assay[a]	Reported results		Comments	Reference
		Without exogenous metabolic system	With exogenous metabolic system		
	Human lymphocytes (sister chromatid exchange)	Negative	Negative	Tested at up to 1000 µg/ml	Obe et al. (1985)
	Chinese hamster ovary cells (micronuclei)	Negative	Negative	Tested at up to 1 mM	Douglas et al. (1985)
	Chinese hamster liver cells (aneuploidy)	Negative	Not tested	Tested at up to 2000 µg/ml	Danford (1985)
	Chinese hamster lung cells (polyploidy)	Not tested	Positive	At 6000-12 000 µg/ml	Ishidate & Sofuni (1985)
	Rat liver RL4 cells (polyploidy)	Negative	Not tested	Tested at up to 1000 µg/ml	Priston & Dean (1985)
Cell transformation	Syrian hamster embryo cells (morphological)	Positive	Not tested	At 10-100 µg/ml	Barrett, J.C. & Lamb (1985)
	Syrian hamster embryo cells (morphological)	Uncertain	Not tested	Tested at up to 300 µg/ml	Sanner & Rivedal (1985)
	Mouse C3H 10T1/2 cells (morphological)	Positive	Uncertain	At 4570 µg/ml	Lawrence & McGregor (1985)
	Mouse C3H 10T1/2 cells (morphological)	Negative	Not tested	Tested at up to 1000 µg/ml	Nesnow et al. (1985)
	Mouse BALB/c 3T3 A31-1-13 cells (morphological)	Negative	Positive	At 2500-7500 µg/ml; metabolic system was rat-liver cells plus 12-0-tetradecanoyl-phorbol 13-acetate	Matthews et al. (1985)

Table 2 (contd)

Test system	Organism/assay[a]	Reported results		Comments	Reference
		Without exogenous metabolic system	With exogenous metabolic system		
	Rat embryo (retrovirus-infected) cells (anchorage independence)	Negative	Not tested	Tested at up to 50 μg/ml	Suk & Humphreys (1985)
	Syrian hamster embryo cells/SA7 virus (enhancement of viral transformation)	Negative	Not tested	Tested at up to 44 mM	Hatch & Anderson (1985)
Inhibition of metabolic cooperation	Chinese hamster V79 cells (6TG^r/6TG^s; 8AG^r/8AG^s)	Negative	Not tested	Tested at up to 3.6 mM	Elmore et al. (1985); Scott et al. (1985); Umeda et al. (1985)

[a]Abbreviations: his, histidine; trp, tryptophan; arg, arginine; 6TG, 6-thioguanine; r, resistant; s, sensitive; 8AG, 8-azaguanine; Oua, ouabain; TFT, trifluorothymidine; BrdUrd, bromodeoxyuridine

Caprolactam showed no activity in the majority of the tests; however, consistently positive results were obtained in tests for somatic mutations in *Drosophila melanogaster*. In tests in which positive results were indicated, the Working Group re-examined the data as described. Caprolactam was reported by two laboratories to induce reverse mutations in *Saccharomyces cerevisiae* XV185-14C. [Although the Working Group confirmed the positive evaluation of the data from one laboratory, close examination of the data from the second laboratory revealed no consistent or dose-related increase in the number of revertants at the loci examined.] Caprolactam was reported by one laboratory to induce gene conversions, but less than a two-fold increase over the level seen in controls was shown.

In two laboratories, statistically-significant positive results were obtained in an eye-spot assay which detects somatic mutations in *D. melanogaster*. In a wing-spot assay for somatic mutation, different larval stages of *D. melanogaster* were fed several doses of caprolactam for 6 or 72 h. Clearly positive results were obtained in the 6-h studies, but results in the 72-h study were only marginally positive.

The significant increase in the incidence of chromosomal aberrations in cultured Chinese hamster lung cells reported by one laboratory was obtained only with the highest dose tested (12 mg/ml) [an extremely high concentration]. In a second laboratory, caprolactam (270-2750 ug/ml) induced statistically significant increases in the incidence of chromosomal aberrations in cultured human lymphocytes obtained from two separate donors.

In a single experiment, positive results were reported with two (10 and 100 μg/ml) of five doses tested in the Syrian hamster embryo transformation assay, but the effect was not clearly dose-related. In the BALB/c 3T3 cell transformation assay, caprolactam (2500-7500 μg/ml) induced a dose-related increase only in the presence of primary rat hepatocytes and 12-*O*-tetradecanoylphorbol 13-acetate. One laboratory reported a weak transforming ability of caprolactam (4570 μg/ml) in C3H 10T1/2 cells. [The Working Group noted that this evaluation was based on only one Type-II and one Type-III focus in 12 flasks.]

(b)   Humans

Toxic effects

Caprolactam causes dermal irritation and sensitization (Antoniev & Gerasimov, 1971; Ferguson & Wheeler, 1973). Functional disorders of the nervous system, genitourinary tract and cardiovascular system have been reported among exposed female workers (Petrov, 1975).

Effects on reproduction and prenatal toxicity

Of 320 workers exposed to caprolactam, cyclohexanone and a mixture of 1,1'-biphenyl and 1,1'-oxybis(benzene) (dinil), 62% showed dyspermia (46% with oligospermia [not defined], 12% with azoospermia and 4% with necrospermia [method of determination not reported]), as compared with 43% of 237 workers exposed only to caprolactam and cyclohexanone (31% with oligospermia, 10% with azoospermia and 2% with necrospermia) and with 25% of 67 controls (22% with oligospermia, 3% with azoospermia and 0 with necrospermia) (Kuchukhidze & Dolidze, 1975). [The Working Group noted that details of sample collection and processing were not reported, and that possible confounding factors, such as abstinence time, mixed chemical exposures, age and smoking habits, were not controlled for.]

Women exposed occupationally to caprolactam were reported to have an increased frequency of a variety of complications during pregnancy (Martynova *et al.*, 1972).

Absorption, distribution, excretion and metabolism
No data were available to the Working Group.

Mutagenicity and chromosomal effects
No data were available to the Working Group.

3.3 Case reports and epidemiological studies of carcinogenicity to humans

No data were available to the Working Group.

4. Summary of Data Reported and Evaluation

4.1 Exposure data

Caprolactam has been used widely since the 1950s in the production of nylon fibres. Occupational exposure to caprolactam occurs in the manufacture of the monomer, during polymerization and in fibre spinning plants.

4.2 Experimental data

Caprolactam was tested for carcinogenicity in mice and rats by oral administration in the diet. No carcinogenic effect was observed.

Caprolactam has not been adequately evaluated for its effects on reproductive and prenatal toxicity.

Caprolactam gave negative results in a wide range of in-vitro short-term tests. It did not induce mutation in *Salmonella typhimurium* in the presence or absence of an exogenous metabolic system, recombination or aneuploidy in fungi, or DNA damage, DNA repair, point mutation, sister chromatid exchange, micronuclei, aneuploidy or polyploidy in cultured mammalian cells. Results of borderline positivity were obtained in tests for gene conversion in yeast and for morphological transformation in cultured mammalian cells. Caprolactam induced somatic-cell mutations in *Drosophila melanogaster*. There is some evidence that it induced point mutations in yeast and chromosomal aberrations in cultured human cells.

Overall assessment of data from short-term tests: Caprolactam[a]

	Genetic activity			Cell transformation
	DNA damage	Mutation	Chromosomal effects	
Prokaryotes		−		
Fungi/Green plants		?	−	
Insects		+[b]		
Mammalian cells (*in vitro*)	−	−	?	?
Mammals (*in vivo*)				
Humans (*in vivo*)				
Degree of evidence in short-term tests for genetic activity: **Inadequate**				Cell transformation: inadequate

[a]The groups into which the table is divided and the symbols '−', '+' and '?' are defined on pp. 19-20 of the Preamble; the degrees of evidence are defined on pp. 20-21.

[b]Somatic mutations

4.3 Human data

No data were available to evaluate the reproductive effects or prenatal toxicity of caprolactam to humans.

No case report or epidemiological study was available to evaluate the carcinogenicity of caprolactam to humans.

4.4 Evaluation[1]

There is *no evidence* for the carcinogenicity of caprolactam to experimental animals.

No data on humans are available.

In the absence of epidemiological data, no evaluation of the carcinogenicity of caprolactam to humans could be made.

---

[1]For definition of the italicized term, see Preamble, p. 18.

5. References

Allied Corp. (1982) *Caprolactam, Nylon 6 monomer* (*Product Data and Material Safety Data Sheet*), Morristown, NJ

Amacher, D.E. & Turner, G.N. (1985) *Tests of gene mutational activity in the L5178Y/TK assay system*. In: Ashby, J., de Serres, F.J., Draper, M., Ishidate, M., Jr, Margolin, B.H., Matter, B.E. & Shelby, M.D., eds, *Progress in Mutation Research*, Vol. 5, *Evaluation of Short-Term Tests for Carcinogens. Report of the International Programme on Chemical Safety's Collaborative Study on In Vitro Assays*, Amsterdam, Elsevier, pp. 487-496

American Conference of Governmental Industrial Hygienists (1984) *Threshold Limit Values for Chemical Substances and Physical Agents in the Work Environment and Biological Exposure Indices with Intended Changes for 1984-85*, Cincinnati, OH, p. 12

Anon. (1985) Caprolactam makers buffetted by aromatics pricing shifts and downstream competition. *Chem. Mark. Rep.*, 15 April, pp. 5, 15

Antoniev, A.A. & Gerasimov, B.S. (1971) Occupational diseases of the skin in the production of caprolactam (Russ.). *Klin. Med.*, *49*, 116-122

Arni, P. (1985) *Induction of various genetic effects in the yeast* Saccharomyces cerevisiae *strain D7*. In: Ashby, J., de Serres, F.J., Draper, M., Ishidate, M., Jr, Margolin, B.H., Matter, B.E. & Shelby, M.D., eds, *Progress in Mutation Research*, Vol. 5, *Evaluation of Short-Term Tests for Carcinogens. Report of the International Programme on Chemical Safety's Collaborative Study on In Vitro Assays*, Amsterdam, Elsevier, pp. 217-224

Ashby, J., de Serres, F.J., Draper, M., Ishidate, M., Jr, Margolin, B.H., Matter, B.E. & Shelby, M.D., eds (1985) *Progress in Mutation Research*, Vol. 5, *Evaluation of Short-Term Tests for Carcinogens. Report of the International Programme on Chemical Safety's Collaborative Study on In Vitro Assays*, Amsterdam, Elsevier

Baker, R.S.U. & Bonin, A.M. (1985) *Tests with the plate-incorporation assay*. In: Ashby, J., de Serres, F.J., Draper, M., Ishidate, M., Jr, Margolin, B.H., Matter, B.E. & Shelby, M.D., eds, *Progress in Mutation Research*, Vol. 5, *Evaluation of Short-Term Tests for Carcinogens. Report of the International Programme on Chemical Safety's Collaborative Study on In Vitro Assays*, Amsterdam, Elsevier, pp. 177-180

Barrett, J.C. & Lamb, P.W. (1985) *Tests with the Syrian hamster embryo cell transformation assay*. In: Ashby, J., de Serres, F.J., Draper, M., Ishidate, M., Jr, Margolin, B.H., Matter, B.E. & Shelby, M.D., eds, *Progress in Mutation Research*, Vol. 5, *Evaluation of Short-Term Tests for Carcinogens. Report of the International Programme on Chemical Safety's Collaborative Study on In Vitro Assays*, Amsterdam, Elsevier, pp. 623-628

Barrett, R.H. (1985) *Assays for unscheduled DNA synthesis in HeLa S3 cells.* In: Ashby, J., de Serres, F.J., Draper, M., Ishidate, M., Jr, Margolin, B.H., Matter, B.E. & Shelby, M.D., eds, *Progress in Mutation Research*, Vol. 5, *Evaluation of Short-Term Tests for Carcinogens. Report of the International Programme on Chemical Safety's Collaborative Study on In Vitro Assays*, Amsterdam, Elsevier, pp. 347-352

Bradley, M.O. (1985) *Measurement of DNA single-strand breaks by alkaline elution in rat hepatocytes.* In: Ashby, J., de Serres, F.J., Draper, M., Ishidate, M., Jr, Margolin, B.H., Matter, B.E. & Shelby, M.D., eds, *Progress in Mutation Research*, Vol. 5, *Evaluation of Short-Term Tests for Carcinogens. Report of the International Programme on Chemical Safety's Collaborative Study on In Vitro Assays*, Amsterdam, Elsevier, pp. 353-357

Brooks, T.M., Gonzalez, L.P., Calvert, R. & Parry, J.M. (1985) *The induction of mitotic gene conversion in the yeast* Saccharomyces cerevisiae *strain JD1.* In: Ashby, J., de Serres, F.J., Draper, M., Ishidate, M., Jr, Margolin, B.H., Matter, B.E. & Shelby, M.D., eds, *Progress in Mutation Research*, Vol. 5, *Evaluation of Short-Term Tests for Carcinogens. Report of the International Programme on Chemical Safety's Collaborative Study on In Vitro Assays*, Amsterdam, Elsevier, pp. 225-228

Carere, A., Conti, G., Conti, L. & Crebelli, R. (1985) *Assays in Aspergillus nidulans for the induction of forward-mutation in haploid strain 35 and for mitotic nondisjunction, haploidization and crossing-over in diploid strain P1.* In: Ashby, J., de Serres, F.J., Draper, M., Ishidate, M., Jr, Margolin, B.H., Matter, B.E. & Shelby, M.D., eds, *Progress in Mutation Research*, Vol. 5, *Evaluation of Short-Term Tests for Carcinogens. Report of the International Programme on Chemical Safety's Collaborative Study on In Vitro Assays*, Amsterdam, Elsevier, pp. 307-312

Crespi, C.L., Ryan, C.G., Seixas, G.M., Turner, T.R. & Penman, B.W. (1985) *Tests for mutagenic activity using mutation assays at two loci in the human lymphoblast cell lines TK6 and AHH-1.* In: Ashby, J., de Serres, F.J., Draper, M., Ishidate, M., Jr, Margolin, B.H., Matter, B.E. & Shelby, M.D., eds, *Progress in Mutation Research*, Vol. 5, *Evaluation of Short-Term Tests for Carcinogens. Report of the International Programme on Chemical Safety's Collaborative Study on In Vitro Assays*, Amsterdam, Elsevier, pp. 497-516

Danford, N. (1985) *Tests for chromosome aberrations and aneuploidy in the Chinese hamster fibroblast cell line CH1-L.* In: Ashby, J., de Serres, F.J., Draper, M., Ishidate, M., Jr, Margolin, B.H., Matter, B.E. & Shelby, M.D., eds, *Progress in Mutation Research*, Vol. 5, *Evaluation of Short-Term Tests for Carcinogens. Report of the International Programme on Chemical Safety's Collaborative Study on In Vitro Assays*, Amsterdam, Elsevier, pp. 397-411

Deutsche Forschungsgemeinschaft (1984) *Maximal Concentrations in the Workplace and Biological Occupational Limit Value* (Ger.), Part XX, Weinheim, Verlag Chemie GmbH, p.22

Douglas, G.R., Blakey, D.H., Liu-Lee, V.W., Bell, R.D.L. & Bayley, J.M. (1985) *Alkaline sucrose sedimentation, sister-chromatid exchange and micronucleus assays in CHO cells.* In: Ashby, J., de Serres, F.J., Draper, M., Ishidate, M., Jr, Margolin, B.H., Matter, B.E. & Shelby, M.D., eds, *Progress in Mutation Research*, Vol. 5, *Evaluation of Short-Term Tests for Carcinogens. Report of the International Programme on Chemical Safety's Collaborative Study on In Vitro Assays*, Amsterdam, Elsevier, pp. 359-366

Elmore, E., Korytynski, E.A. & Smith, M.P. (1985) *Tests with Chinese hamster V79 inhibition of metabolic cooperation assay.* In: Ashby, J., de Serres, F.J., Draper, M., Ishidate, M., Jr, Margolin, B.H., Matter, B.E. & Shelby, M.D., eds, *Progress in Mutation Research*, Vol. 5, *Evaluation of Short-Term Tests for Carcinogens. Report of the International Programme on Chemical Safety's Collaborative Study on In Vitro Assays*, Amsterdam, Elsevier, pp. 597-612

Fajen, J.M., Jones, J., McCammon, C., Phillips, R., Blade, L., Boyle, T. & Childs, D. (1982) *In-Depth Industrial Hygiene Report of the American ENKA Company*, Cincinnati, OH, National Institute for Occupational Safety and Health, Industrial Hygiene Section, Industrywide Studies Branch, p. 17, Appendix 10

Ferguson, L.R. (1985) *Petite mutagenesis in* Saccharomyces cerevisiae *strain D5.* In: Ashby, J., de Serres, F.J., Draper, M., Ishidate, M., Jr, Margolin, B.H., Matter, B.E. & Shelby, M.D., eds, *Progress in Mutation Research*, Vol. 5, *Evaluation of Short-Term Tests for Carcinogens. Report of the International Programme on Chemical Safety's Collaborative Study on In Vitro Assays*, Amsterdam, Elsevier, pp. 229-234

Ferguson, W.S. & Wheeler, D.D. (1973) Caprolactam vapor exposures. *Am. ind. Hyg. Assoc. J., 34*, 384-389

Fisher, W.B. & Crescentini, L. (1982) *Caprolactam.* In: Mark, H.F., Othmer, D.F., Overberger, C.G. & Seaborg, G.T., eds, *Kirk-Othmer Encyclopedia of Chemical Technology*, 3rd ed., Vol. 18, New York, John Wiley & Sons, pp. 425-436

Fox, M. & Delow, G.F. (1985) *Tests for mutagenic activity at the HGPRT locus in Chinese hamster V79 cells in culture.* In: Ashby, J., de Serres, F.J., Draper, M., Ishidate, M., Jr, Margolin, B.H., Matter, B.E. & Shelby, M.D., eds, *Progress in Mutation Research*, Vol. 5, *Evaluation of Short-Term Tests for Carcinogens. Report of the International Programme on Chemical Safety's Collaborative Study on In Vitro Assays*, Amsterdam, Elsevier, pp. 517-523

Fujikawa, K., Ryo, H. & Kondo, S. (1985) *The* Drosophila *reversion assay using the unstable* zeste-white *somatic eye color system.* In: Ashby, J., de Serres, F.J., Draper, M., Ishidate, M., Jr, Margolin, B.H., Matter, B.E. & Shelby, M.D., eds, *Progress in Mutation Research*, Vol. 5, *Evaluation of Short-Term Tests for Carcinogens. Report of the International Programme on Chemical Safety's Collaborative Study on In Vitro Assays*, Amsterdam, Elsevier, pp. 319-324

Gabrielyan, N.I., Kuchukhidze, G.E. & Chirkova, E.M. (1975) Characterization of the general and gonadotropic action of caprolactam (Russ.). *Gig. Tr. prof. Zabol.*, *10*, 40-42

Games, L.M. & Hites, R.A. (1977) Composition, treatment efficiency, and environmental significance of dye manufacturing plant effluents. *Anal. Chem.*, *49*, 1433-1440

Garner, R.C. & Campbell, J. (1985) *Tests for the induction of mutations to ouabain or 6-thioguanine resistance in mouse lymphoma L5178Y cells*. In: Ashby, J., de Serres, F.J., Draper, M., Ishidate, M., Jr, Margolin, B.H., Matter, B.E. & Shelby, M.D., eds, *Progress in Mutation Research*, Vol. 5, *Evaluation of Short-Term Tests for Carcinogens. Report of the International Programme on Chemical Safety's Collaborative Study on In Vitro Assays*, Amsterdam, Elsevier, pp. 525-529

Glauert, H.P., Kennan, W.S., Sattler, G.L. & Pitot, H.C. (1985) *Assays to measure the induction of unscheduled DNA synthesis in cultured hepatocytes*. In: Ashby, J., de Serres, F.J., Draper, M., Ishidate, M., Jr, Margolin, B.H., Matter, B.E. & Shelby, M.D., eds, *Progress in Mutation Research*, Vol. 5, *Evaluation of Short-Term Tests for Carcinogens. Report of the International Programme on Chemical Safety's Collaborative Study on In Vitro Assays*, Amsterdam, Elsevier, pp. 371-373

Goldblatt, M.W., Farguharson, M.E., Bennett, G. & Askew, B.M. (1954) ϵ-Caprolactam. *Br. J. ind. Med.*, *11*, 1-10

Grasselli, J.G. & Ritchey, W.M., eds (1975) *CRC Atlas of Spectral Data and Physical Constants for Organic Compounds*, Vol. 3, Cleveland, OH, CRC Press, Inc., p. 444

Greene, E.J., Friedman, M.A. & Sherrod, J.A. (1979) In vitro mutagenicity and cell transformation screening of caprolactam. *Environ. Mutagenesis*, *1*, 399-407

Gulati, D.K., Sabharwal, P.S. & Shelby, M.D. (1985) *Tests for the induction of chromosomal aberrations and sister chromatid exchanges in cultured Chinese hamster ovary (CHO) cells*. In: Ashby, J., de Serres, F.J., Draper, M., Ishidate, M., Jr, Margolin, B.H., Matter, B.E. & Shelby, M.D., eds, *Progress in Mutation Research*, Vol. 5, *Evaluation of Short-Term Tests for Carcinogens. Report of the International Programme on Chemical Safety's Collaborative Study on In Vitro Assays*, Amsterdam, Elsevier, pp. 413-426

Gutiérrez Jodra, L., García-Ochoa Soria, F. & Aracil Mira, J. (1980) *Determination of traces of ϵ-caprolactam in the environment* (Sp.). In: *Third Symposium de Higiene Industrial, Madrid 1979*, Madrid, MAPFRE, SA, pp. 81-92

Harrington, T.R. & Nestmann, E.R. (1985) *Tests for mutagenic activity in growing cells of the yeast* Saccharomyces cerevisiae *strain XV185-14C*. In: Ashby, J., de Serres, F.J., Draper, M., Ishidate, M., Jr, Margolin, B.H., Matter, B.E. & Shelby, M.D., eds, *Progress in Mutation Research*, Vol. 5, *Evaluation of Short-Term Tests for Carcinogens. Report of the International Programme on Chemical Safety's Collaborative Study on In Vitro Assays*, Amsterdam, Elsevier, pp. 257-260

Hatch, G.G. & Anderson, T.M. (1985) *Assays for enhanced DNA viral transformation of primary Syrian hamster embryo (SHE) cells.* In: Ashby, J., de Serres, F.J., Draper, M., Ishidate, M., Jr, Margolin, B.H., Matter, B.E. & Shelby, M.D., eds, *Progress in Mutation Research*, Vol. 5, *Evaluation of Short-Term Tests for Carcinogens. Report of the International Programme on Chemical Safety's Collaborative Study on In Vitro Assays*, Amsterdam, Elsevier, pp. 629-638

Hawley, G.G., ed. (1981) *The Condensed Chemical Dictionary*, 10th ed., New York, Van Nostrand Reinhold Co., p. 191

Health and Safety Executive (1985) *Occupational Exposure Limits* (*Guidance Note EH 40/85*), London, Her Majesty's Stationery Office, p. 9

Hohensee, F. (1951) On pharmacological and physiological action of ϵ-caprolactam (Ger.). *Faserforsch. Textiltech.*, *8*, 299-303

Howard, C.A., Sheldon, T. & Richardson, C.R. (1985) *Tests for the induction of chromosomal aberrations in human peripheral lymphocytes in culture.* In: Ashby, J., de Serres, F.J., Draper, M., Ishidate, M., Jr, Margolin, B.H., Matter, B.E. & Shelby, M.D., eds, *Progress in Mutation Research*, Vol. 5, *Evaluation of Short-Term Tests for Carcinogens. Report of the International Programme on Chemical Safety's Collaborative Study on In Vitro Assays*, Amsterdam, Elsevier, pp. 457-467

IARC (1979) *IARC Monographs on the Evaluation of the Carcinogenic Risk of Chemicals to Humans*, Vol. 19, *Some Monomers, Plastics and Synthetic Elastomers, and Acrolein*, Lyon, France, pp. 115-130

Inge-Vechtomov, S.G., Pavlov, Y.I., Noskov, V.N., Repnevskaya, M.V., Karpova, T.S., Khromov-Borisov, N.N., Chekuolene, J. & Chitavichus, D. (1985) *Tests for genetic activity in the yeast* Saccharomyces cerevisiae: *Study of forward and reverse mutation, mitotic recombination and illegitimate mating induction.* In: Ashby, J., de Serres, F.J., Draper, M., Ishidate, M., Jr, Margolin, B.H., Matter, B.E. & Shelby, M.D., eds, *Progress in Mutation Research*, Vol. 5, *Evaluation of Short-Term Tests for Carcinogens. Report of the International Programme on Chemical Safety's Collaborative Study on In Vitro Assays*, Amsterdam, Elsevier, pp. 243-255

International Labour Office (1980) *Occupational Exposure Limits for Airborne Toxic Substances. A Tabular Compilation of Values from Selected Countries*, 2nd (rev.) ed. (*Occupational Safety and Health Services No. 37*), Geneva, pp. 62-65

Ishidate, M., Jr & Sofuni, T. (1985) *The in vitro chromosomal aberration test using Chinese hamster lung (CHL) fibroblast cells in culture.* In: Ashby, J., de Serres, F.J., Draper, M., Ishidate, M., Jr, Margolin, B.H., Matter, B.E. & Shelby, M.D., eds, *Progress in Mutation Research*, Vol. 5, *Evaluation of Short-Term Tests for Carcinogens. Report of the International Programme on Chemical Safety's Collaborative Study on In Vitro Assays*, Amsterdam, Elsevier, pp. 427-432

Izmerov, N.F., ed. (1983) *Scientific Reviews of Soviet Literature on Toxicity and Hazards of Chemicals, Caprolactum* (*No. 35*), Moscow, International Register of Potentially Toxic Chemicals, Centre of International Projects

Khadzhieva, E.D. (1969a) The effect of caprolactam on the sexual cycle (experimental investigation) (Russ.). *Gig. Tr. prof. Zabol.*, *13*, 22-25

Khadzhieva, E.D. (1969b) Effect of caprolactam on the reproductive functions of albino rats. *Hyg. Sanit.*, *34*, 28-32

Knaap, A.G.A.C. & Langebroek, P.B. (1985) *Assays for the induction of gene mutations at the thymidine kinase locus and the hypoxanthine guanine phosphoribosyltransferase locus in L5178Y mouse lymphoma cells in culture.* In: Ashby, J., de Serres, F.J., Draper, M., Ishidate, M., Jr, Margolin, B.H., Matter, B.E. & Shelby, M.D., eds, *Progress in Mutation Research*, Vol. 5, *Evaluation of Short-Term Tests for Carcinogens. Report of the International Programme on Chemical Safety's Collaborative Study on In Vitro Assays*, Amsterdam, Elsevier, pp. 531-536

Kuchukhidze, G.E. & Dolidze, T.G. (1975) Effect of cyclohexanone, caprolactam, and dinil on the reproductive function of workers in industry (Russ.). *Sb. Tr. Nauchno-Issled. Inst. Gig. Tr. prof. Zabol. Tiflis*, *14*, 188-198

Kuroda, Y., Yokoiyama, A. & Kada, T. (1985) *Assays for the induction of mutations to 6-thioguanine resistance in Chinese hamster V79 cells in culture.* In: Ashby, J., de Serres, F.J., Draper, M., Ishidate, M., Jr, Margolin, B.H., Matter, B.E. & Shelby, M.D., eds, *Progress in Mutation Research*, Vol. 5, *Evaluation of Short-Term Tests for Carcinogens. Report of the International Programme on Chemical Safety's Collaborative Study on In Vitro Assays*, Amsterdam, Elsevier, pp. 537-542

Kuroki, T. & Munakata, K. (1985) *Assays for the induction of mutations to ouabain resistance in V79 Chinese hamster cells in culture with cell- or microsome-mediated metabolic activation.* In: Ashby, J., de Serres, F.J., Draper, M., Ishidate, M., Jr, Margolin, B.H., Matter, B.E. & Shelby, M.D., eds, *Progress in Mutation Research*, Vol. 5, *Evaluation of Short-Term Tests for Carcinogens. Report of the International Programme on Chemical Safety's Collaborative Study on In Vitro Assays*, Amsterdam, Elsevier, pp. 543-545

Lakhanisky, T. & Hendrickx, B. (1985) *Induction of DNA single-strand breaks in CHO cells in culture.* In: Ashby, J., de Serres, F.J., Draper, M., Ishidate, M., Jr, Margolin, B.H., Matter, B.E. & Shelby, M.D., eds, *Progress in Mutation Research*, Vol. 5, *Evaluation of Short-Term Tests for Carcinogens. Report of the International Programme on Chemical Safety's Collaborative Study on In Vitro Assays*, Amsterdam, Elsevier, pp. 367-370

Lane, A.M., Phillips, B.J. & Anderson, D. (1985) *Tests for the induction of sister chromatid exchanges in Chinese hamster ovary (CHO) cells in culture.* In: Ashby, J., de Serres, F.J., Draper, M., Ishidate, M., Jr, Margolin, B.H., Matter, B.E. & Shelby, M.D., eds, *Progress in Mutation Research*, Vol. 5, *Evaluation of Short-Term Tests for Carcinogens. Report of the International Programme on Chemical Safety's Collaborative Study on In Vitro Assays*, Amsterdam, Elsevier, pp. 451-455

Lawrence, N. & McGregor, D.B. (1985) *Assays for the induction of morphological transformation in C3H/10T1/2 cells in culture with and without S9-mediated metabolic activation.* In: Ashby, J., de Serres, F.J., Draper, M., Ishidate, M., Jr, Margolin, B.H., Matter, B.E. & Shelby, M.D., eds, *Progress in Mutation Research*, Vol. 5, *Evaluation of Short-Term Tests for Carcinogens. Report of the International Programme on Chemical Safety's Collaborative Study on In Vitro Assays*, Amsterdam, Elsevier, pp. 651-658

Lee, C.G. & Webber, T.D. (1985) *The induction of gene mutations in the mouse lymphoma L5178Y/TK⁺/⁻ assay and the Chinese hamster V79/HGPRT assay.* In: Ashby, J., de Serres, F.J., Draper, M., Ishidate, M., Jr, Margolin, B.H., Matter, B.E. & Shelby, M.D., eds, *Progress in Mutation Research*, Vol. 5, *Evaluation of Short-Term Tests for Carcinogens. Report of the International Programme on Chemical Safety's Collaborative Study on In Vitro Assays*, Amsterdam, Elsevier, pp. 547-554

Lefaux, R. (1968) *Practical Toxicology of Plastics*, Cleveland, OH, CRC Press, pp. 90-92

Liber, H.L. (1985) *Mutation tests with* Salmonella *using 8-azaguanine resistance as the genetic marker.* In: Ashby, J., de Serres, F.J., Draper, M., Ishidate, M., Jr, Margolin, B.H., Matter, B.E. & Shelby, M.D., eds, *Progress in Mutation Research*, Vol. 5, *Evaluation of Short-Term Tests for Carcinogens. Report of the International Programme on Chemical Safety's Collaborative Study on In Vitro Assays*, Amsterdam, Elsevier, pp. 213-216

Lomonova, G.V. (1966) Toxicity of caprolactam (Russ.). *Gig. Tr. prof. Zabol.*, *10*, 54-57

Loprieno, N., Boncristiani, G., Forster, R. & Goldstein, B. (1985) *Assays for forward mutation in* Schizosaccharomyces pombe *strain P1.* In: Ashby, J., de Serres, F.J., Draper, M., Ishidate, M., Jr, Margolin, B.H., Matter, B.E. & Shelby, M.D., eds, *Progress in Mutation Research*, Vol. 5, *Evaluation of Short-Term Tests for Carcinogens. Report of the International Programme on Chemical Safety's Collaborative Study on In Vitro Assays*, Amsterdam, Elsevier, pp. 297-306

Martin, C.N. & Campbell, J. (1985) *Tests for the induction of unscheduled DNA repair synthesis in HeLa cells.* In: Ashby, J., de Serres, F.J., Draper, M., Ishidate, M., Jr, Margolin, B.H., Matter, B.E. & Shelby, M.D., eds, *Progress in Mutation Research*, Vol. 5, *Evaluation of Short-Term Tests for Carcinogens. Report of the International Programme on Chemical Safety's Collaborative Study on n Vitro Assays*, Amsterdam, lsevier, pp. 375-379

Martynova, A.P., Lotis, V.M., Khadzhieva, E.D. & Gaidova, E.S. (1972) Occupational hygiene of women engaged in the production of capron (6-handecanone) fibre (Russ.). *Gig. Tr. prof. Zabol.*, *11*, 9-13

Matsushima, T., Muramatsu, M. & Haresaku, M. (1985) *Mutation tests on* Salmonella typhimurium *by the preincubation method.* In: Ashby, J., de Serres, F.J., Draper, M., Ishidate, M., Jr, Margolin, B.H., Matter, B.E. & Shelby, M.D., eds, *Progress in Mutation Research*, Vol. 5, *Evaluation of Short-Term Tests for Carcinogens. Report of the International Programme on Chemical Safety's Collaborative Study on In Vitro Assays*, Amsterdam, Elsevier, pp. 181-186

Matthews, E.J., DelBalzo, T. & Rundell, J.O. (1985) *Assays for morphological transformation and mutation to ouabain resistance of Balb/c-3T3 cells in culture.* In: Ashby, J., de Serres, F.J., Draper, M., Ishidate, M., Jr, Margolin, B.H., Matter, B.E. & Shelby, M.D., eds, *Progress in Mutation Research*, Vol. 5, *Evaluation of Short-Term Tests for Carcinogens. Report of the International Programme on Chemical Safety's Collaborative Study on In Vitro Assays*, Amsterdam, Elsevier, pp. 639-650

Mehta, R.D. & von Borstel, R.C. (1985) *Tests for genetic activity in the yeast* Saccharomyces cerevisiae *using strains D7-144, XV185-14C and RM52.* In: Ashby, J., de Serres, F.J., Draper, M., Ishidate, M., Jr, Margolin, B.H., Matter, B.E. & Shelby, M.D., eds, *Progress in Mutation Research*, Vol. 5, *Evaluation of Short-Term Tests for Report of the International Programme on Chemical Safety's Collaborative Study on In Vitro Assays*, Amsterdam, Elsevier, pp. 271-284

Myhr, B., Bowers, L. & Caspary, W.J. (1985) *Assays for the induction of gene mutations at the thymidine kinase locus of L5178Y mouse lymphoma cells in culture.* In: Ashby, J., de Serres, F.J., Draper, M., Ishidate, M., Jr, Margolin, B.H., Matter, B.E. & Shelby, M.D., eds, *Progress in Mutation Research*, Vol. 5, *Evaluation of Short-Term Tests for Carcinogens. Report of the International Programme on Chemical Safety's Collaborative Study on In Vitro Assays*, Amsterdam, Elsevier, pp. 555-568

Natarajan, A.T., Bussmann, C.J.M., van Kesteren-van Leeuwen, A.C., Meijers, M. & van Rijn, J.L.S. (1985) *Tests for chromosome aberrations and sister-chromatid exchanges in Chinese hamster ovary (CHO) cells in culture.* In: Ashby, J., de Serres, F.J., Draper, M., Ishidate, M., Jr, Margolin, B.H., Matter, B.E. & Shelby, M.D., eds, *Progress in Mutation Research*, Vol. 5, *Evaluation of Short-Term Tests for Carcinogens. Report of the International Programme on Chemical Safety's Collaborative Study on In Vitro Assays*, Amsterdam, Elsevier, pp. 433-437

National Toxicology Program (1982) *Carcinogenesis Bioassay of Caprolactam (CAS No. 105-60-2) in F344 Rats and B6C3F1 Mice (Feed Study) (Technical Report Series No. 214)*, Research Triangle Park, NC

Nelson, J.H. (1980) *Special Analytical Measurements and Short-term Method Development (US NTIS PB82-114802)*, Cincinnati, OH, National Institute for Occupational Safety and Health, pp. 8-9

Nesnow, S., Curtis, G. & Garland, H. (1985) *Tests with the C3H/10T1/2 clone 8 morphological transformation bioassay.* In: Ashby, J., de Serres, F.J., Draper, M., Ishidate, M., Jr, Margolin, B.H., Matter, B.E. & Shelby, M.D., eds, *Progress in Mutation Research*, Vol. 5, *Evaluation of Short-Term Tests for Carcinogens. Report of the International Programme on Chemical Safety's Collaborative Study on In Vitro Assays*, Amsterdam, Elsevier, pp. 659-664

NIH/EPA Chemical Information System (1983) *Carbon-13 NMR Spectral Search System, Mass Spectral Search System,* and *Infrared Spectral Search System*, Arlington, VA, Information Consultants, Inc.

Obe, G., Hille, A., Jonas, R., Schmidt, S. & Thenhaus, U. (1985) *Tests for the induction of sister-chromatid exchanges in human peripheral lymphocytes in culture.* In: Ashby, J., de Serres, F.J., Draper, M., Ishidate, M., Jr, Margolin, B.H., Matter, B.E. & Shelby, M.D., eds, *Progress in Mutation Research*, Vol. 5, *Evaluation of Short-Term Tests for Carcinogens. Report of the International Programme on Chemical Safety's Collaborative Study on In Vitro Assays*, Amsterdam, Elsevier, pp. 439-442

Oberly, T.J., Bewsey, B.J. & Probst, G.S. (1985) *Tests for the induction of forward mutation at the thymidine kinase locus of L5178Y mouse lymphoma cells in culture.* In: Ashby, J., de Serres, F.J., Draper, M., Ishidate, M., Jr, Margolin, B.H., Matter, B.E. & Shelby, M.D., eds, *Progress in Mutation Research*, Vol. 5, *Evaluation of Short-Term Tests for Carcinogens. Report of the International Programme on Chemical Safety's Collaborative Study on In Vitro Assays*, Amsterdam, Elsevier, pp. 569-582

Otsubo, T., Tajiri, H. & Shinpo, Y. (1974) Spectrophotometric determination of trace amounts of Σ-caprolactam in waste water with iron(III) chloride (Jpn.). *Bunseki Kagaku, 23*, 163-166 [*Chem. Abstr., 81*, 41128p]

Palitti, F., Fiore, M., De Salvia, R., Tanzarella, C., Ricordy, R., Forster, R., Mosesso, P., Astolfi, S. & Loprieno, N. (1985) *Tests for the induction of chromosomal aberrations in Chinese hamster ovary (CHO) cells in culture.* In: Ashby, J., de Serres, F.J., Draper, M., Ishidate, M., Jr, Margolin, B.H., Matter, B.E. & Shelby, M.D., eds, *Progress in Mutation Research*, Vol. 5, *Evaluation of Short-Term Tests for Carcinogens. Report of the International Programme on Chemical Safety's Collaborative Study on In Vitro Assays*, Amsterdam, Elsevier, pp. 443-450

Parry, J.M. & Eckardt, F. (1985a) *The detection of mitotic gene conversion, point mutation and mitotic segregation using the yeast* Saccharomyces cerevisiae *strain D7.* In: Ashby, J., de Serres, F.J., Draper, M., Ishidate, M., Jr, Margolin, B.H., Matter, B.E. & Shelby, M.D., eds, *Progress in Mutation Research*, Vol. 5, *Evaluation of Short-Term Tests for Carcinogens. Report of the International Programme on Chemical Safety's Collaborative Study on In Vitro Assays*, Amsterdam, Elsevier, pp. 261-269

Parry, J.M. & Eckardt, F. (1985b) *The induction of mitotic aneuploidy, point mutation and mitotic crossing-over in the yeast* Saccharomyces cerevisiae *strains D61-M and D6.* In: Ashby, J., de Serres, F.J., Draper, M., Ishidate, M., Jr, Margolin, B.H., Matter, B.E. & Shelby, M.D., eds, *Progress in Mutation Research*, Vol. 5, *Evaluation of Short-Term Tests for Carcinogens. Report of the International Programme on Chemical Safety's Collaborative Study on In Vitro Assays*, Amsterdam, Elsevier, pp. 285-295

Petrov, N.V. (1975) Health status of women working in the chemical fibre industry according to data of medical examinations (Russ.). *Vrach. Delo, 10*, 145-148

Pevzner, I.D. & Melent'eva, N.D. (1975) Analysis of waste waters during production of polyamides (Russ.). *Plast. Massy, 5*, 67-68 [*Chem. Abstr., 83*, 102794t]

Priston, R.A.J. & Dean, B.J. (1985) *Tests for the induction of chromosome aberrations, polyploidy and sister-chromatid exchanges in rat liver (RL₂).* In: Ashby, J., de Serres, F.J., Draper, M., Ishidate, M., Jr, Margolin, B.H., Matter, B.E. & Shelby, M.D., eds, *Progress in Mutation Research*, Vol. 5, *Evaluation of Short-Term Tests for Carcinogens. Report of the International Programme on Chemical Safety's Collaborative Study on In Vitro Assays*, Amsterdam, Elsevier, pp. 387-395

Probst, G.S. & Hill, L.E. (1985) *Tests for the induction of DNA-repair synthesis in primary cultures of adult rat hepatocytes.* In: Ashby, J., de Serres, F.J., Draper, M., Ishidate, M., Jr, Margolin, B.H., Matter, B.E. & Shelby, M.D., eds, *Progress in Mutation Research*, Vol. 5, *Evaluation of Short-Term Tests for Carcinogens. Report of the International Programme on Chemical Safety's Collaborative Study on In Vitro Assays*, Amsterdam, Elsevier, pp. 381-386

Rexroat, M.A. & Probst, G.S. (1985) *Mutation tests with* Salmonella *using the plate-incorporation assay.* In: Ashby, J., de Serres, F.J., Draper, M., Ishidate, M., Jr, Margolin, B.H., Matter, B.E. & Shelby, M.D., eds, *Progress in Mutation Research*, Vol. 5, *Evaluation of Short-Term Tests for Carcinogens. Report of the International Programme on Chemical Safety's Collaborative Study on In Vitro Assays*, Amsterdam, Elsevier, pp. 201-212

Sadtler Research Laboratories (1980) *The Sadtler Standard Spectra Collection, Cumulative Index*, Philadelphia, PA

Safe Drinking Water Committee (1977) *Drinking Water and Health*, Washington DC, National Academy of Sciences, pp. 698-700, 798

Sanner, T. & Rivedal, E. (1985) *Tests with the Syrian hamster embryo (SHE) cell transformation assay.* In: Ashby, J., de Serres, F.J., Draper, M., Ishidate, M., Jr, Margolin, B.H., Matter, B.E. & Shelby, M.D., eds, *Progress in Mutation Research*, Vol. 5, *Evaluation of Short-Term Tests for Carcinogens. Report of the International Programme on Chemical Safety's Collaborative Study on In Vitro Assays*, Amsterdam, Elsevier, pp. 665-671

Saunders, J.H. (1982) *Nylon-6 and Nylon-6,6.* In: Mark, H.F., Othmer, D.F., Overberger, C.G. & Seaborg, G.T., eds, *Kirk-Othmer Encyclopedia of Chemical Technology*, 3rd ed., Vol. 18, New York, John Wiley & Sons, pp. 372-405

Sax, N.I. (1984) *Dangerous Properties of Industrial Materials*, 6th ed., New York, Van Nostrand Reinhold Co., p. 1515

Scott, J.K., Davidson, H. & Nelmes, A.J. (1985) *Assays for inhibition of metabolic cooperation between mammalian cells in culture.* In: Ashby, J., de Serres, F.J., Draper, M., Ishidate, M., Jr, Margolin, B.H., Matter, B.E. & Shelby, M.D., eds, *Progress in Mutation Research*, Vol. 5, *Evaluation of Short-Term Tests for Carcinogens. Report of the International Programme on Chemical Safety's Collaborative Study on In Vitro Assays*, Amsterdam, Elsevier, pp. 613-618

Shackelford, W.M. & Keith, L.H. (1976) *Frequency of Organic Compounds Identified in Water (EPA-600/4-76-062)*, Athens, GA, US Environmental Protection Agency, pp. 96-97

Sheftel, V.O. & Sova, R.E. (1974) Sanitary-chemical study of the migration of a monomer from Kaprolon to water (Russ.). *Gig. Sanit.*, *6*, 93-94 [*Chem. Abstr.*, *81*, 122046n]

Statsek, N.K. & Ivanova, T.P. (1978) Hygienic investigations of synthetic polyamide fabrics and clothing made thereof (Russ.). *Gig. Sanit.*, *10*, 38-41

Styles, J.A., Clay, P. & Cross, M.F. (1985) *Assays for the induction of gene mutations at the thymidine kinase and the Na^+/K^+ ATPase loci in two different mouse lymphoma cell lines in culture*. In: Ashby, J., de Serres, F.J., Draper, M., Ishidate, M., Jr, Margolin, B.H., Matter, B.E. & Shelby, M.D., eds, *Progress in Mutation Research*, Vol. 5, *Evaluation of Short-Term Tests for Carcinogens. Report of the International Programme on Chemical Safety's Collaborative Study on In Vitro Assays*, Amsterdam, Elsevier, pp. 587-596

Suk, W.A. & Humphreys, J.E. (1985) *Assay for the carcinogenicity of chemical agents using enhancement or anchorage-independent survival of retrovirus-infected Fischer rat embryo cells*. In: Ashby, J., de Serres, F.J., Draper, M., Ishidate, M., Jr, Margolin, B.H., Matter, B.E. & Shelby, M.D., eds, *Progress in Mutation Research*, Vol. 5, *Evaluation of Short-Term Tests for Carcinogens. Report of the International Programme on Chemical Safety's Collaborative Study on In Vitro Assays*, Amsterdam, Elsevier, pp. 673-783

Sweeny, W. (1968) *Polyamides (general)*. In: Kirk, R.E. & Othmer, D.F., eds, *Encyclopedia of Chemical Technology*, 2nd ed., Vol. 16, New York, John Wiley & Sons, pp. 29-32

Toste, A.P., Kirby, L.T. & Pahl, T.R. (1984) *Role of organics in the subsurface migration of radionuclides in groundwater*. In: Barney, G.S., Schultz, W.W. & Navratil, J.D., eds, *Geochemical Behaviour of Disposed Radioactive Waste (ACS Symposium Series No. 246)*, Washington DC, American Chemical Society, pp. 251-270

Työsuojeluhallitus (National Finnish Board of Occupational Safety and Health) (1981) *Airborne Contaminants in the Workplace (Safety Bull. 3)* (Finn.), Tampere, p. 16

Umeda, M., Noda, K. & Tanaka, K. (1985) *Assays for inhibition of metabolic cooperation in a microassay method*. In: Ashby, J., de Serres, F.J., Draper, M., Ishidate, M., Jr, Margolin, B.H., Matter, B.E. & Shelby, M.D., eds, *Progress in Mutation Research*, Vol. 5, *Evaluation of Short-Term Tests for Carcinogens. Report of the International Programme on Chemical Safety's Collaborative Study on In Vitro Assays*, Amsterdam, Elsevier, pp. 619-622

US Food and Drug Administration (1984) Food and drugs. *US Code Fed. Regul.*, *Title 21*, Parts 175.105, 177.1500, pp. 126, 234

Verschueren, K. (1983) *Handbook of Environmental Data on Organic Chemicals*, 2nd ed., New York, Van Nostrand Reinhold, pp. 332-333

Vogel, E.W. (1985) *The* Drosophila *somatic recombination and mutation assay (SRM) using the* white-coral *somatic eye color system*. In: Ashby, J., de Serres, F.J., Draper, M., Ishidate, M., Jr, Margolin, B.H., Matter, B.E. & Shelby, M.D., eds, *Progress in Mutation Research*, Vol. 5, *Evaluation of Short-Term Tests for Carcinogens. Report of the International Programme on Chemical Safety's Collaborative Study on In Vitro Assays*, Amsterdam, Elsevier, pp. 313-317

Waddell, W.J., Marlowe, C. & Friedman, M.A. (1984) The distribution of [^{14}C]caprolactam in male, female and pregnant mice. *Food chem. Toxicol.*, *22*, 293-303

Weast, R.C., ed. (1984) *CRC Handbook of Chemistry and Physics*, 65th ed., Boca Raton, FL, CRC Press, p. C-216

van Went, G.F. (1985) *The test for sister-chromatid exchanges in Chinese hamster V79 cells in culture*. In: Ashby, J., de Serres, F.J., Draper, M., Ishidate, M., Jr, Margolin, B.H., Matter, B.E. & Shelby, M.D., eds, *Progress in Mutation Research*, Vol. 5, *Evaluation of Short-Term Tests for Carcinogens. Report of the International Programme on Chemical Safety's Collaborative Study on In Vitro Assays*, Amsterdam, Elsevier, pp. 469-477

Williams, G.M., Tong, C. & Ved Brat, S. (1985) *Tests with the rat hepatocyte primary culture/DNA-repair test*. In: Ashby, J., de Serres, F.J., Draper, M., Ishidate, M., Jr, Margolin, B.H., Matter, B.E. & Shelby, M.D., eds, *Progress in Mutation Research*, Vol. 5, *Evaluation of Short-Term Tests for Carcinogens. Report of the International Programme on Chemical Safety's Collaborative Study on In Vitro Assays*, Amsterdam, Elsevier, pp. 341-345

Windholz, M., ed. (1983) *The Merck Index*, 10th ed., Rahway, NJ, Merck & Co., p. 243

Würgler, F.E., Graf, U. & Frei, H. (1985) *Somatic mutation and recombination test in wings of* Drosophila melanogaster. In: Ashby, J., de Serres, F.J., Draper, M., Ishidate, M., Jr, Margolin, B.H., Matter, B.E. & Shelby, M.D., eds, *Progress in Mutation Research*, Vol. 5, *Evaluation of Short-Term Tests for Carcinogens. Report of the International Programme on Chemical Safety's Collaborative Study on In Vitro Assays*, Amsterdam, Elsevier, pp. 325-340

Zdzienicka, M.Z. & Simons, J.W.I.M. (1985) *Assays for the induction of mutations to 6-thioguanine and ouabain resistance in Chinese hamster ovary (CHO) cells in culture*. In: Ashby, J., de Serres, F.J., Draper, M., Ishidate, M., Jr, Margolin, B.H., Matter, B.E. & Shelby, M.D., eds, *Progress in Mutation Research*, Vol. 5, *Evaluation of Short-Term Tests for Carcinogens. Report of the International Programme on Chemical Safety's Collaborative Study on In Vitro Assays*, Amsterdam, Elsevier, pp. 583-586

Zeiger, E. & Haworth, S. (1985) *Tests with preincubation modification of the* Salmonella/-microsome assay. In: Ashby, J., de Serres, F.J., Draper, M., Ishidate, M., Jr, Margolin, B.H., Matter, B.E. & Shelby, M.D., eds, *Progress in Mutation Research*, Vol. 5, *Evaluation of Short-Term Tests for Carcinogens. Report of the International Programme on Chemical Safety's Collaborative Study on In Vitro Assays*, Amsterdam, Elsevier, pp. 187-199

Zimmermann, F.K., Heinisch, J. & Scheel, I. (1985) *Tests for the induction of mitotic aneuploidy in the yeast* Saccharomyces cerevisiae *strain D61.M*. In: Ashby, J., de Serres, F.J., Draper, M., Ishidate, M., Jr, Margolin, B.H., Matter, B.E. & Shelby, M.D., eds, *Progress in Mutation Research*, Vol. 5, *Evaluation of Short-Term Tests for Carcinogens. Report of the International Programme on Chemical Safety's Collaborative Study on In Vitro Assays*, Amsterdam, Elsevier, pp. 235-242

OTHER MONOMERS

3,3'-DIMETHOXYBENZIDINE-4,4'-DIISOCYANATE

3,3'-Dimethoxybenzidine (*ortho*-dianisidine), the immediate hydrolysis product of 3,3'-dimethoxybenzidine-4,4'-diisocyanate, was considered by two previous Working Groups, in June 1973 and February 1982 (IARC, 1974, 1982).

1. Chemical and Physical Data

1.1 Synonyms and trade names

Chem. Abstr. Services Reg. No.: 91-93-0

Chem. Abstr. Name: 1,1'-Biphenyl, 4,4'-diisocyanato-3,3'-dimethoxy-

IUPAC Systematic Name: 3,3'-Dimethoxy-4,4'-biphenylylene diisocyanate

Synonyms: DADI; dianisidine diisocyanate; 3,3'-dimethoxy-4,4'-biphenyl diisocyanate; 3,3'-dimethoxy-4,4'-biphenylene diisocyanate; 3,3'-dimethoxy-4,4'-biphenylylene isocyanate; 3,3'-dimethoxy-4,4'-biphenylene isocyanic acid ester; 3,3'-dimethoxy-4,4'-diphenylylisocyanate; isocyanic acid, 3,3'-dimethoxy-4,4'-biphenylene ester; NCI-CO2175

1.2 Structural and molecular formulae and molecular weight

$C_{16}H_{12}N_2O_4$

Mol. wt: 296.30

1.3 Chemical and physical properties of the pure substance

(a) *Description*: Grey to brown powder (Hawley, 1981)

(b) *Melting-point*: 112°C (Hawley, 1981)

(c) *Spectroscopy data*: Ultraviolet (National Cancer Institute, 1979a), infrared, nuclear magnetic resonance and mass spectral data (NIH/EPA Chemical Information System, 1983) have been reported.

(d) *Solubility*: Soluble in ketones and esters (Hawley, 1981)

(e) *Stability*: Emits toxic fumes of nitric oxide when heated to decomposition (Sax, 1984); hydrolysed to 3,3'-dimethoxybenzidine

(f) *Conversion factor:* mg/m^3 = 12.1 × ppm^a

1.4 Technical products and impurities

No technical product containing 3,3'-dimethoxybenzidine-4,4'-diisocyanate is available commercially.

2. Production, Use, Occurrence and Analysis

2.1 Production and use

(a) *Production*

3,3'-Dimethoxybenzidine-4,4'-diisocyanate has been prepared by the reaction of dimethoxybenzidine dihydrochloride with phosgene in an aromatic solvent (Shriner *et al.*, 1978). One US company produced 3,3'-dimethoxybenzidine-4,4'-diisocyanate in the 1970s. There is presently no known producer.

(b) *Use*

3,3'-Dimethoxybenzidine-4,4'-diisocyanate can be used in isocyanate-based adhesive systems and as a component of polyurethane elastomers. It provides a high-strength

---

^{a}Calculated from: mg/m^3 = (molecular weight/24.45) × ppm, assuming standard temperature (25°C) and pressure (760 mm Hg)

backbone and acts as a cross-linking intermediate (Hawley, 1981). The US National Cancer Institute (1979b) has characterized 3,3'-dimethoxybenzidine-4,4'-diisocyanate as an experimental chemical with possible uses in coatings, gaskets and shock absorbers.

(*c*) *Regulatory status and guidelines*

Regulatory action has been taken on occupational and environmental exposure to 3,3'-dimethoxybenzidine (especially dimethoxybenzidine-based dyes), but no standard has been set for the diisocyanate. The US National Institute for Occupational Safety and Health (1978) recommended occupational exposure limits for diisocyanates as a class of 0.06 mg/m^3 time-weighted average and 0.24 mg/m^3 ceiling.

2.2 Occurrence

(*a*) *Natural occurrence*

It is not known whether 3,3'-dimethoxybenzidine-4,4'-diisocyanate occurs as a natural product.

(*b*) *Occupational exposure*

No data were available to the Working Group.

2.3 Analysis

In developing an apparatus for generating standard aerosol atmospheres containing 3,3'-dimethoxybenzidine-4,4'-diisocyanate, Meddle and Wood (1968) monitored concentrations of the aerosol by (1) collecting on No. 42 Whatman filter paper, eluting with a standard volume of carbon tetrachloride, and analysing by infrared spectroscopy, or (2) collecting in an absorbing solution, developing a colour, and measuring colorimetrically [details not given].

3. Biological Data Relevant to the Evaluation of Carcinogenic Risk to Humans

3.1 Carcinogenicity studies in animals

(*a*) *Oral administration*

Mouse: Groups of 50 male and 50 female B6C3F1 mice, six weeks old, were given dietary concentrations of 22 000 or 44 000 mg/kg 3,3'-dimethoxybenzidine-4,4'-diisocyanate [purity unspecified, but containing at least two impurities] *ad libitum* for 78 weeks, followed by basal diet for a further 25 weeks, at which time all animals were killed. Diets were prepared daily and a check of stability in the diet showed no decomposition. Groups of 20 male and 20 female mice receiving basal diet only for 103 weeks served as controls. There was no significant difference in survival of treated and control animals: 18/20 (90%) control, 40/50 (80%) low-dose and 46/50 (92%) high-dose males; 18/20 (90%) control, 36/50 (72%) low-dose and 31/50 (62%) high-dose females survived to the end of the experiment. There was no increased incidence of treatment-related tumours (National Cancer Institute, 1979a).

Rat: Groups of 50 male and 50 female Fischer 344/N rats, six weeks of age, received 1500 or 3000 mg/kg bw 3,3'-dimethoxybenzidine-4,4'-diisocyanate (of the same purity as described above) as a 15-30% aqueous suspension containing 9 g sodium chloride, 5 g carboxymethylcellulose, 4 ml polysorbate 80 and 9 mg benzyl alcohol/l, by gavage on five days per week for 22 weeks. Animals were subsequently fed diets containing concentrations of 22 000 or 44 000 mg/kg 3,3'-dimethoxybenzidine-4,4'-diisocyanate for a further 56 weeks and were then kept on basal diet and observed for a further 26 weeks prior to sacrifice. Control groups of 20 male and 20 female rats received the suspending vehicle alone for 22 weeks followed by 82 weeks of basal diet. Survival of both male and female rats at termination of the study (104 weeks) was dose-related: 15/20 (75%) control, 22/50 (44%) low-dose and 16/50 (32%) high-dose males; 15/20 (75%) control, 21/50 (42%) low-dose and 21/50 (42%) high-dose females. A significant increase in the combined incidence of leukaemias and malignant lymphomas was observed: 0/18 control, 18/48 low-dose and 16/46 high-dose males [$p = 0.022$, trend test; $p = 0.001$ (low-dose) and $p = 0.002$ (high-dose), Fisher exact test]; 1/20 control, 8/50 low-dose and 15/48 high-dose females [$p = 0.007$, trend test; $p = 0.016$ (high-dose) Fisher exact test]. Increased incidences of various types of skin tumours were observed on the head, back and inguinal areas in males and females. This increase was statistically significant in both high-dose (14/46; $p = 0.005$, Fisher exact test) and low-dose (17/48; $p = 0.002$, Fisher exact test) males as compared to controls (0/18). A treatment-related increase in the incidence of Zymbal-gland tumours was observed: 1/18 control, 6/48 low-dose and 9/46 high-dose males; 0/20 control, 9/50 low-dose and 6/48 high-dose females. The historical incidence of these neoplasms in untreated Fischer 344/N rats from the same laboratory was 1/300 males and 0/298 females. A dose-related incidence of endometrial stromal polyps was observed in females: 0/20 control, 5/48 low-dose and 10/48 high-dose animals [$p = 0.013$, trend test; $p = 0.022$ (high-dose), Fisher exact test] (National Cancer Institute, 1979a). [The Working Group noted the limited biological significance attached to these lesions by the authors.]

(b) Carcinogenicity of breakdown products

There is *sufficient evidence* for the carcinogenicity of 3,3'-dimethoxybenzidine to experimental animals (IARC, 1982).

3.2 Other relevant biological data

(a) *Experimental systems*

Toxic effects

No data were available to the Working Group.

Effects on reproduction and prenatal toxicity

No data were available to the Working Group.

Absorption, distribution, excretion and metabolism

No data were available to the Working Group.

3,3′-Dimethoxybenzidine-4,4′-diisocyanate undergoes hydrolysis to yield 3,3′-dimethoxybenzidine (IARC, 1974) and may bind to cellular components; however no specific data are available.

Mutagenicity and other short-term tests

In a preincubation assay, 3,3′-dimethoxybenzidine-4,4′-diisocyanate was mutagenic to *Salmonella typhimurium* TA98 in the presence but not in the absence of an exogenous metabolic system (S9) from Aroclor-induced rats or Syrian hamsters; it was not mutagenic to strains TA1535, TA1537 or TA100 (Haworth *et al.*, 1983).

(b) *Humans*

No data were available to the Working Group.

3.3 Case reports and epidemiological studies of carcinogenicity to humans

No data were available to the Working Group.

4. Summary of Data Reported and Evaluation

4.1 Exposure data

3,3′-Dimethoxybenzidine-4,4′-diisocyanate has been used in isocyanate-based adhesives and as a component of polyurethane elastomers. There is no evidence of current exposure.

4.2 Experimental data

3,3′-Dimethoxybenzidine-4,4′-diisocyanate was tested for carcinogenicity in one study in mice by administration in the diet and in one study in rats by gavage followed by dietary administration. No treatment-related tumour was observed in mice. A statistically significant increase in the combined incidence of leukaemia and malignant lymphomas was observed in both male and female rats, together with a treatment-related increase in the incidence of tumours of the skin and Zymbal gland. Increases in the incidence of endometrial stromal polyps were observed in female rats.

No data were available to evaluate the reproductive effects or prenatal toxicity of 3,3′-dimethoxybenzidine-4,4′-diisocyanate to experimental animals.

3,3′-Dimethoxybenzidine-4,4′-diisocyanate was mutagenic to *Salmonella typhimurium* in the presence of an exogenous metabolic system.

Overall assessment of data from short-term tests: 3,3′-Dimethoxybenzidine-4,4′-diisocyanate[a]

	Genetic activity			Cell transformation
	DNA damage	Mutation	Chromosomal effects	
Prokaryotes		+		
Fungi/Green plants				
Insects				
Mammalian cells (*in vitro*)				
Mammals (*in vivo*)				
Humans (*in vivo*)				
Degree of evidence in short-term tests for genetic activity: **Inadequate**				Cell transformation: No data

[a]The groups into which the table is divided and the symbol + are defined on pp. 19-20 of the Preamble; the degrees of evidence are defined on pp. 20-21.

4.3 Human data

No data were available to evaluate the reproductive effects or prenatal toxicity of 3,3′-dimethoxybenzidine-4,4′-diisocyanate to humans.

No case report or epidemiological study was available to evaluate the carcinogenicity of 3,3′-dimethoxybenzidine-4,4′-diisocyanate to humans.

4.4 Evaluation[1]

There is *limited evidence* for the carcinogenicity of 3,3'-dimethoxybenzidine-4,4'-diisocyanate to experimental animals.

No data on humans were available.

In the absence of epidemiological data, no evaluation of the carcinogenicity of 3,3'-dimethoxybenzidine-4,4'-diisocyanate to humans could be made.

5. References

Hawley, G.G., ed. (1981) *The Condensed Chemical Dictionary*, 10th ed., New York, Van Nostrand Reinhold Co., p. 321

Haworth, S., Lawlor, T., Mortelmans, K., Speck, W. & Zeiger, E. (1983) *Salmonella* mutagenicity test results for 250 chemicals. *Environ. Mutagenesis, Suppl. 1*, 3-142

IARC (1974) *IARC Monographs on the Evaluation of Carcinogenic Risk of Chemicals to Man*, Vol. 4, *Some Aromatic Amines, Hydrazine and Related Substances*, N-*Nitroso Compounds and Miscellaneous Alkylating Agents*, Lyon, pp. 41-47

IARC (1982) *IARC Monographs on the Evaluation of the Carcinogenic Risk of Chemicals to Humans*, Suppl. 4, *Chemicals, Industrial Processes and Industries Associated with Cancer in Humans, IARC Monographs Volumes 1 to 29*, Lyon, pp. 116-118

Meddle, D.W. & Wood, R. (1968) Apparatus for preparing standard aerosol atmospheres. *Chem. Ind.*, November, pp. 1635-1637

National Cancer Institute (1979a) *Bioassay of 3,3'-Dimethoxybenzidine-4,4'-diisocyanate for Possible Carcinogenicity (CAS No. 91-93-0) (Technical Report No. 128)*, Bethesda, MD

National Cancer Institute (1979b) Report on bioassay of 3,3'-dimethoxybenzidine-4,4'-diisocyanate for possible carcinogenicity. Availability. *Fed. Regist., 44*, 2026

National Institute for Occupational Safety and Health (1978) *Criteria for a Recommended Standard for Occupational Exposure to Diisocyanates (DHEW (NIOSH) Pub. No. 78-215)*, Cincinnati, OH, p. 2

NIH/EPA Chemical Information System (1983) *Carbon-13 NMR Spectral Search System, Mass Spectral Search System*, and *Infrared Spectral Search System*, Arlington, VA, Information Consultants, Inc.

---

[1]For definition of the italicized term, see Preamble, p. 18.

Sax, N.I. (1984) *Dangerous Properties of Industrial Materials*, 6th ed., New York, Van Nostrand Reinhold Co., p. 894

Shriner, C.R., Drury, J.S., Hammons, A.S., Towill, L.E., Lewis, E.B. & Opresko, D.M. (1978) *Reviews of the Environmental Effects of Pollutants: II. Benzidine* (*EPA-600/1-78-024; US NTIS PB-281076*), Oak Ridge, TN, Oak Ridge National Laboratory, p. 37

TOLUENE DIISOCYANATE[1]

This substance was considered by a previous Working Group, in February 1978 (IARC, 1979). Since that time, new data have become available and these have been incorporated into the monograph and taken into consideration in the present evaluation. 2,4-Diaminotoluene, the immediate hydrolysis product of 2,4-toluene diisocyanate, was considered by a Working Group in June 1977 (IARC, 1978).

1. Chemical and Physical Data

2,4-Toluene diisocyanate

1.1 Synonyms and trade names

Chem. Abstr. Services Reg. No.: 584-84-9

Chem. Abstr. Name: Benzene, 2,4-diisocyanato-1-methyl-

IUPAC Systematic Name: 4-Methyl-*meta*-phenylene diisocyanate

Synonyms: Cresorcinol diisocyanate; 2,4-diisocyanato-1-methylbenzene; diisocyanatotoluene; 2,4-diisocyanatotoluene; isocyanic acid, methyl phenylene ester; 4-methyl-*meta*-phenylene isocyanate; TDI; 2,4-TDI; toluene diisocyanate; toluene 2,4-diisocyanate; *meta*-toluene diisocyanate; tolylene diisocyanate; tolylene 2,4-diisocyanate; 2,4-tolylene diisocyanate; *meta*-tolylene diisocyanate

Trade Names: Desmodur T80; Hylene T; Mondur TDS

1.2 Structural and molecular formulae and molecular weight

$C_9H_6N_2O_2$

Mol. wt: 174.15

---

[1]2,4-Toluene diisocyanate, 2,6-toluene diisocyanate and their commercial mixtures

1.3 Chemical and physical properties of the pure substance

(a) *Description*: Clear water-white to pale-yellow liquid with a sharp pungent odour (Hawley, 1981; Verschueren, 1983; Windholz, 1983; Sax, 1984)

(b) *Boiling-point*: 251°C at 760 mm Hg; 124-126°C at 18 mm Hg (Hawley, 1981; Buckingham, 1982; Verschueren, 1983; Windholz, 1983; National Fire Protection Association, 1984)

(c) *Melting-point*: Freezing-point, 22°C (International Isocyanate Institute Inc., 1980; Mobay Chemical Corp., 1984a)

(d) *Density*: $d_{15.5}^{25}$ 1.22 (Hawley, 1981; Mobay Chemical Corp., 1984a)

(e) *Spectroscopy data*: Ultraviolet (Sadtler Research Laboratories, 1980 [15732[a]]), infrared (Sadtler Research Laboratories, 1980; prism [148], grating [29893]), nuclear magnetic resonance (Sadtler Research Laboratories, 1980; proton [17271], C-13 [2001]) and mass spectral data (NIH/EPA Chemical Information System, 1983) have been reported.

(f) *Solubility*: Soluble in diethyl ether and acetone (Hawley, 1981); miscible with diglycol monomethyl ether, carbon tetrachloride, benzene, chlorobenzene, kerosene and olive oil (Windholz, 1983).

(g) *Volatility*: Vapour pressure, 0.01 mm Hg at 20°C (Hawley, 1981); relative vapour density (air = 1), 6.0 (Verschueren, 1983)

(h) *Stability*: Flash-point, 132°C (Hawley, 1981; Windholz, 1983); combustible when exposed to heat or flame (Sax, 1984); darkens on exposure to sunlight (Windholz, 1983)

(i) *Reactivity*: Reacts readily with compounds containing active hydrogens, such as water, acids and alcohols; contact with bases, such as caustic soda and tertiary amines, may cause uncontrollable polymerization and the rapid evolution of heat; high temperatures can cause formation of dimer (Hawley, 1981; Olin Chemicals, 1982; Windholz, 1983; BASF Wyandotte Corp., 1984). In the liquid product or in concentrated solutions, hydrolysis of a single isocyanate function to the amine is followed by rapid reaction of the amine with an isocyanate function in the second molecule, resulting in the formation of dimers, oligomers and polymers. The formation of free diaminotoluene is unlikely under these conditions. In dilute solutions, the formation of free diaminotoluene is more probable (Chadwick & Cleveland, 1981; Ulrich, 1983)

---

[a]Spectrum number in Sadtler compilation

(j)   *Conversion factor:* $mg/m^3 = 7.12 \times ppm^a$

2,6-Toluene diisocyanate

1.1 Synonyms and trade names

Chem. Abstr. Services Reg. No.: 91-08-7

Chem. Abstr. Name: Benzene, 1,3-diisocyanato-2-methyl-

IUPAC Systematic Name: 2-Methyl-*meta*-phenylene diisocyanate

Synonyms: 2,6-Diisocyanato-1-methylbenzene; 2,6-diisocyanatotoluene; 2-methyl-*meta*-phenylene isocyanate; 2,6-TDI; toluene 2,6-diisocyanate; tolylene 2,6-diisocyanate; *meta*-tolylene diisocyanate

Trade Names: Hylene TCPA; Hylene TIC; Hylene TM; Hylene TM-65; Hylene TRF; Niax TDI; Niax TDI-P

1.2 Structural and molecular formulae and molecular weight

$$O = C = N \overset{\underset{\displaystyle CH_3}{}}{\bigcirc} N = C = O$$

$C_9H_6N_2O_2$ Mol. wt: 174.15

1.3 Chemical and physical properties of the pure substance

(a)   *Description:* Liquid (Buckingham, 1982)

(b)   *Boiling-point:* 129-133°C at 18 mm Hg (Buckingham, 1982)

(c)   *Melting-point:* Freezing-point, 7.2°C (Olin Chemicals, 1982)

---

[a]Calculated from: $mg/m^3 = $ (molecular weight$/24.45) \times$ ppm, assuming standard temperature (25°C) and pressure (760 mm Hg)

(d)   *Density*: 1.22 (Aldrich Chemical Co., 1984)

(e)   *Spectroscopy data*: Infrared (Pouchert, 1981 [1144C[a]]) and nuclear magnetic resonance spectral data (Pouchert, 1983 [445C]) have been reported.

(f)   *Reactivity*: In the liquid product or in concentrated solutions, hydrolysis of a single isocyanate function to the amine is followed by rapid reaction of the amine with an isocyanate function in a second molecule, resulting in the formation of dimers, oligomers and polymers. The formation of free diaminotoluene is unlikely under these conditions. In dilute solutions, the formation of free diaminotoluene is more probable (Chadwick & Cleveland, 1981; Ulrich, 1983)

(g)   *Conversion factor*: mg/m³ = 7.12 × ppm[b]

Commercial toluene diisocyanate mixtures

1.1 Synonyms and trade names

Chem. Abstr. Services Reg. No.: 26471-62-5

Chem. Abstr. Name: Benzene, 1,3-diisocyanatomethyl-

IUPAC Systematic Name: Methyl-*meta*-phenylene diisocyanate

Synonyms: Benzene, diisocyanatomethyl-; diisocyanatotoluene; isocyanic acid, methylphenylene ester; methylphenylene isocyanate; methyl-*meta*-phenylene isocyanate; TDI; toluene 2,4- and 2,6-diisocyanate; toluene 2,4- and 2,6-diisocyanate, 80/20 mixture; toluenediisocyanates; tolylene diisocyanate; tolylene isocyanate

Trade Names: Desmodur T100; Hylene-T; Hylene-T organic isocyanate; Nacconate-100; Mondur-TD; Mondur-TD-80; Rubinate® TDI; Rubinate® TDI 80/20; T100; TDI-80; TDI 80-20

1.2 Structural and molecular formulae and molecular weight

[see isomers]

$C_9H_6N_2O_2$ Mol. wt: 174.15

---

[a]Spectrum number in Pouchert compilation

[b]Calculated from: mg/m³ = (molecular weight/24.45) × ppm, assuming standard temperature (25°C) and pressure (760 mm Hg)

1.3 Chemical and physical properties of the mixtures (2,4:2,6-isomers, 80:20 and 65:35; data refer to the 80:20 mixture, except when noted)

(a) *Description*: Colourless to pale-yellow liquid with a sharp pungent odour (both mixtures) (International Isocyanate Institute Inc., 1980; Olin Chemicals, 1982; Rubicon Chemicals Inc., 1983; BASF Wyandotte Corp., 1984; Mobay Chemical Corp., 1984b)

(b) *Boiling-point*: 251°C (both mixtures) (International Isocyanate Institute Inc., 1980; Olin Chemicals, 1982; Rubicon Chemicals Inc., 1983; BASF Wyandotte Corp., 1984; Mobay Chemical Corp., 1984b)

(c) *Melting-point*: Freezing-point, <15°C (80:20 mixture); <8 (65:35 mixture) (International Isocyanate Institute Inc., 1980); 11.5-13.5°C (Olin Chemicals, 1982); 13°C (Mobay Chemical Corp., 1984b)

(d) *Density*: d_{15}^{25} 1.22 (both mixtures) (Chadwick & Cleveland, 1981)

(e) *Spectroscopy data*: Infrared (Craver, 1977a [10269[a]]; Craver, 1977b [10108]) and mass spectral data (NIH/EPA Chemical Information System, 1983) have been reported.

(f) *Solubility*: Reacts with water; soluble in diethyl ether, acetone and other organic solvents (both mixtures) (Hawley, 1981); miscible with diglycol monomethyl ether, carbon tetrachloride, benzene, chlorobenzene, kerosene and olive oil (Windholz, 1983)

(g) *Volatility*: Vapour pressure, 0.01 mm Hg at 20°C (Olin Chemicals, 1982; BASF Wyandotte Corp., 1984); 0.02 mm Hg at 25°C (Rubicon Chemicals Inc., 1983); relative vapour density (air = 1), 6.0 (International Isocyanate Institute, 1980; Olin Chemicals, 1982; Rubicon Chemicals Inc., 1983; Mobay Chemical Corp., 1984b)

(h) *Stability*: Flash-point, 132°C (open-cup) (Rubicon Chemicals Inc., 1983; BASF Wyandotte Corp., 1984)

(i) *Reactivity*: Reacts readily with compounds containing active hydrogens, such as water, acids and alcohols; contact with bases, such as caustic soda and tertiary amines, may cause uncontrollable polymerization and the rapid evolution of heat; high temperatures can cause formation of dimer (Olin Chemicals, 1982; BASF Wyandotte Corp., 1984). In the liquid product or in concentrated solutions, hydrolysis of a single isocyanate function to the amine is followed by rapid reaction of the amine with an isocyanate function in a second molecule, resulting in the

----

[a]Spectrum number in Craver compilations

formation of dimers, oligomers and polymers. The formation of free diaminotoluene is unlikely under these conditions. In dilute solutions, the formation of free diaminotoluene is more probable (Chadwick & Cleveland, 1981; Ulrich, 1983). At ambient temperatures, the 2,4-toluene diisocyanate is more reactive than the 2,6-isomer, which may lead to relatively more off-gassing of 2,6-toluene diisocyanate during foam production (Rando *et al.*, 1984).

(*j*)   *Conversion factor:* mg/m³ = 7.12 x ppm[a]

1.4 Technical products and impurities

Toluene diisocyanate (TDI) is available commercially as a clear to pale-yellow liquid containing a mixture of 80% 2,4-isomer and 20% 2,6-isomer. A mixture of 65% 2,4-isomer and 35% 2,6-isomer and >99.5% pure 2,4-toluene diisocyanate are also available (Mobay Chemical Corp., 1984b,c).

Toluene diisocyanate in the 80:20 isomer ratio is produced in the USA in two forms, designated as type I and type II, which differ slightly in acidity and hydrolysable chloride content (BASF Wyandotte Corp., 1981). A typical analysis of this 80:20 toluene diiso--cyanate is as follows: purity, 99.5% min; 2,4-isomer, 80 ± 1%; 2,6-isomer, 20 ± 1%; acidity (as hydrochloric acid), 0.001-0.011% (varies); hydrolysable chloride, 0.010-0.014% max; and total chlorine, 0.01-0.2% max.

In Japan, commercially available pure 2,4-toluene diisocyanate has the following specifications: purity, 99.5% min; 2,4-isomer, 97.5% min; 2,6-isomer, 2.5% max; acidity (as hydrochloric acid), 0.010-0.013%; hydrolytic hydrochloric acid, 0.010-0.013%; total hydrochloric acid, 0.05% max; and freezing-point, 21.0°C min. The commercially available 80:20 toluene diisocyanate mixture has the following specifications: purity, 99.6% min; 2,4-isomer, 78.0-81.0%; 2,6-isomer, 19.0-22.0%; acidity (as hydrochloric acid), 0.004% max; hydrolytic hydrochloric acid, 0.01% max; total hydrochloric acid, 0.07% max; freezing-point, 11.8-13.4°C. A commercially available 65:35 toluene diisocyanate mixture has the following specifications: purity, 99.5% min; 2,4-isomer, 63-67%; 2,6-isomer, 33-37%; acidity (as hydrochloric acid), 0.010-0.013% max; hydrolytic hydrochloric acid, 0.01-0.013% max; and total hydrochloric acid, 0.05% max.

2. Production, Use, Occurrence and Analysis

2.1 Production and use

(*a*)   Production

Toluene diisocyanate has been produced commercially since the late 1930s. It is manufactured primarily by the reaction of phosgene with toluenediamine (Mannsville

---

[a]Calculated from: mg/m³ = (molecular weight/24.45) × ppm, assuming standard temperature (25°C) and pressure (760 mm Hg)

Chemical Products Corp., 1983). Initially, dinitrotoluene is produced by the nitration of toluene using a nitric acid-sulphonic acid mixture, which yields 76% 2,4-dinitrotoluene and 24% of the 2,6-isomer. The nitration product is reduced catalytically to the diamine. Diaminotoluene is dissolved in an organic solvent, usually mono- or dichlorobenzene, and reacted with a phosgene solution for several hours at gradually increasing temperatures. The crude isomer solution is fractionated to recover hydrogen chloride, unreacted phosgene and the final toluene diisocyanate product (Chadwick & Cleveland, 1981).

A non-phosgene process developed in Japan involves the carbonylation of dinitrotoluene. The product of this reaction, a diurethane, is converted thermally to toluene diisocyanate and alcohol.

Toluene diisocyanate is most commonly formulated as the 80:20 mixture of the 2,4- and 2,6-isomers. US production of toluene diisocyanate increased from 20 000 tonnes in 1960 to 139 000 tonnes in 1970 and had reached 290 000 tonnes by 1983 (Mannsville Chemical Products Corp., 1983; US International Trade Commission, 1984). The effective annual production capacity in the USA in 1982 was 313 000 tonnes; 261 000 tonnes were produced. During this period, the USA imported about 90 tonnes and exported 77 200 tonnes (Mannsville Chemical Products Corp., 1983). Exports of toluene diisocyanate from the USA in 1982 were to the following countries (hundred thousand tonnes): Canada (10.8), The Netherlands (6.1), Federal Republic of Germany (5.8), Japan (5.6), Belgium (5.2), Republic of Korea (5.1) and other countries (38.3).

All US producers of toluene diisocyanate manufacture the 80:20 isomer mixture. One firm markets the 80:20 mixture, the 65:35 mixture, as well as the pure 2,4-isomer (Mobay Chemical Corp., 1984a,b,c).

A plant in Brazil had the capacity to produce 20 000 tonnes toluene diisocyanate in 1982. The sole Mexican plant had a capacity of 12 000 tonnes (Ulrich, 1983)

Western European nations had an annual toluene diisocyanate production capacity in 1983 of 344 000 tonnes. The Federal Republic of Germany had the greatest capacity, at 145 000 tonnes. The capacity of other major European producers are (in hundred thousand tonnes): France (80), Italy (60), Belgium (30) and Spain (24). Of the 265 million kg produced in western Europe, 175 million were used and 90 million were exported, primarily to eastern Europe, North Africa, and the Middle East. The Netherlands, Portugal and the UK did not report their production capacity in 1983.

The COMECON nations had the capacity to produce 46 000 tonnes toluene diisocyanate in 1982. Two firms in Yugoslavia had a combined production capacity of 38 000 tonnes. The capacity for the sole plant in the German Democratic Republic was 8000 tonnes (Ulrich, 1983).

Four firms in Japan reported a combined toluene diisocyanate production capacity of 77 000 tonnes in 1982; commercial production was 67 000 tonnes in that year. During 1982, Japan imported approximately 5000 tonnes and exported 9000 tonnes of toluene diisocyanate. The sole plant in the Republic of Korea in operation in 1982 had a capacity of 10 000 tonnes (Ulrich, 1983).

(b)   *Use* (Table 1)

Polyurethane foams account for approximately 90% of the total supply of toluene diisocyanate. They can be made from toluene diisocyanate by one of two synthetic methods. The 'one-shot' technique involves reaction of toluene diisocyanate with a di- or polyfunctional alcohol to form the polyurethane backbone of the polymer. Excess toluene diisocyanate reacts with water to form amines, which further react with toluene diisocyanate to introduce urea groups into the polymer chain. Cross-linking of the chain is accomplished by the interaction of toluene diisocyanate with these urea groups. The second method, the prepolymer process, involves reaction of toluene diisocyanate with a polyl to form a polymer with isocyanate end groups. Glycols or diamines are then reacted with this prepolymer to cross-link the polymeric chain and complete the synthetic process.

Polyurethane coatings have abrasion resistance, good adhesion, chemical resistance and skin flexibility and are fast curing (Ulrich, 1983). Toluene diisocyanate is used to a lesser degree as a component of coatings and elastomer systems. See Table 1.

Table 1. Use of toluene diisocyanate[a]

Application	Percent
Flexible polyurethane foams	90
Furniture	43
Transportation	21
Carpet underlay	14
Bedding	12
Polyurethane coatings	5
Elastomers	3
Other	2

[a]From Anon. (1984a)

Polyurethane foams

Flexible polyurethane foam is used mainly in the furniture and bedding industry. In the USA, a typical modern housing unit of 167 m² floor space, including furniture, carpet underlay and bedding, contains 136 kg flexible polyurethane foam. Automotive seating and padding can result in the use of 11-14 kg polyurethane per automobile (Anon. 1984b).

Rigid polyurethane foams are primarily used as insulation. Toluene diisocyanate-based rigid polyurethane foam is used in household refrigerators and, in board or laminate form, for residential sheathing or commercial roofing. 'Pour-in-place' or 'spray-in' rigid foam is used as insulation for truck tailers, railroad freight cars and cargo containers (Ulrich, 1983).

Polyurethane coatings

Urethane-modified alkyds contain approximately 6-7% isocyanate, mostly toluene diisocyanate, and are used as floor finishes, wood finishes and paints. Moisture-curing coatings are used as wood and concrete sealants and floor finishes. Aircraft, truck and passenger-car coatings are often comprised of toluene diisocyanate prepolymer systems.

Elastomers

Castable urethane elastomers are used in applications requiring strength, flexibility and shock-absorption, and are resistant to oil, solvents and ultraviolet radiation (Ulrich, 1983). They are used in adhesive and sealant compounds (Mannsville Chemical Products Corp., 1983) and in automobile parts, shoe soles, roller skate wheels, pond liners and blood bags (Ulrich, 1983). They are also used in oil fields and mines. Certain elastomer products are produced from the pure 2,4-isomer rather than the 80:20 mixture (Mannsville Chemical Products Corp., 1983).

(*c*) *Regulatory status and guidelines*

Occupational exposure limits to toluene diisocyanate have been set by 18 countries by regulation or recommended guideline (Table 2).

The US Food and Drug Administration (1984) has determined that 2,4- and 2,6-toluene diisocyanate isomers may be used as components of adhesives that come in contact with food, and that toluene diisocyanate may be used as a component of polyurethane resins that form a surface in contact with food.

Toluene diisocyanate has been designated by the US Environmental Protection Agency (1984) as a hazardous waste under the Resource Conservation and Recovery Act of 1976, because of its toxicity and reactivity.

2.2 Occurrence

(*a*) *Natural occurrence*

It is not known whether 2,4- and 2,6-toluene diisocyanates occur as natural products.

(*b*) *Occupational exposure*

The occurrence of toluene diisocyanate in the work environment, primarily in air, has been reported in association with its commercial production, its handling and processing prior to polyurethane foam production, the manufacturing of polyurethane foam products and coatings, its release in stack exhaust from plants, and its release into the air from sprays, insulation materials and polyurethane foam coated fabrics. Available representative information on the occurrence of toluene diisocyanate in these areas of activity is summarized in Table 3. No data were available on ambient air levels of toluene diisocyanate in the production of elastomers and adhesives.

Table 2. Occupational exposure limits for 2,4-toluene diisocyanate[a]

Country	Year	Concentration (mg/m³)	Interpretation[b]
Australia	1978	0.14	Ceiling
Belgium	1978	0.12	Ceiling
Council of Europe	1974	0.14	
Czechoslovakia	1976	0.07	TWA
		0.14	Ceiling
Denmark (toluene diisocyanate)	1980	0.07	Ceiling
Finland (toluene diisocyanate)	1981	0.14	Ceiling
German Democratic Republic	1979	0.1	TWA
		0.1	Ceiling
Hungary	1974	0.5	TWA
Italy	1978	0.5	Ceiling
Japan	1978	0.14	TWA
Netherlands	1978	0.14	TWA
Norway (toluene diisocyanate)	1980	0.07	Ceiling
Romania	1975	0.1	TWA
		0.3	Ceiling
Sweden (toluene diisocyanate)	1984	0.04	TWA
		0.07	Ceiling
Switzerland (also for 2,6-toluene diisocyanate)	1978	0.14	TWA
USA			
ACGIH	1984	0.04	TWA
		0.15	STEL
NIOSH (toluene diisocyanate)	1978	0.035	TWA
		0.14	Ceiling
OSHA	1983	0.14	Ceiling
USSR	1977	0.5	Ceiling
Yugoslavia	1971	0.14	Ceiling

[a]From National Institute for Occupational Safety and Health (NIOSH) (1978); International Isocyanate Institute, Inc. (1980); International Labour Office (1980); Työsuojeluhallitus (1981); US Occupational Safety and Health Administration (OSHA) (1983); American Conference of Governmental Industrial Hygienists (ACGIH) (1984); Arbetarskyddsstyrelsens Författningssamling (1984)

[b]TWA, time-weighted average; STEL, short-term exposure limit

Table 3. Mean and maximum air concentrations of toluene diisocyanate[a] in the workplace

Exposure type Year of study	Country	Concentration[b]		References
		Mean/Range (μg/m³)	Maximum (μg/m³)	
Toluene diisocyanate production				
1962-1964	UK	360-710		Adams (1975)
1966-1970	UK		about 140	Adams (1975)
1956-1974	USA	<30-430	1420	Porter et al. (1975)
1973-1978	USA	0.7-180		Diem et al. (1982)
Polyurethane foam production				
1955	USA	1490	2705	Walworth & Virchow (1959)
1957	USA	350	710	Walworth & Virchow (1959)
1964	New Zealand	21-875		Glass & Thom (1964)
1965	USA	140-210		Peters et al. (1968)
1966	USA	20-60		Peters et al. (1968, 1969)
1967	USA	64-85		Peters et al. (1969)
1968	USSR		3400	Tonkoshkurov (1969)
1969	Poland		90	Ciosek et al. (1969)
1972	USA	14-90*		Wegman et al. (1974)
1972-1974	USA	7-120*		Wegman et al. (1982)
1974-1976	USA	35-280*		Wegman et al. (1982)
1974	USA	30-230*		Gunter & Lucas (1975)
1975	USA	230-540* 340-470		Gunter (1975)
1973-1976	USA (plant 1)	3-11*		Musk et al. (1982)
1973-1976	USA (plant 2)	9-16*		Musk et al. (1982)
1973	USA	ND-40 ND-32		Vandervort & Shama (1973)
1974-1975	USA	2-50*		Roper & Cromer (1975)
1978	USA	ND[c]-230* 100-514		White & Wegman (1978)
1980-1981	USA		12*	Burroughs & Moody (1982)
1981	USA	0[d]-7*	40	Almaguer et al. (1982)
1981	Sweden	63-159		Andersson et al. (1982)
Elastomer production				
1974	Czechoslovakia	70 000-140 000		Sova (1974)

Table 3 (contd)

Exposure type Year of study	Country	Concentration[b]		References
		Mean/Range (μg/m^3)	Maximum (μg/m^3)	
Polyurethane: Spray foam use				
1970 (2,4-isomer)	USA	2-1220* 13-28		Chrostek & Cromer(1975)
1979	Canada	7-570* 14-1050		Hosein & Farkas (1981)
Polyurethane: Spray paint use				
1960	USA	570-710		Maxon (1964)
1975	USA	10-<50	40*	Hervin & Thoburn (1975)
Toluene diisocyanate release from insulation (in a ship's hold)				
1983	Japan	120-150		Hobara *et al.* (1984)
Toluene diisocyanate release from coated fabric (in a work area)				
1979	USA	2-20		White *et al.* (1980)

[a]Unidentified mixtures of primarily 2,4- and 2,6-toluene diisocyanate reported in association with the production of toluene diisocyanate, its use in the manufacturing of polyurethane products, or the use of these products

[b]All concentrations were reported as concentrations in ambient air of work areas, except for those indicated with an asterisk (*), which are personal samples.

[c]Limit of detection, 0.3 μg 2,4-toluene diisocyanate per sample

[d]Limit of detection, 0.2 μg/ml of absorbed solution

Analyses of the isomeric composition of atmospheric toluene diisocyanate in a plant producing polyurethane foam demonstrated a large increase in the level of 2,6-isomer relative to that of the 2,4-isomer, particularly at the finishing end of the production process. Median air concentrations of 2,4-isomer were 5.0 and 2.3 μg/m^3 for the initial mixing and finishing ends of the process, respectively; the respective median values for the 2,6-isomer were 6.4 and 7.8 μg/m^3, with a maximum value >450 μg/m^3 at the finishing end. These findings were attributed to enhanced emission of the less chemically active 2,6-isomer from the cured foam bats and retention of the 2,4-isomer as a polymer (Rando *et al.*, 1984).

Aniline and the 2,4 and 2,6 isomers of toluene diisocyanate and toluenediamine were detected under controlled experimental conditions in the thermodegradation fumes of polyurethane varnish used in the insulation of copper wire. Consistent with these findings, the compounds were also detected in workplace atmosphere during the industrial production of polyurethane-coated wire. Under these conditions, the concentration of the combined 2,4 and 2,6 isomers of toluene diisocyanate varied from $<$1-740 μg/m^3 and that of the two isomers of toluenediamine from $<$0.5-4900 μg/m^3. The highest concentrations, 6500 and 17 800 μg/m^3 for toluene diisocyanate and toluene diamine, respectively, were detected in a ventilation exhaust. The compounds and their isomers were also identified and quantified by high-performance liquid chromatography, gas chromatography and mass spectrometry (Rosenberg, 1984).

(c) Water

Toluene diisocyanate has been reported in the waste-water of a furniture manufacturing area in a concentration range of 0.1-4.1 mg/l. The colorimetric method used did not differentiate between the possible diisocyanates or the corresponding amines (De Rosa *et al.*, 1980).

(d) Soil

Ten days after an accident resulting in the spillage of 13 tonnes of toluene diisocyanate from a lorry on a swampy wet forest area, toluene diisocyanate and toluenediamine were in the soil. After six years, only toluene diisocyanate-derived polyureas were found in soil samples taken at the same site (Duff, 1983).

(e) Other

Levels of 100-17 700 μg/m^3 toluene diisocyanate were reported in samples from the stack exhaust of a polyurethane foam production plant (Grieveson & Reeve, 1983).

Toluene diisocyanate has been reported to be present as the free monomer in a urethane foam fabric coating at concentrations of less than 200 mg/kg (Scott & Carey, 1976). The formation of amines, as well as ureas, from toluene diisocyanate under environmental or manufacturing conditions has been discussed in several reports (Walker & Pinches, 1981; Sandridge, 1982; Walker, 1982; Duff, 1983; Rosenberg, 1984).

2.3 Analysis

Selected methods for the analysis of toluene diisocyanate in air and polymer products are listed in Table 4.

A number of methods have been developed for the analysis of toluene diisocyanate in air. The method developed by Marcali (1957), modified by Grim and Linch (1964) for lower concentrations, was adopted by the US National Institute for Occupational Safety and

Table 4. Methods for the analysis of toluene diisocyanate

Sample matrix	Sample preparation	Assay procedure[a]	Limit of detection	Reference
Air	Draw air through impinger containing aqueous acid; diazotize (NaNO$_2$/NaBr); decompose excess nitrous acid; react with N-(1-naphthyl)-ethylenediamine	Colorimetric	50 μg/m^3	Taylor (1977)
	Draw air through tube containing glass wool coated with N-para-nitrobenzyl-N-propylamine; extract (dichloro-methane)	HPLC/UV	4 μg/m^3	Taylor (1980)
	Draw air through impinger containing 1-(2-methoxyphenyl)-piperazine in toluene; evaporate toluene; dissolve in methanol	HPLC/ECh	0.2 μg/m^3	Warwick et al.(1981)
	Draw air through impinger containing ethanol	HPLC/UV	1-5 μ/m^3	Bagon & Purnell (1980); Davey & Edwards (1983); Nieminen et al. (1983)
	Draw air through impinger containing aqueous acid; neutralize; extract (chloroform or toluene); react with trifluoroacetic anhydride or heptafluorobutyric anhydride	GC/ECD	1-5 μg/m^3	Ebell et al. (1980); Bishop et al. (1983)
Polymer	Extract (ortho-dichlorobenzene)	GC/FID	5 μg/g	Conte & Cossi (1981)

[a]Abbreviations: HPLC/UV, high-performance liquid chromatography/ultraviolet detection; HPLC/ECh, high-performance liquid chromatography/electrochemical detection; GC/ECD, gas chromatography/electron capture detection; GC/FID, gas chromatography/flame ionization detection

Health as the recommended method in 1974. The method involves collection and simultaneous hydrolysis to diaminotoluene, diazotization and coupling with N-(1-naphthyl)-ethylenediamine to form a coloured product that is analysed colorimetrically at 550 nm. The range is reported as 50-1000 μg/m^3 (Dharmarajan, 1977; Taylor; 1977). A modification has been suggested recently which eliminates the different responses from the 2,4 and 2,6 isomers (Rando & Hammad, 1985). The method of Marcali (1957) does not differentiate airborne toluene diisocyanate from its hydrolysis product diaminotoluene, and other free amines may also give a positive interference.

As the recommended limits for occupational exposure to toluene diisocyanate decreased, more sensitive and selective methods were required. The current analytical method of the US National Institute for Occupational Safety and Health has been validated for the 2,4 isomer over the range 17-580 $\mu g/m^3$, with a calculated limit of detection of 4 $\mu g/m^3$ (Taylor, 1980). The method has also been used successfully for higher concentrations [Graham, 1980 (2,4 and 2,6 isomers); Tucker & Arnold, 1982 (2,4 isomer)]. This method takes advantage of the selective reaction of organic isocyanates with N-para-nitrobenzyl-N-propylamine (PNBPA) coated on glass wool to form urea derivatives that can be determined quantitatively by high-performance liquid chromatography with ultraviolet detection at 254 nm (HPLC/UV). The principal drawbacks are the instability of PNBPA and the necessity for washing the HPLC column at intervals to remove PNBPA and its degradation products (Vogt et al., 1976; National Institute for Occupational Safety and Health, 1977; Taylor, 1980). Acetylation of excess PNBPA prior to HPLC analysis has been suggested (Bagon & Purnell, 1980).

A number of variants of the HPLC/UV method have been reported. Other reagents that form substituted urea derivatives with toluene diisocyanate have been used in impingers for HPLC/UV or HPLC/fluorescence analysis (Sangö & Zimerson, 1980; Kormos et al., 1981) or coated on cross-linked polystyrene (Andersson et al., 1982). Another urea-forming reagent, 1-(2-pyridyl)piperazine, is reported to have the advantages of increased stability, compared to PNBPA, when coated on a solid support and of increased sensitivity of its isocyanate reaction products to UV detection (Goldberg et al., 1981; Warwick et al., 1981; Chang & Burg, 1982). Electrochemical detection of HPLC-separated isocyanate derivatives of 1-(2-methoxyphenyl)piperazine or para-aminophenol offers a further increase in sensitivity (to 200 ng/m^3 or less) and simplified sample handling by eliminating the preconcentration step (Warwick et al., 1981; Meyer & Tallman, 1983).

Another simple method involves the collection of airborne toluene diisocyanate in an impinger containing ethanol; the resultant ethyl urethane derivatives are reportedly formed quantitatively and are analysed by HPLC/UV, with a detection limit in the range of 1-5 $\mu g/m^3$ (Bagon & Purnell, 1980; Davey & Edwards, 1983; Nieminen et al., 1983). This method has also been used to determine free monomeric toluene diisocyanate in prepolymer samples (Bagon & Hardy, 1978).

Air samples containing toluene diisocyanate have been collected in an impinger containing aqueous acid in which toluene diisocyanate hydrolyses rapidly to 2,4- and 2,6-toluenediamine (Taylor, 1977). When the neutralized solution is extracted (dichloromethane) and the diamines are separated and analysed directly by HPLC/UV (240 nm), detection limits of 2.6 and 1.4 $\mu g/m^3$ for the 2,4 and 2,6 isomers, respectively, are reported for a 50-l air sample (Peng & Muzal, 1984). Again, this method does not distinguish between toluene diisocyanate and its hydrolysis products.

It is noteworthy that the HPLC retention volume of the 2,4 isomer derivative differs from that of the 2,6 isomer derivative in virtually every HPLC method reported for toluene diisocyanate, making possible the separate determination of the individual isomers.

Gas chromatographic methods have also been developed for toluene diisocyanate in air and in polyurethane products. Air samples (20-60 l) containing toluene diisocyanate are drawn through an aqueous acid impinger solution, and the resultant diamines are extracted and converted to the bis(trifluoroacetamide) or bis(heptafluorobutyramide) derivatives. Analysis by gas chromatography with electron capture detection gives lower quantifiable limits, in the range of 1-5 $\mu g/m^3$. The 2,4- and 2,6-bis(heptafluorobutyramide) derivatives are not separated under these conditions (Ebell *et al.*, 1980; Bishop *et al.*, 1983). Extraction of polyurethane foam with *ortho*-dichlorobenzene and direct gas chromatography/flame ionization detection for toluene diisocyanate has been reported to detect as little as 5 $\mu g/g$ residual toluene diisocyanate in a polyurethane product (Conte & Cossi, 1981).

A paper-tape monitor developed by Reilly (1968) has been used for personal sampling of toluene diisocyanate exposures in the workplace. The monitor, available commercially as the MCM (miniature continuous monitor) 4000 (MDA Scientific Ltd), is based on the colour-forming reaction of toluene diisocyanate with a complex amine [Brenthol GB (2-hydroxy-11*H*-benzo[*a*]carbazole-3-carboxy-*para*-anisidide)], sodium nitrite, ammonium acetate and diethylphthalate, and is reportedly sensitive to concentrations as low as 14 $\mu g/m^3$ at a sampling rate of 0.2 l/min (Nutt, 1983). However, if toluenediamine is present in the sampled air at concentrations similar to those of toluene diisocyanate, it interferes significantly with the colour-forming reaction (Walker & Pinches, 1981).

3. Biological Data Relevant to the Evaluation of Carcinogenic Risk to Humans

3.1 Carcinogenicity studies in animals

(a) Oral administration

Mouse: Groups of 50 male and 50 female B6C3F$_1$ mice, 12 weeks of age, were administered 120 or 240 mg/kg bw (males) or 60 or 120 mg/kg bw (females) commercial-grade (86% 2,4 isomer; 14% 2,6 isomer) toluene diisocyanate in corn oil by gavage on five days per week for 105 weeks. The concentration of toluene diisocyanate in corn oil was equivalent to 36 or 72 mg/ml and 18 or 36 mg/ml. Groups of 50 male and 50 female mice received corn oil only and served as vehicle controls. There was a significant dose-related reduction in the mean body weight of treated males throughout the study; in females, this effect was seen only after 56 weeks in those receiving the high dose. There was a reduction in survival in high-dose males, with 26/50 (52%) animals still alive at termination (week 119), compared to 46/50 (92%) in the control group and 40/50 (80%) in the low-dose group. No treatment-related tumour was seen in male mice. The survival rate in females was: 34/50 (68%) control, 43/50 (86%) low-dose and 33/50 (66%) high-dose animals. In females, haemangiomas (in the spleen and subcutaneous tissues) and haemangiosarcomas (in the liver, ovaries and peritoneum) occurred in 0/50 (0%) control, 1/50 (2%) low-dose and 5/50 (10%) high-dose animals, giving a statistically significant positive trend ($p = 0.01$, Cochran-Armitage trend test). The incidence of hepatocellular adenomas was also significantly increased in females: 2/50 (4%) control, 3/50 (6%) low-dose and 12/50 (24%) high-dose animals ($p = 0.001$, Cochran-Armitage trend test) (National Toxicology Program, 1983). [The Working Group noted the poor survival of male mice.]

Rat: Groups of 50 male and 50 female Fischer 344/N rats, 11 weeks old, were administered 30 or 60 mg/kg bw (males) or 60 or 120 mg/kg bw (females) commercial-grade toluene diisocyanate (86% 2,4 isomer; 14% 2,6 isomer) in corn oil by gavage on five days per week for 106 weeks. The concentration of toluene diisocyanate in corn oil was 9 or 18 mg/ml and 18 or 36 mg/ml. Groups of 50 male and 50 female rats received corn oil only and served as vehicle controls. Males and females showed dose-related decreases in mean body weights from weeks 10 and 20, respectively. There was also a marked reduction in survival in treated animals: 36/50 (72%) control, 14/50 (28%) low-dose and 8/50 (16%) high-dose males, and 36/50 (72%) control, 19/50 (38%) low-dose and 6/50 (12%) high-dose females were alive at the termination of the study (119 weeks). A treatment-related increase in the incidence of subcutaneous fibromas and fibrosarcomas individually and combined was observed in males. The incidence of fibrosarcomas was 0/50 control, 3/50 low-dose and 3/50 high-dose animals; the combined incidence was 3/50 (6%) control, 6/50 (12%) low-dose and 12/50 (24%) high-dose animals ($p = 0.007$, Cochran-Armitage trend test). The terminal rates for the combined incidence were 3/36 control, 3/14 low-dose and 3/8 high-dose animals. The overall rate of mammary fibroadenomas in female rats was: 15/50 (30%) controls, 21/50 (42%) low-dose and 18/50 (36%) high-dose and was not significant using the Fisher exact test, but was significant by incidental tumour or life-table analysis ($p < 0.001$). The terminal tumour rate for mammary fibroadenomas was: 13/36 (36%) controls, 15/19 (79%) low-dose and 4/6 (67%) high-dose animals. The dose-related incidence of pancreatic acinar-cell adenomas in males [1/47 (2%) control, 3/47 (6%) low-dose and 7/49 (14%) high-dose animals] was significantly increased in the high-dose group compared to controls ($p = 0.034$). In females, pancreatic islet-cell adenomas were found at terminal sacrifice in 0/36 controls, 3/19 low-dose and 2/6 high-dose animals ($p \leqslant 0.01$, tests for incidental tumours comparing each dose group to controls). In addition, one islet-cell carcinoma was observed in one low-dose female. A dose-related increase in the incidence of neoplastic nodules in the liver of female rats was also noted (National Toxicology Program, 1983). [The Working Group noted the poor survival rates of both male and female treated animals.]

(b) Inhalation exposure

Mouse: Groups of 120 male and 120 female CD-1 mice, three to four weeks old, were exposed to 0, 0.05 ppm or 0.15 ppm [0, 0.36 or 1.07 mg/m³] production-grade toluene diisocyanate (approximately 80% 2,4 isomer and 20% 2,6 isomer) in an inhalation chamber for 6 h per day on five days per week for 104 weeks. There was a significant reduction in body weight in the high-dose group [sex not stated] and a significant increase in mortality in both high- and low-dose females by the termination of the study (controls, 60%; low-dose, 77%; high-dose, 74%). No such effect was seen in males. Neither the types of tumour observed nor their incidences were dose-related, and both corresponded to those seen in historical controls for this strain of mice. However, dose-related pathological changes were observed in the nasal cavity (chronic or necrotic rhinitis), together with changes in the lower respiratory tract (interstitial pneumonia, catarrhal bronchitis) in both groups [see also section 3.2(a)] (Loeser, 1983).

Rat: Groups of 126 male and 126 female Sprague-Dawley CD rats, six to nine weeks old, were exposed to 0, 0.05 or 0.15 ppm [0, 0.36 or 1.07 mg/m³] production-grade toluene diisocyanate (approximately 80% 2,4 isomer and 20% 2,6 isomer) in an inhalation chamber for 6 h per day on five days per week for 108 weeks (females) or 110 weeks (males). A significant reduction in weight gain was observed during the first 12 weeks of the study among the high-dose animals of each sex, but body-weight gain was similar in all groups thereafter. No significant difference in mortality between treated and control groups of either sex was reported. Tumour incidences and types were reported to be similar in control and treated groups (Loeser, 1983). [The Working Group noted that, although no macroscopic change was reported in the upper respiratory tract, histopathological examination of the nasal turbinates was still in progress.]

(c)   Carcinogenicity of breakdown products

On contact with water, toluene diisocyanates may be converted to the corresponding diaminotoluenes.

2,4-Diaminotoluene

2,4-Diaminotoluene was evaluated previously in the *IARC Monographs* (IARC, 1978), and there was found to be *sufficient evidence* of its carcinogenicity in experimental animals (IARC, 1982). Since that time, new data have become available.

Oral administration

Mouse: Groups of 50 male and 50 female B6C3F$_1$ mice, six weeks of age, received 2,4-diaminotoluene (>99.9% pure) in the diet *ad libitum* at concentrations of either 100 (low dose) or 200 (high dose) mg/kg of diet for 101 weeks. A group of 20 males and 20 females fed the basal diet served as controls. A reduction in mean body weight occurred in the high-dose males and in both low- and high-dose females compared to controls, but there was no significant difference in survival at 101 weeks. Hepatocellular carcinomas occurred in female mice with a positive dose-related trend ($p = 0.002$) at an incidence that was statistically significant when each dose group was compared directly to controls [controls, 0/19; low-dose, 13/41 ($p = 0.007$); high-dose, 18/46 ($p = 0.001$)]. In addition, a statistically significant ($p < 0.001$) increase in the incidence of lymphomas occurred in low-dose female mice (controls, 2/19; low-dose, 29/47; high-dose, 11/46). There was no statistically significant increase in tumours in treated male mice (National Cancer Institute, 1979).

Rat: Groups of 50 male and 50 female Fischer 344/N rats, six weeks of age, were given 2,4-diaminotoluene (>99.9% pure) in the diet *ad libitum* at concentrations of 125 (low dose) or 250 (high dose) mg/kg of diet for 40 weeks, at which time the low dose was reduced to 50 mg/kg of diet and the high dose to 100 mg/kg of diet due to excessive weight loss of the animals. Treatment was continued for a further 63 weeks for the low-dose group and for a further 39 (males) and 44 (females) weeks for the high-dose groups, at which time the animals were killed. The time-weighted average doses were 79 mg/kg of diet for low-dose rats, 176 mg/kg of diet for high-dose males and 171 mg/kg of diet for high-dose females. Groups of 20 male and 20 female rats were fed the basal diet and served as controls. At 78 weeks, survival in males was: controls, 18/20 (90%); low-dose, 42/50 (84%); and high-dose, 32/50 (64%). Of the females, all of 20 controls and 46/50 (92%) in the low- and high-dose groups were still alive. A positive dose-related trend in the combined incidence of hepatocellular carcinomas and neoplastic nodules was observed in both males [controls, 0/20 (0%); low-dose, 5/49 (10%); and high-dose, 10/50 (20%); $p = 0.014$] and females [controls, 0/20 (0%); low-dose, 0/50 (0%); and high-dose, 6/49 (12%); $p = 0.008$]. However, the differences in the incidences between individual treatment groups and controls were not statistically significant when tested directly by the Fisher exact test, except in high-dose males ($p = 0.026$). The combined incidence of mammary-gland carcinomas and adenomas in females was statistically significant ($p < 0.001$) when compared to controls [controls, 1/20 (5%); low-dose, 38/50 (74%); and high-dose, 41/50 (82%)]. In male rats, there was a positive dose-related trend ($p = 0.009$) in the incidence of subcutaneous-tissue fibromas: controls, 1/20 (5%); low-dose, 15/50 (30%); and high dose, 19/50 (38%) (National Cancer Institute, 1979).

2,6-Diaminotoluene dihydrochloride

Oral administration

Mouse: Groups of 50 male and 50 female B6C3F1 mice, six to seven weeks of age, received 50 or 100 mg/kg 2,6-diaminotoluene dihydrochloride (>99% pure) in the diet *ad libitum* for 103 weeks, after which they were maintained on basal diet for a further week prior to sacrifice and autopsy. Groups of 50 males and 50 females fed the basal diet alone served as controls. There was no significant difference in survival between treated and control animals either during or at termination of the study. An increase in the incidence of lymphomas in low-dose males was not statistically significant (males: control, 2/50; low-dose, 8/50; and high-dose, 2/50), nor was that of hepatocellular carcinomas in female mice (0/50 control, 0/49 low-dose and 3/49 high-dose) (National Cancer Institute, 1980).

Rat: Groups of 50 male and 50 female Fischer 344/N rats, five weeks of age, were fed diets containing 250 or 500 mg/kg 2,6-diaminotoluene dihydrochloride (>99% pure) *ad libitum* for 103 weeks, after which they were maintained on basal diet for a further week prior to sacrifice and autopsy. Groups of 50 males and 50 females were fed basal diet only and served as controls. A variety of tumours was found in both control and treated animals, but there was no evidence that these were related to treatment, and the incidence and histological type were those commonly found in ageing Fischer 344/N rats (National Cancer Institute, 1980).

3.2 Other relevant biological data

Reviews of the toxicity of 2,4- and 2,6-toluene diisocyanates are available (National Institute for Occupational Safety and Health, 1973; Gustavsson, 1977). Almost none of the published papers on toluene diisocyanate specify which isomer was used or its purity; in many studies, commercial-grade toluene diisocyanate (approximately 80% 2,4 and 20% 2,6 isomer) was used.

(a) Experimental systems

Toxic effects

Reported oral LD_{50} values for toluene diisocyanate in rats are 5.8 g/kg bw (Zapp, 1957) and 7.5 g/kg bw (Union Carbide Corp., 1967).

The LC_{50} following exposure to toluene diisocyanate for 4 h per day for 14 days was: mouse, 70 mg/m³ (10 ppm); guinea-pig, 90 mg/m³ (13 ppm); and rat, 100 mg/m³ (14 ppm). The LC_{50} following exposure for seven days was 80 mg/m³ (11 ppm) in rabbits. During exposure, mice, rats and guinea-pigs exhibited lachrymation, salivation, restlessness and hyperactivity (Duncan et al., 1962).

Rats receiving up to 240 mg/kg bw toluene diisocyanate by gavage daily on five days per week for 13 weeks were found to suffer from mild to moderate bronchopneumonia (National Toxicology Program, 1983).

Single or repeated exposure to concentrations of 2,4-toluene diisocyanate ranging from 0.05-14 mg/m³ (0.007-2 ppm) for periods of up to 3 h resulted in reductions in respiratory rate in Swiss mice (Sangha & Alarie, 1979). The concentration of toluene diisocyanate that caused a 50% decrease in the respiratory rate in mice was reported to be 3 mg/m³ (0.39 ppm); pulmonary injury was characterized principally by squamous metaplasia of the respiratory epithelium (Buckley et al., 1984).

Guinea-pigs exposed by inhalation to 14-35 mg/m³ (2-5 ppm) toluene diisocyanate in air for 6 h per day for three days were sensitized, as shown three weeks later when they were exposed to 0.14 mg/m³ (0.02 ppm) for 5 h: a more pronounced reduction in respiratory rate was observed in pretreated animals than in those that had not been previously exposed (Stevens & Palmer, 1970). Respiratory hypersensitivity developed in guinea-pigs receiving skin applications of various doses of toluene diisocyanate (Karol et al., 1981). The concentration dependence of this phenomenon has been examined in terms of the sensitizing dose and the challenge exposure to toluene diisocyanate, with complex results (Koschier et al., 1983).

Rats and rabbits were exposed to 0.7 mg/m³ (0.1 ppm) toluene diisocyanate for 6 h on one day per week for 38 weeks; rats, rabbits and guinea-pigs were exposed to the same dose level for 6 h per day on five days per week for a total of 58 exposures. In rabbits and guinea-pigs, no proliferation of fibrous tissue was seen in response to toluene diisocyanate. Rats showed proliferation of fibrous tissue in the walls of the bronchioles as well as pneumonitis, tracheitis and bronchitis (Niewenhuis et al., 1965). Similar effects were noted in rats receiving toluene diisocyanate by gavage in the course of a two-year bioassay for carcinogenic activity (National Toxicology Program, 1983). Among mice, chronic or necrotic rhinitis was common in exposed groups, with lesser lesions of the lower respiratory tract (bronchitis) and eyes (Loeser, 1983; see section 3.1).

Antibodies to toluene diisocyanate were produced in guinea-pigs exposed by inhalation, dermal contact or intraperitoneal injection (Karol, 1980). Relationships between antibody production, pulmonary sensitivity, dermal sensitivity and airborne concentration of toluene diisocyanate have been examined, with complex results (Karol, 1983).

In dogs, a correlation has been made between immunological and respiratory responses to toluene diisocyanate. Dogs exposed once every second week for 41 weeks to 1 mg/kg bw toluene diisocyanate delivered as an aerosol intratracheally developed a systemic immune response to toluene diisocyanate conjugated with dog serum albumin as well as immediate-type airway responses (Patterson *et al.*, 1983).

Effects on reproduction and prenatal toxicity
No data were available to the Working Group.

Absorption, distribution, excretion and metabolism
No data were available to the Working Group.

Because of its known chemical reactivity (see section 1), toluene diisocyanate may undergo hydrolysis to yield the corresponding diaminotoluene (IARC, 1979) and may bind to cellular components; however, no specific data are available.

Mutagenicity and other short-term tests
2,4-Toluene diisocyanate [purity unspecified], tested at up to 2500 ug/plate, was not mutagenic to *Salmonella typhimurium* TA1535, TA1538, TA98 or TA100 in the presence of a metabolic system (S9) from the liver of Aroclor-induced rats [details not given] (Anderson & Styles, 1978). Commercial-grade toluene diisocyanate (2,4- and 2,6-toluene diisocyanates, 80:20; Desmodur T80) was mutagenic at concentrations of 125-500 μg/plate in strains TA1538, TA98 and TA100, but not in TA1537, in the presence of phenobarbital-induced rat-liver S9 [data reported for strain TA98 only] (Andersen *et al.*, 1980).

Groups of five male and five female Sprague-Dawley CD rats and CD-1 mice were exposed by inhalation to the vapours of production-grade toluene diisocyanate (2,4- and 2,6-toluene diisocyanates, 80:20) at doses of 0.05 or 0.15 ppm (0.36 or 1.07 mg/m^3) for 6 h per day on five days per week for four weeks. There was no dose- or treatment-related increase in the number of micronucleated polychromatic erythrocytes in bone marrow recovered from exposed animals (Loeser, 1983). [The Working Group noted the inadequate reporting of this study.]

Mutagenicity of breakdown products

2,4-Diaminotoluene

The activity in short-term tests of 2,4-diaminotoluene, a breakdown product of 2,4-toluene diisocyanate, has been reviewed (IARC, 1978).

Irreversible DNA-binding was not detected when [³H]-2,4-diaminotoluene was incubated with calf-thymus DNA in the presence of a rat-liver microsomal metabolic system (Aune *et al.*, 1979).

2,4-Diaminotoluene is mutagenic to several strains of *Salmonella typhimurium* in the presence of an exogenous metabolic system. The frameshift strains TA1538 and TA98 are the most sensitive and positive results have been obtained with metabolic systems (S9) from livers of uninduced rats (Aune *et al.*, 1979; Dybing *et al.*, 1981); rats induced with Aroclor (Ames *et al.*, 1975; Pienta *et al.*, 1977a; Shahin *et al.*, 1980; Parodi *et al.*, 1981; Haworth *et al.*, 1983; Kawalek *et al.*, 1983), Kanechlor-500 (Nishi & Nishioka, 1982), phenobarbital (Andersen *et al.*, 1980; Dybing *et al.*, 1981; Kawalek *et al.*, 1983) and β-naphthoflavone (Aune *et al.*, 1979; Dybing *et al.*, 1981); uninduced and β-naphthoflavone-induced mice (Dybing & Thorgeirsson, 1977); and Aroclor-induced Syrian hamsters (Haworth *et al.*, 1983).

In a summary paper, 2,4-diaminotoluene was reported not to induce meiotic aneuploidy in *Neurospora crassa* in the absence of an exogenous metabolic system (Griffiths, 1981).

2,4-Diaminotoluene induced sex-linked recessive lethal mutations when fed as 5.9 or 15.2 mM solutions to adult male *Drosophila melanogaster*; mutagenic activity was highest in metabolically active germ cells (spermatids and spermatocytes) (Blijleven, 1977). Injection of adult male *Drosophila melanogaster* with 0.25 μl of 5-20 mM 2,4-diaminotoluene resulted in the induction of X-chromosome recessive mutations (lethal and visible) and rDNA mutations (Fahmy & Fahmy, 1977).

2,4-Diaminotoluene (0.3-3 mM) induced DNA strand breaks (detected by alkaline elution analysis) in Chinese hamster V79 cells cultured in the presence of rat-liver S9 [details of induction not given]; unequivocally positive results were seen only with the highest dose (Swenberg, 1981). Negative results were obtained by Sina *et al.* (1983) using alkaline-elution analysis of freshly prepared uninduced rat hepatocytes treated with 0.03-3 mM 2,4-diaminotoluene.

Nontoxic doses of 2,4-diaminotoluene ($<10^{-4}$ M) induced unscheduled DNA synthesis in cultured primary rat hepatocytes (Bermudez *et al.*, 1979).

Single-strand DNA breaks, detected by hydroxylapatite chromatography, were induced in cultured human skin fibroblasts by 0.1 mM 2,4-diaminotoluene in the presence of an exogenous metabolic system consisting of microsomes from sheep seminal vesicles supplemented with arachidonic acid; this system supplies prostaglandin synthetase. Inhibitors of this activity (indomethacin or acetylsalicylic acid) abolished the effect. Negative results were obtained when microsomes from livers of phenobarbital- or 3-methyl--cholanthrene-induced rats were used as the metabolic system (Nordenskjöld *et al.*, 1984).

2,4-Diaminotoluene induced trifluorothymidine-resistant mutants in L5178Y mouse lymphoma cells only in the absence of S9. Mutants resistant to 6-thioguanine were not detected. In Chinese hamster ovary cells, 5-fluorodeoxyuridine- but not 6-thioguanine-resistant mutants were induced by 2,4-diaminotoluene in both the presence and absence of liver S9 from Aroclor-induced rats (Coppinger *et al.*, 1984).

2,4-Diaminotoluene induced morphological transformation in secondary Syrian hamster embryo cells (Pienta *et al.*, 1977a,b; Pienta & Kawalek, 1981). 2,4-Diaminotoluene enhanced the transformation of primary Syrian hamster embryo cells by simian adenovirus 7 (SA7) when given subsequently. It was reported to induce morphological transformation of secondary Syrian hamster embryo cells, but good dose-responses were rare in this study, and it was reported to be inactive in three of six separate experiments [figures given for only two experiments] (Greene & Friedman, 1980).

Male Wister rats (untreated or pretreated with phenobarbital or β-naphthoflavone) were given intraperitoneal injections of 100 mg/kg bw [^{3}H]-2,4-diaminotoluene and killed 4 h later. Irreversible binding of radiolabel was not detected in DNA extracted from the liver, kidneys or femoral muscle of treated rats, although there was significant binding to protein and RNA (Aune *et al.*, 1979).

Alkaline-elution analysis of liver DNA extracted 4 or 24 h after male Sprague-Dawley rats were given an intraperitoneal injection of 4.1 mmol/kg bw 2,4-diaminotoluene (twice the LD_{50} dose) revealed the presence of significant levels of single-strand DNA breaks (Parodi *et al.*, 1981).

In an in-vivo/in-vitro DNA-repair assay, 2,4-diaminotoluene (150 mg/kg bw) was administered by gavage to male Fischer 344/N rats. Two or 12 h after treatment, hepatocytes were isolated and cultured with radiolabelled thymidine for assay of unscheduled DNA synthesis as a measure of DNA repair. 2,4-Diaminotoluene induced significant levels of unscheduled DNA synthesis in hepatocytes recovered 2 and 12 h after treatment *in vivo* (Mirsalis *et al.*, 1982).

Groups of five CBA x BALB/c F$_1$ mice were given five daily intraperitoneal injections of 2,4-diaminotoluene at doses ranging from 50-500 mg/kg bw per day. No increase in the incidence of sperm-head abnormalities was seen (Topham, 1980).

In order to test effects on testicular DNA synthesis, groups of ten C57B1/6 x C3H mice were given intraperitoneal injections of 111-375 mg/kg bw 2,4-diaminotoluene. Statistically significant dose-related decreases in the incorporation of ^{125}I-iododeoxyuridine into testicular DNA were observed (Greene *et al.*, 1981).

Dominant lethal mutations were not induced in groups of 20 male DBA/2J mice treated on two successive days by gavage or by intraperitoneal injection with 40 mg/kg bw 2,4-diaminotoluene. Sperm collected from ten mice from each group eight weeks after treatment showed no significant increase in the incidence of abnormal morphology when compared with appropriate controls (Soares & Lock, 1980).

Male Swiss mice received an intraperitoneal injection of 9 or 18 mg/kg bw 2,4-diaminotoluene and the incidence of sister chromatid exchange in bone-marrow cells was determined 24 h after treatment. Both dose levels induced statistically significant increases (1.53- and 1.39-fold at the low and high dose, respectively) (Parodi *et al.*, 1983).

2,6-Diaminotoluene

2,6-Diaminotoluene (1.5-5 μmol/plate) was mutagenic to *S. typhimurium* TA98 and TA100 in the presence of Aroclor-induced rat-liver S9 (Florin *et al.*, 1980).

2,6-Diaminotoluene enhanced the transformation of primary Syrian hamster embryo cells by simian adenovirus 7. It was reported to induce morphological transformation of secondary Syrian hamster embryo cells, but good dose-responses were rare in this study, and it was inactive in three of six separate experiments [figures given for only two experiments] (Greene & Friedman, 1980).

In an in-vivo/in-vitro DNA-repair assay, 2,6-diaminotoluene (150 mg/kg bw) was administered by gavage to male Fischer 344/N rats. Two or 12 h after treatment, hepatocytes were isolated and cultured with radiolabelled thymidine for assay of unscheduled DNA synthesis as a measure of DNA repair. 2,6-Diaminotoluene did not induce significant levels of unscheduled DNA synthesis in hepatocytes recovered 2 and 12 hours after treatment *in vivo* (Mirsalis *et al.*, 1982).

In order to test effects on testicular DNA synthesis, groups of ten C57Bl/6 × C3H mice were given intraperitoneal injections of 30-100 mg/kg bw 2,6-diaminotoluene. Statistically significant dose-related decreases in the incorporation of ^{125}I-iodeoxyuridine into testicular DNA were observed. The authors did not exclude the possibility that 2,6-diaminotoluene inhibited testicular DNA synthesis indirectly by inducing a marked drop in body temperature in treated animals (Greene *et al.*, 1981).

(b) Humans

Toxic effects

The toxic effects of toluene diisocyanate in humans have been reviewed (National Institute for Occupational Health, 1973, 1981; Izmerov, 1983).

Toluene diisocyanate is a powerful irritant to mucous membranes of the eye and upper and lower respiratory tract (National Institute for Occupational Safety and Health, 1973). Bronchial hypersensitivity developed in 2-5% of workers exposed to 0.02 ppm (0.14 mg/m³) or less (Elkins *et al.*, 1962; Peters & Wegman, 1975; National Institute for Occupational Safety and Health, 1981). Further exposure resulted in severe respiratory symptoms in individuals 'sensitized' to toluene diisocyanate; improvement occurs usually, but not always, when exposure is discontinued (National Institute for Occupational Safety and Health, 1973; Peters & Wegman, 1975; National Institute for Occupational Safety and Health, 1981; Moller *et al.*, 1984).

Acute changes in pulmonary function have been observed in exposed workers during the course of a work shift (Gandevia, 1963; Peters *et al.*, 1968). Such changes have been reported to be dose-related (Wegman *et al.*, 1974; Holness *et al.*, 1984). An increased rate of loss of pulmonary function has been observed in cohorts of workers exposed to low levels of toluene diisocyanate (Peters *et al.*, 1969; Adams, 1970; Peters, 1970); this has been found to be dose-related, with an excess rate occurring at about 0.002 or 0.003 ppm (0.014 or 0.021 mg/m³) (Wegman *et al.*, 1977; Diem *et al.*, 1982; Wegman *et al.*, 1982). Exposure to levels of approximately 0.001 ppm (0.007 mg/m³) for five to ten years produced no apparent respiratory effect (Musk *et al.*, 1982; Gee & Morgan, 1985).

Exposure to toluene diisocyanate may cause chronic restrictive pulmonary disease (Pham *et al.*, 1978a,b; Oleru, 1980), and hypersensitivity pneumonitis has also been associated with exposure to isocyanates (Charles *et al.*, 1976). Chronic bronchitis has been reported to be more frequent in workers exposed to high concentrations or repeatedly to low concentrations of toluene diisocyanate (McKerrow *et al.*, 1970). Persistent respiratory symptoms have been observed in sensitized workers not further exposed to toluene diisocyanate (Adams, 1975).

Exposure to very high concentrations of toluene diisocyanate results in long-term sequelae that affect the central nervous system, and symptoms such as headache, poor memory, difficulty in concentrating, confusion, changes in personality, irritability and depression have been reported (Le Quesne *et al.*, 1976).

Effects on reproduction and prenatal toxicity
No data were available to the Working Group.

Absorption, distribution, excretion and metabolism
No data were available to the Working Group.

Mutagenicity and chromosomal effects
No data were available to the Working Group.

3.3 Case reports and epidemiological studies of carcinogenicity to humans

Mortillaro and Schiavon (1982) described a 47-year-old nonsmoking spray-painter who had an adenocarcinoma of the lung. He had been exposed to toluene diisocyanate and 4,4'-methylenediphenyl diisocyanate (IARC, 1979) for 15 years and had had a ten-year history of lung disease thought to be caused by exposure to isocyanates.

4. Summary of Data Reported and Evaluation

4.1 Exposure data

Toluene diisocyanate has been available commercially since the late 1930s. Occupational exposure to toluene diisocyanate occurs during its production and in the processing and handling of polyurethane foam products.

4.2 Experimental data

Commercial mixtures of 2,4- and 2,6-toluene diisocyanate were tested for carcinogenicity in mice and rats by intragastric administration and by inhalation exposure. Intragastric administration induced a dose-related increase in the incidence of subcutaneous fibromas and fibrosarcomas (combined) in male rats, together with an increase in the incidence of pancreatic acinar-cell adenomas in male rats and in pancreatic islet-cell adenomas, neoplastic nodules of the liver and mammary gland fibroadenomas in female rats. In female mice, dose-related increases in the combined incidence of haemangiomas and haemangiosarcomas and of hepatocellular adenomas were observed; no treatment-related tumour was seen in male mice, possibly due to poor survival. No treatment-related tumour was observed after exposure of mice or rats to commercial toluene diisocyanate by inhalation, although the results of the study with rats have not been reported fully.

The Working Group noted the similarity in tumour response of mice and rats to toluene diisocyanate and 2,4-diaminotoluene.

No data were available to evaluate the reproductive or prenatal toxicity of toluene diisocyanate to experimental animals.

The available data were inadequate to assess the mutagenicity of toluene diisocyanate. 2,4- and 2,6-Diaminotoluenes (breakdown products of 2,4- and 2,6-toluene diisocyanates) were mutagenic to *Salmonella typhimurium* in the presence of an exogenous metabolic system. 2,4-Diaminotoluene induced mutation in *Drosophila melanogaster* and DNA damage, DNA repair and mutation in cultured mammalian cells. It also induced morphological transformation in cultured mammalian cells. It induced DNA damage and DNA repair in the liver of rats, and increases in the frequency of sister chromatid exchanges in bone-marrow cells of mice treated *in vivo*. 2,4-Diaminotoluene did not induce dominant lethal mutations in mice.

Overall assessment of data from short-term tests: Toluene diisocyanate[a]

	Genetic activity			Cell transformation
	DNA damage	Mutation	Chromosomal effects	
Prokaryotes		?		
Fungi/Green plants				
Insects				
Mammalian cells (*in vitro*)				
Mammals (*in vivo*)				
Humans (*in vivo*)				
Degree of evidence in short-term tests for genetic activity: **Inadequate**				Cell transformation: No data

[a]The groups into which the table is divided and the symbol ? are defined on pp. 19-20 of the Preamble; the degrees of evidence are defined on pp. 20-21.

4.3 Human data

Toluene diisocyanate is a potent respiratory irritant and sensitizer even at low airborne concentrations.

No data were available to evaluate the reproductive effects or prenatal toxicity of toluene diisocyanate to humans.

The one case report of an adenocarcinoma of the lung associated with exposure to isocyanates was inadequate for evaluation of the carcinogenicity of toluene diisocyanate.

4.4 Evaluation[1]

There is *sufficient evidence*[2] for the carcinogenicity of toluene diisocyanate to experimental animals.

There is *inadequate evidence* for the carcinogenicity of toluene diisocyanate to humans.

5. References

Adams, W.G.F. (1970) Lung function of men engaged in the manufacture of tolylene diisocyanate (TDI). *Proc. R. Soc. Med., 63*, 378-379

Adams, W.G.F. (1975) Long-term effects on the health of men engaged in the manufacture of tolylene di-isocyanate. *Br. J. ind. Med., 32*, 72-78

Aldrich Chemical Co. (1984) *1984-1985 Aldrich Catalog/Handbook of Fine Chemicals*, Milwaukee, WI, p. 1048

Almaguer, D., Orris, P. & Kramkowski, R. (1982) *Health Hazard Evaluation Report No. HETA-81-128-1107, Janesville Products, Bradhead, WI (US NTIS PB84-141845)*, Cincinnati, OH, National Institute for Occupational Safety and Health

American Conference of Governmental Industrial Hygienists (1984) *Threshold Limit Values for Chemical Substances and Physical Agents in the Work Environment and Biological Exposure Indices with Intended Changes for 1984-85*, Cincinnati, OH, p. 31

Ames, B.N., Kammen, H.O. & Yamasaki, E. (1975) Hair dyes are mutagenic: Identification of a variety of mutagenic ingredients. *Proc. natl Acad. Sci. USA, 72*, 2423-2427

---

[1]For definition of the italicized terms, see preamble, pp. 18 and 22.

[2]In the absence of adequate data in humans, it is reasonable, for practical purposes, to regard chemicals for which there is sufficient evidence of carcinogenicity in animals as if they represented a carcinogenic risk to humans.

Andersen, M., Binderup, M.-L., Kiel, P., Larsen, H. & Maxild, J. (1980) Mutagenic action of isocyanates used in the production of polyurethanes. *Scand. J. Work Environ. Health, 6*, 221-226

Anderson, D. & Styles, J.A. (1978) Appendix II. The bacterial mutation test. *Br. J. Cancer, 37*, 924-929

Andersson, K., Gudéhn, A., Levin, J.-O., & Nilsson, C.-A. (1982) Analysis of gaseous diisocyanates in air using chemosorption sampling. *Chemosphere, 11*, 3-10

Anon. (1984a) Chemical profile: TDI. *Chem. Mark. Rep., 226*, 66

Anon. (1984b) TDI. *Chem. Mark. Rep., 225*, 14

Arbetarskyddsstyrelsens Författningssamling (National Swedish Board of Occupational Safety and Health) (1984) *Hygienic Limit Values (AFS 1984:5)* (Swed.), Stockholm, p. 34

Aune, T., Nelson, S.D. & Dybing, E. (1979) Mutagenicity and irreversible binding of the hepatocarcinogen, 2,4-diaminotoluene. *Chem.-biol. Interactions, 25*, 23-33

Bagon, D.A. & Hardy, H.L. (1978) Determination of free monomeric toluene diisocyanate (TDI) and 4,4'-diisocyanatodiphenylmethane (MDI) in TDI and MDI prepolymers, respectively, by high-performance liquid chromatography. *J. Chromatogr., 152*, 560-564

Bagon, D.A. & Purnell, C.J. (1980) Determination of airborne free monomeric aromatic and aliphatic isocyanates by high-performance liquid chromatography. *J. Chromatogr., 190*, 175-182

BASF Wyandotte Corp. (1981) *Technical Service Report: Toluene Diisocyanate*, Parsippany, NJ

BASF Wyandotte Corp. (1984) *Material Safety Data Sheet: Toluene Diisocyanate (Report No. 585621)*, Parsippany, NJ

Bermudez, E., Tillery, D. & Butterworth, B.E. (1979) The effect of 2,4-diaminotoluene and isomers of dinitrotoluene on unscheduled DNA synthesis in primary rat hepatocytes. *Environ. Mutagenesis, 1*, 391-398

Bishop, R.W., Ayers, T.A. & Esposito, G.G. (1983) A gas chromatographic procedure for the determination of airborne MDI and TDI. *Am. ind. Hyg. Assoc. J., 44*, 151-155

Blijleven, W.G.H. (1977) Mutagenicity of four hair dyes in *Drosophila melanogaster*. *Mutat. Res., 48*, 181-186

Buckingham, J., ed. (1982) *Dictionary of Organic Compounds*, 5th ed., 1st Suppl. New York, Chapman and Hall, p. 196

Buckley, L.A., Jiang, X.Z., James, R.A., Morgan, K.T. & Barrow, C.S. (1984) Respiratory tract lesions induced by sensory irritants at the RD50 concentration. *Toxicol. appl. Pharmacol., 74*, 417-429

Burroughs, G.E. & Moody, P.L. (1982) *Health Hazard Evaluation Report No. HETA-81-029-1088 Industrial Plastics, Valley City, OH (US NTIS PB83-198390)*, Cincinnati, OH, National Institute for Occupational Safety and Health

Chadwick, D.H. & Cleveland, T.H. (1981) *Isocyanates, organic.* In: Mark, H.F., Othmer, D.F., Overberger, C.G. & Seaborg, G.T., eds, *Kirk-Othmer Encyclopedia of Chemical Technology*, 3rd ed., Vol. 13, New York, John Wiley & Sons, pp. 789-818

Chang, S.-N. & Burg, W.R. (1982) Determination of airborne 2,4-toluenediisocyanate vapors. *J. Chromatogr.*, *246*, 113-120

Charles, J., Bernstein, A., Jones, B., Jones, D.J., Edwards, J.H., Seal, R.M.E. & Seaton, A. (1976) Hypersensitivity pneumonitis after exposure to isocyanates. *Thorax*, *31*, 127-136

Chrostek, W.J. & Cromer, J.W., Jr (1975) *Health Hazard Evaluation Determination Report No. 74-42-168, Trionic Industries, Incorporated, Harrisburg, PA*, Cincinnati, OH, National Institute for Occupational Safety and Health

Ciosek, A., Gesicka, E. & Kesy-Dabrowska, I. (1969) The evaluation of the occupational exposure of workers employed at the production of polyurethane foam (Pol.). *Med. Pracy*, *20*, 417-424

Conte, A. & Cossi, G. (1981) Gas chromatographic determination of free toluene diisocyanate in flexible urethane foams. *J. Chromatogr.*, *213*, 162-165

Coppinger, W.J., Brennan, S.A., Carver, J.H. & Thompson, E.D. (1984) Locus specificity of mutagenicity of 2,4-diaminotoluene in both L5178Y mouse lymphoma and AT3-2 Chinese hamster ovary cells. *Mutat. Res.*, *135*, 115-123

Craver, C.D., ed. (1977a) *The Coblentz Society Desk Book of Infrared Spectra*, Kirkwood, MO, The Coblentz Society, Inc.

Craver, C.D., ed. (1977b) *Plasticizers and Other Additives*, Kirkwood, MO, The Coblentz Society, Inc.

Davey, J.E. & Edwards, A.D. (1983) Determination of toluene-2,4-diisocyanate in rubber fumes. *Analyst*, *108*, 407-411

De Rosa, F., Rivali, F., Dardanelli, C., Salvadori, P., Capriotti, L. & Polidori, G. (1980) The furniture industry and wastewater pollution (Ital.). *Inquinamento*, *22*, 43-45

Dharmarajan, V. (1977) Analysis of toluene diisocyanate (TDI) and p,p'-diphenylmethane diisocyanate (MDI) in air. *Am. ind. Hyg. Assoc. J.*, *38*, 725-726

Diem, J.E., Jones, R.N., Hendrick, D.J., Glindmeyer, H.W., Dharmarajam, V., Butcher, B.T., Salvaggio, J.E. & Weill, H. (1982) Five-year longitudinal study of workers employed in a new toluene diisocyanate manufacturing plant. *Am. Rev. resp. Dis.*, *126*, 420-428

Duff, P.B. (1983) *The fate of TDI in the environment.* In: *Polyurethane: New Paths to Progress, Marketing, Technology; Proceedings of the 6th SPI International Technical Marketing Conference, San Diego, CA, November 2-4 1983*, New York, Society of the Plastic Industry, pp. 408-412

Duncan, B., Scheel, L.D., Fairchild, E.J., Killens, R. & Graham, S. (1962) Toluene diisocyanate inhalation toxicity: Pathology and mortality. *Am. ind. Hyg. Assoc. J.*, *19*, 447-456

Dybing, E. & Thorgeirsson, S.S. (1977) Metabolic activation of 2,4-diaminoanisole, a hair-dye component. I. Role of cytochrome P-450 metabolism in mutagenicity *in vitro. Biochem. Pharmacol., 26*, 729-734

Dybing, E., Saxholm, H.J.K., Aune, T., Wirth, P.J. & Thorgeisson, S.S. (1981) Studies on mutagenic and carcinogenic *N*-substituted aryl compounds: Cosmetics and drugs. *Natl Cancer Inst. Monogr., 58*, 21-26

Ebell, G.F., Fleming, D.E., Genovese, J.H. & Taylor, G.A. (1980) Simultaneous determination of 2,4- and 2,6-diisocyanotoluene (TDI) and 3,3'-dichloro-4,4'-diamino-diphenylmethane (MOCA) in air. *Ann. occup. Hyg., 23*, 185-188

Elkins, H.B., McCarl, G.W., Brugsch, H.G. & Fahy, J.P. (1962) Massachusetts experience with toluene di-isocyanate. *Am. ind. Hyg. Assoc. J., 23*, 265-272

Fahmy, M.J. & Fahmy, O.G. (1977) Mutagenicity of hair dye components relative to the carcinogen benzidine in *Drosophila melanogaster. Mutat. Res., 56*, 31-38

Florin, I., Rutberg, L., Curvall, M. & Enzell, C.R. (1980) Screening of tobacco smoke constituents for mutagenicity using the Ames' test. *Toxicology, 18*, 219-232

Gandevia, B. (1963) Studies of ventilatory capacity and histamine response during exposure to isocyanate vapour in polyurethane foam manufacture. *Br. J. ind. Med., 20*, 204-209

Gee, J.B. & Morgan, W.K.C. (1985) A 10-year follow-up study of a group of workers exposed to isocyanates. *J. occup. Med., 27*, 15-18

Glass, W.I. & Thom, N.G. (1964) Respiratory hazards associated with toluene di-isocyanate in polyurethane foam production. *N. Z. med. J., 63*, 642-647

Goldberg, P.A., Walker, R.F., Ellwood, P.A. & Hardy, H.L. (1981) Determination of trace atmospheric isocyanate concentrations by reversed-phase high-performance liquid chromatography using 1-(2-pyridyl)piperazine reagent. *J. Chromatogr., 212*, 93-104

Graham, J.D. (1980) Simplified sample handling procedure for monitoring industrial isocyanates in air. *J. chromatogr. Sci., 18*, 384-387

Greene, E.J. & Friedman, M.A. (1980) In vitro cell transformation screening of 4 toluene diamine isomers. *Mutat. Res., 79*, 363-375

Greene, E.J., Salerno, A.J. & Friedman, M.A. (1981) Effect of 4 toluene diamine isomers on murine testicular DNA synthesis. *Mutat. Res., 91*, 75-79

Grieveson, B.M. & Reeve, B. (1983) Isocyanate emissions: A review of work on environmental aspects of handling toluene diisocyanate. *Cell. Polymers, 2*, 165-175

Griffiths, A.J.F. (1981) *Neurospora and environmentally aneuploidy.* In: Stich, H.F. & San, R.H.C., eds, *Short-Term Tests For Chemical Carcinogens*, New York, Springer-Verlag, pp. 187-199

Grim, K.E. & Linch, A.L. (1964) Recent isocyanate-in-air analysis studies. *Am. ind. Hyg. Assoc. J., 25*, 285-290

Gunter, B.J. (1975) *Health Hazard Evaluation Determination Report No. 74-148-239, Lange Company, Broomfield, CO*, Cincinnati, OH, National Institute for Occupational Safety and Health

Gunter, B.J. & Lucas, J.B. (1975) *Health Hazard Evaluation Determination Report No. 74-73-233, Gates Rubber Company, Denver, CO*, Cincinnati, OH, National Institute for Occupational Safety and Health

Gustavsson, P. (1977) *Diisocyanates. A Review of the Literature on Medical and Toxicological Observations (Arbete och Hälsa, Vetenskaplig Skriftserie 1977:11)* (Swed.), Stockholm, Liber Tryck

Hawley, G.G., ed. (1981) *The Condensed Chemical Dictionary*, 10th ed., New York, Van Nostrand Reinhold Co., p. 1030

Haworth, S., Lawlor, T., Mortelmans, K., Speck, W. & Zeiger, E. (1983) *Salmonella* mutagenicity test results for 250 chemicals. *Environ. Mutagenesis, Suppl. 1*, 3-142

Hervin, R.L. & Thoburn, T.W. (1975) *Health Hazard Evaluation/Toxicity Determination Report No. HHE-72-96-237, Trans World Airlines Main Overhaul Facility, Kansas City International Airport, Kansas City, Missouri (US NTIS PB-249417)*, Cincinnati, OH, National Institute for Occupational Safety and Health

Hobara, T., Kobayashi, H., Higashihara, E., Kawamoto, T., Iwamoto, S., Shimazu, W. & Sakai, T. (1984) Health hazard by exposure to toluene-diisocyanate in the shipyard. *Bull. environ. Contam. Toxicol., 32*, 134-139

Holness, D.L., Broder, I., Corey, P.N., Booth, N., Mozzon, D., Nazar, M.A. & Guirguis, S. (1984) Respiratory variables and exposure-effect relationships in isocyanate-exposed workers. *J. occup. Med., 26*, 449-455

Hosein, H.R. & Farkas, S. (1981) Risk associated with the spray application of polyurethane foam. *Am. ind. Hyg. Assoc. J., 42*, 663-665

IARC (1978) *IARC Monographs on the Evaluation of the Carcinogenic Risk of Chemicals to Man*, Vol. 16, *Some Aromatic Amines and Related Nitro Compounds — Hair Dyes, Colouring Agents and Miscellaneous Industrial Chemicals*, Lyon, pp. 83-95

IARC (1979) *IARC Monographs on the Evaluation of the Carcinogenic Risk of Chemicals to Humans*, Vol. 19, *Some Monomers, Plastics, Synthetic Elastomers, and Acrolein*, Lyon, France, pp. 303-340

IARC (1982) *IARC Monographs on the Evaluation of the Carcinogenic Risk of Chemicals to Humans*, Suppl. 4, *Chemicals, Industrial Processes and Industries Associated with Cancer in Humans, IARC Monographs Volume 1 to 29*, Lyon, p. 268

International Isocyanate Institute, Inc. (1980) *Technical Information. Recommendations for the Handling of Toluene Diisocyanate (TDI)*, New Canaan, CT

International Labour Office (1980) *Occupational Exposure Limits for Airborne Toxic Substances, A Tabular Compilation of Values from Selected Countries*, 2nd (rev.) ed. (*Occupational Safety and Health Series No. 37*), Geneva, pp. 204-205

Izmerov, N.F., ed. (1983) *Scientific Reviews of Soviet Literature on Toxicity and Hazards of Chemicals, Toluylene Diisocyanate* (No. 30), Moscow, International Register of Potentially Toxic Chemicals, Centre of International Projects

Karol, M.H. (1980) Study of guinea pig and human antibodies to toluene diisocyanate. *Am. Rev. resp. Dis., 122*, 965-970

Karol, M.H. (1983) Concentration-dependent immunologic response to toluene diisocyanate (TDI) following inhalation exposure. *Toxicol. appl. Pharmacol.*, *68*, 229-241

Karol, M.H., Hauth, B.A., Riley, E.J. & Magreni, C.M. (1981) Dermal contact with toluene diisocyanate (TDI) produces respiratory tract hypersensitivity in guinea pigs. *Toxicol. appl. Pharmacol.*, *58*, 221-230

Kawalek, J.C., Hallmark, R.K. & Andrews, A.W. (1983) Effect of lithocholic acid on the mutagenicity of some substituted aromatic amines. *J. natl Cancer Inst.*, *71*, 293-298

Kormos, L.H., Sandridge, R.L. & Keller, J. (1981) Determination of isocyanates in air by liquid chromatography with fluorescence detection. *Anal. Chem.*, *53*, 1122-1125

Koschier, F.J., Burden, E.J., Brunkhorst, C.S. & Friedman, M.A. (1983) Concentration-dependent elicitation of dermal sensitization in guinea pigs treated with 2,4-toluene diisocyanate. *Toxicol. appl. Pharmacol.*, *67*, 401-407

Le Quesne, P.M., Axford, A.T., McKerrow, C.B. & Jones, A.J. (1976) Neurological complications after a single severe exposure to toluene di-isocyanate. *Br. J. ind. Med.*, *33*, 72-78

Loeser, E. (1983) Long-term toxicity and carcinogenicity studies with 2,4/2,6-toluenediisocyanate (80/20) in rats and mice. *Toxicol. Lett.*, *15*, 71-81

Mannsville Chemical Products Corp. (1983) *Toluene Diisocyanate (Chemical Products Synopsis)*, Cortland, NY

Marcali, K. (1957) Microdetermination of toluenediisocyanates in atmosphere. *Anal. Chem.*, *29*, 552-558

Maxon, F.C., Jr (1964) Respiratory irritation from toluene diisocyanate. *Arch. environ. Health*, *8*, 755-758

McKerrow, C.B., Davies, H.J. & Jones, A.P. (1970) Symptoms and lung function following acute and chronic exposure to tolylene diisocyanate. *Proc. R. Soc. Med.*, *63*, 376-378

Meyer, S.D. & Tallman, D.E. (1983) The determination of toluene diisocyanate in air by high-performance liquid chromatography with electrochemical detection. *Anal. chim. Acta*, *146*, 227-236

Mirsalis, J.C., Tyson, C.K. & Butterworth, B.E. (1982) Detection of genotoxic carcinogens in the in vivo-in vitro hepatocyte DNA repair assay. *Environ. Mutagenesis*, *4*, 553-562

Mobay Chemical Corp. (1984a) *Material Safety Data Sheet: Mondur® TDS Grade I and II*, Pittsburgh, PA, Code E-003

Mobay Chemical Corp. (1984b) *Material Safety Data Sheet: Mondur® TD-80 (All Grades)*, Pittsburgh, PA, Code E-002

Mobay Chemical Corp. (1984c) *Product Information: Mondur® TDS and Mondur® TD (Technical Bulletin No. EA-8, EA-9)*, Pittsburgh, PA

Moller, D.R., McKay, R.T., Bernstein, I.L. & Brooks, S.M. (1984) Long-term follow-up of workers with TDI asthma (Abstract). *Am. Rev. resp. Dis.*, *129*, A159

Mortillaro, P.T. & Schiavon, M. (1982) One case of lung cancer that developed in the course of a bronchopulmonary disease due to isocyanates (Ital.). *Med. Lav.*, *3*, 207-209

Musk, A.W., Peters, J.M., DiBerardinis, L. & Murphy, R.L.H. (1982) Absence of respiratory effects in subjects exposed to low concentrations of TDI amd MDI. *J. occup. Med., 24,* 746-750

National Cancer Institute (1979) *Bioassay of 2,4-Diaminotoluene for Possible Carcinogenicity (CAS No. 95-80-7),* Bethesda, MD

National Cancer Institute (1980) *Bioassay of 2,6-Toluenediamine Dihydrochloride for Possible Carcinogenicity (CAS No. 15481-70-6) (Tech. Rep. Ser. No. 200),* Bethesda, MD

National Fire Protection Association (1984) *Fire Protection Guide on Hazardous Materials,* 8th ed., Quincy, MA, pp. 325M-87, 49-88

National Institute for Occupational Safety and Health (1973) *Occupational Exposure to Toluene Diisocyanate (HSM 73-11022),* Washington DC, US Department of Health, Education, and Welfare

National Institute for Occupational Safety and Health (1977) *Failure Report No. S344 (NTIS Pub. No. PB81-229007),* Springfield, VA, US Department of Commerce

National Institute for Occupational Safety and Health (1978) *Criteria for a Recommended Standard ... Occupational Exposure to Diisocyanates (DHEW (NIOSH) Pub. No. 78-215),* Washington DC, US Department of Health, Education, and Welfare

National Institute for Occupational Safety and Health (1981) *Respiratory and Immunologic Evaluation of Isocyanate Exposure in a New Manufacturing Plant (DHHS (NIOSH) Publ. No. 81-125),* Washington DC, US Department of Health and Human Services

National Toxicology Program (1983) *NTP Technical Report on the Carcinogenesis Studies of Commercial Grade 2,4 (86%) and 2,6 (14%) Toluene Diisocyanate (CAS No. 26471-62-5) in F344/N Rats and B6C3F$_1$ Mice (Gavage Studies) (Tech. Rep. No. 251),* Research Triangle Park, NC

Nieminen, E.H., Saarinen, L.H. & Laakso, J.T. (1983) Simultaneous determination of aromatic isocyanates and some carcinogenic amines in the work atmosphere by reversed-phase high-performance liquid chromatography. *J. liq. Chromatogr., 6,* 453-469

Niewenhuis, R., Scheel, L., Stemmer, K. & Killens, R. (1965) Toxicity of chronic low level exposures to toluene diisocyanate in animals. *Am. ind. Hyg. Assoc. J., 26,* 143-149

NIH/EPA Chemical Information System (1983) *Carbon-13 NMR Spectral Search System, Mass Spectral Search System,* and *Infrared Spectral Search System,* Arlington, VA, Information Consultants, Inc

Nishi, K. & Nishioka, H. (1982) Light induces mutagenicity of hair-dye *p*-phenylenediamine. *Mutat. Res., 104,* 347-350

Nordenskjöld, M., Andersson, B., Rahimtula, A. & Moldeus, P. (1984) Prostaglandin synthase-catalyzed metabolic activation of some aromatic amines to genotoxic products. *Mutat. Res., 127,* 107-112

Nutt, A. (1983) Determination of isocyanates using a paper tape monitor. *Anal. Proc., 20,* 63-65

Oleru, U.G. (1980) Respiratory function study of Nigerian workers in a TDI-based foam plant. *Am. ind. Hyg. Assoc. J.*, *41*, 595-599

Olin Chemicals (1982) *Toluene Diisocyanate (TDI)*, Stamford, CT

Parodi, S., Taningher, M., Russo, P., Pala, M., Tamaro, M. & Monti-Bragadin, C. (1981) DNA-damaging activity *in vivo* and bacterial mutagenicity of sixteen aromatic amines and azo-derivatives, as related quantitatively to their carcinogenicity. *Carcinogenesis*, *2*, 1317-1326

Parodi, S., Zunino, A., Ottaggio, L., De Ferrari, M. & Santi, L. (1983) Lack of correlation between the capability of inducing sister-chromatid exchanges *in vivo* and carcinogenic potency, for 16 aromatic amines and azo derivatives. *Mutat. Res.*, *108*, 225-238

Patterson, R., Zeiss, C.R. & Harris, K.E. (1983) Immunologic and respiratory responses to airway challenges of dogs with toluene diisocyanate. *J. Allergy clin. Immunol.*, *71*, 604-611

Peng, M. & Muzal, K. (1984) The determination of aromatic diisocyanates in air: A new normal-phase HPLC method. *Liq. Chromatogr.*, *2*, 232-234

Peters, J.M. (1970) Studies of isocyanate toxicity. *Proc. R. Soc. Med.*, *63*, 372-375

Peters, J.M. & Wegman, D.H. (1975) Epidemiology of toluene diisocyanate (TDI)-induced respiratory disease. *Environ. Health Perspect.*, *11*, 97-100

Peters, J.M., Murphy, R.L.H., Pagnotto, L.D. & Van Ganse, W.F. (1968) Acute respiratory effects in workers exposed to low levels of toluene diisocyanate (TDI). *Arch. environ. Health*, *16*, 642-647

Peters, J.M., Murphy, R.L.H. & Ferris, B.G., Jr (1969) Ventilatory function in workers exposed to low levels of toluene diisocyanate: A six-month follow-up. *Br. J. ind. Med.*, *26*, 115-120

Pham, Q.T., Cavelier, C., Mereau, P., Mur, J.M. & Cicolella, A. (1978a) Isocyanates and respiratory function: A study of workers producing polyurethane foam moulding. *Ann. occup. Hyg.*, *21*, 121-129

Pham, Q.T., Cavelier, C., Mur, J.M. & Mereau, P. (1978b) Isocyanates at levels higher than MAC and their effect on respiratory function. *Ann. occup. Hyg.*, *21*, 271-275

Pienta, R.J. & Kawalek, C. (1981) Transformation of hamster embryo cells by aromatic amines. *Natl Cancer Inst. Monogr.*, *58*, 243-251

Pienta, R.J., Shah, M.J., Lebherz, W.B., III & Andrews, A.W. (1977a) Correlation of bacterial mutagenicity and hamster cell transformation with tumorigenicity induced by 2,4-toluenediamine. *Cancer Lett.*, *3*, 45-52

Pienta, R.J., Poiley, J.A. & Lebherz, W.B., III (1977b) Morphological transformation of early passage golden Syrian hamster embryo cells derived from cryopreserved primary cultures as a reliable *in vitro* bioassay for identifying diverse carcinogens. *Br. J. Cancer*, *19*, 642-655

Porter, C.V., Higgins, R.L. & Scheel, L.D. (1975) A retrospective study of clinical, physiologic and immunologic changes in workers exposed to toluene diisocyanate. *Am. ind. Hyg. Assoc. J.*, *36*, 159-168

Pouchert, C.J., ed. (1981) *The Aldrich Library of Infrared Spectra*, 3rd ed., Milwaukee, WI, Aldrich Chemical Co., Inc., p. 1144

Pouchert, C.J., ed. (1983) *The Aldrich Library of NMR Spectra*, 2nd ed., Vol. 2, Milwaukee, WI, Aldrich Chemical Co., pp. 445-446

Rando, R.J. & Hammad, Y.Y. (1985) Modified Marcali method for the determination of total toluene diisocyanate in air. *Am. ind. Hyg. Assoc. J.*, *46*, 206-210

Rando, R.J., Abdel-Kader, H.M. & Hammad, Y.Y. (1984) Isomeric composition of airborne TDI in the polyurethane foam industry. *Am. ind. Hyg. Assoc. J.*, *45*, 199-203

Reilly, D.A. (1968) A test-paper method for the determination of tolylene di-isocyanate vapour in air. *Analyst*, *93*, 178-185

Roper, C.P. & Cromer, J.W., Jr (1975) *Health Hazard Evaluation/Toxicity Determination Report No. HHE-74-118-218, General Tire & Rubber Company, Marion, Indiana (US NTIS PB-249398)*, Cincinnati, OH, National Institute for Occupational Safety and Health

Rosenberg, C. (1984) Direct determination of isocyanates and amines as degradation products in the industrial production of polyurethane-coated wire. *Analyst*, *109*, 859-866

Rubicon Chemicals Inc. (1983) *Material Safety Data Sheet: Rubinate(R) TDI (Toluene Diisocyanate) (Form No. M3779)*, Geismar, LA

Sadtler Research Laboratories (1980) *The Sadtler Standard Spectra Collection, Cumulative Index*, Philadelphia, PA

Sandridge, R.L. (1982) (untitled) *Am. ind. Hyg. Assoc. J.*, *43*, A16-A17

Sangha, G.K. & Alarie, Y. (1979) Sensory irritation by toluene diisocyanate in single and repeated exposures. *Toxicol. appl. Pharmacol.*, *50*, 533-547

Sangö, C. & Zimerson, E. (1980) A new reagent for determination of isocyanates in working atmospheres by HPLC using UV or fluorescence detection. *J. liq. Chromatogr.*, *3*, 971-990

Sax, N.I. (1984) *Dangerous Properties of Industrial Materials*, 6th ed., New York, Van Nostrand Reinhold, p. 2590

Scott, P.H. & Carey, D.A. (1976) Fabrethane, a one component urethane foam fabric coating. *J. coated Fabr.*, *6*, 13-19

Shahin, M.M., Bugaut, A. & Kalopissis, G. (1980) Structure-activity relationship within a series of *m*-diaminobenzene derivatives. *Mutat. Res.*, *78*, 25-31

Sina, J.F., Bean, C.L., Dysart, G.R., Taylor, V.I. & Bradley, M.O. (1983) Evaluation of the alkaline elution/rat hepatocyte assay as a predictor of carcinogenic/mutagenic potential. *Mutat. Res.*, *113*, 357-391

Soares, E.R. & Lock, L.F. (1980) Lack of an indication of mutagenic effects of dinitrotoluenes and diaminotoluenes in mice. *Environ. Mutagenesis*, *2*, 111-124

Sova, B. (1974) Experience with isocyanates in the footwear industry (Czech.). *Kozarstvi*, *24*, 20-22 [*Chem. Abstr.*, *81*, 67963g]

Stevens, M.A. & Palmer, R. (1970) The effect of tolylene diisocyanate on certain laboratory animals. *Proc. R. Soc. Med.*, *63*, 380-382

Swenberg, J.A. (1981) *Utilization of the alkaline elution assay as a short-term test for chemical carcinogens*. In: Stich, H.F. & San, R.H.C., eds, *Short-Term Tests for Chemical Carcinogens*, New York, Springer-Verlag, pp. 48-58

Taylor, D.G. (1977) *NIOSH Manual of Analytical Methods*, 2nd ed., Vol. 1 (*DHEW (NIOSH) Publication No. 77-157-A*), Washington DC, US Government Printing Office, pp. 141-1 - 141-8

Taylor, D.G. (1980) *NIOSH Manual of Analytical Methods*, Vol. 6 (*DHHS (NIOSH) Publication No. 80-125*), Washington DC, US Government Printing Office, pp. 326-1 — 326-11

Tonkoshkurov, Y.S. (1969) Sanitary and hygienic conditions during the preparation and use of the polymer cement 'Polief' (Russ.). *Gig. Tr. prof. Zabol.*, *13*, 41 [*Chem. Abstr.*, *72*, 70364g]

Topham, J.C. (1980) Do induced sperm-head abnormalities in mice specifically identify mammalian mutagens rather than carcinogens? *Mutat. Res.*, *74*, 379-387

Tucker, S.P. & Arnold, J.E. (1982) Sampling and determination of 2,4-bis(carbonyl-amino)toluene and 4,4'-bis(carbonylamino)-diphenylmethane in air. *Anal. Chem.*, *54*, 1137-1141

Työsuojeluhallitus (National Finnish Board of Occupational Safety and Health) (1981) Bull. *3*) (Finn.), Tampere, p. 25

Ulrich, H. (1983) *Urethane polymers*: In: Mark, H.F., Othmer, D.F., Overberger, C.G. & Seaborg, G.T., eds, *Kirk-Othmer Encyclopedia of Chemical Technology*, 3rd ed., Vol. 13, New York, John Wiley & Sons, pp. 576-608

Union Carbide Corp. (1967) *Toxicological Studies: 'Niax' Isocyanate TDI*, New York, Industrial Medicine and Toxicology Department

US Environmental Protection Agency (1984) Protection of environment. *US Code Fed. Regul.*, *Title 40*, Part 261.33, p. 364

US Food and Drug Administration (1984) Food and drugs. *US Code Fed. Regul.*, *Title 21*, Parts 175.105, 177.1680, pp. 137, 256

US International Trade Commission (1984) *Synthetic Organic Chemicals, US Production and Sales, 1983* (*USITC Publication 1588*), Washington DC, US Government Printing Office, p. 27

US Occupational Safety and Health Administration (1983) *General Industry. OSHA Safety and Health Standards (29 CFR 1910), OSHA 2206* (revised), Washington DC, p. 602

Vandervort, R. & Shama, S.K. (1973) *Health Hazard Evaluation Determination Report No. 73-30-90, King Seeley Thermos Company, Macomb, IL*, Cincinnati, OH, National Institute for Occupational Safety and Health

Verschueren, K. (1983) *Handbook of Environmental Data on Organic Chemicals*, 2nd ed., New York, Van Nostrand Reinhold, pp. 1108-1109

Vogt, C.R.H., Ko, C.Y. & Ryan, T.R. (1976) *Modification of an Analytical Procedure for Isocyanates to High Speed Liquid Chromatography* (*US NTIS PB-262675*), Springfield, VA, US Department of Commerce

Walker, R.F. (1982) (untitled) *Am. ind. Hyg. Assoc. J.*, *43*, A17, A20, A22, A24

Walker, R.F. & Pinches, M.A. (1981) Chemical interference effects in the measurement of atmospheric toluene diisocyanate concentrations when sampling with an impregnated paper tape. *Am. ind. Hyg. Assoc. J.*, *42*, 392-397

Walworth, H.T. & Virchow, W.E. (1959) Industrial hygiene experiences with toluene diisocyanate. *Am. ind. Hyg. Assoc. J.*, *20*, 205-210

Warwick, C.J., Bagon, D.A. & Purnell, C.J. (1981) Application of electrochemical detection to the measurement of free monomeric aromatic and aliphatic isocyanates in air by high-performance liquid chromatography. *Analyst*, *106*, 676-685

Wegman, D.H., Pagnotto, L.D., Fine, L.J. & Peters, J.M. (1974) A dose-response relationship in TDI workers. *J. occup. Med.*, *16*, 258-260

Wegman, D.H., Peters, J.M., Pagnotto, L. & Fine, L.J. (1977) Chronic pulmonary function loss from exposure to toluene diisocyanate. *Br. J. ind. Med.*, *34*, 196-200

Wegman, D.H., Musk, A.W., Main, D.M. & Pagnotto, L.D. (1982) Accelerated loss of FEV-1 in polyurethane production workers: A four-year prospective study. *Am. J. ind. Med.*, *3*, 209-215

White, G.L. & Wegman, D.H. (1978) *Health Hazard Evaluation Determination Report HE 78-68-546, Lear Siegler, Inc., Marblehead, MA*, Cincinnati, OH, National Institute for Occupational Safety and Health

White, W.G., Sugden, E., Morris, M.J. & Zapata, E. (1980) Isocyanate-induced asthma in a car factory. *Lancet*, *i*, 756-760

Windholz, M., ed., (1983) *The Merck Index*, 10th ed., Rahway, NJ, Merck & Co., p. 1364 [9358]

Zapp, J.A., Jr (1957) Hazards of isocyanates in polyurethane foam plastic production. *Arch. ind. Health*, *15*, 324-330

2,6-DICHLORO-*para*-PHENYLENEDIAMINE

1. Chemical and Physical Data

1.1 Synonyms and trade names

Chem. Abstr. Services Reg. No.: 609-20-1

Chem. Abstr. Name: 1,4-Benzenediamine, 2,6-dichloro-

IUPAC Systematic Name: 2,6-Dichloro-*para*-phenylenediamine

Synonyms: 1,4-Diamino-2,6-dichlorobenzene; 2,5-diamino-1,3-dichlorobenzene; 2,6-dichloro-1,4-benzenediamine; 2,6-dichloro-1,4-phenylenediamine; 3,5-dichloro-1,4-phenylenediamine; NCI-C50260

Trade Names: C.I. 37020; Daito Brown Salt RR; Fast Brown RR Salt

1.2 Structural and molecular formulae and molecular weight

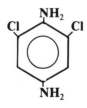

$C_6H_6Cl_2N_2$

Mol. wt: 177.03

1.3 Chemical and physical properties of the pure substance

(*a*) *Description*: Gray, microcrystalline powder (National Toxicology Program, 1982); needles or prisms (from diluted ethanol) (Weast, 1984)

(*b*) *Melting-point*: 124-126°C (Weast, 1984)

(c) *Spectroscopy data*: Ultraviolet (Sadtler Research Laboratories, 1980 [7843[a]]), infrared (Sadtler Research Laboratories, 1980, prism [19962], grating [21479]), nuclear magnetic resonance (Sadtler Research Laboratories, 1980, proton [27280], C-13 [5438]) and mass spectral data (NIH/EPA Chemical Information System, 1983) have been reported.

(d) *Solubility*: Soluble in ethanol, diethyl ether, acetone and benzene (Weast, 1984)

(e) *Stability*: Emits very toxic vapours of chlorine and nitric oxide when heated to decomposition (Sax, 1984)

(f) *Conversion factor:* $mg/m^3 = 7.24 \times ppm$[b]

1.4 Technical products and impurities

2,6-Dichloro-*para*-phenylenediamine is not available in commercial bulk quantities. No information on technical products was available to the Working Group.

2. Production, Use, Occurrence and Analysis

2.1 Production and use

(a) Production

2,6-Dichloro-*para*-phenylenediamine is synthesized by reduction of 2,6-dichloro-4-nitroaniline (Toxicology Data Base, 1985). No current producer of this chemical has been identified; the sole US manufacturer ceased production in 1978 (National Toxicology Program, 1982).

(b) Use

This compound has been used as a chemical intermediate for C.I. Azoic Diazo Component 117 (Toxicology Data Base, 1985) and, to a limited extent, in the preparation of certain polyamide fibres and as a curing agent for polyurethane (National Toxicology Program, 1982).

(c) Regulatory status and guidelines

No data were available to the Working Group.

---

[a]Spectrum number in Sadtler compilation

[b]Calculated from: $mg/m^3 = $ (molecular weight$/24.45) \times$ ppm, assuming standard temperature (25°C) and pressure (760 mm Hg)

2.2 Occurrence

(a) Natural occurrence

It is not known whether 2,6-dichloro-*para*-phenylenediamine occurs as a natural product. It is a metabolite of the herbicide-fungicide 2,6-dichloro-4-nitroaniline in humans, rhesus monkeys, goats, dogs, rats, mice and bacteria (Van Alfen & Kosuge, 1974; Gallo *et al.*, 1976; Van Alfen & Kosuge, 1976; Jaglan & Arnold, 1982).

(b) Occupational exposure

No data were available to the Working Group.

2.3 Analysis

2,6-Dichloro-*para*-phenylenediamine has been isolated from soil or plant material by acetone or benzene extraction and thin-layer chromatography (von Stryk, 1967; Van Alfen & Kosuge, 1976). Spots can be detected under ultraviolet light (von Stryk, 1967) or by characteristic colour reactions with various electron acceptors (Hutzinger, 1969).

A method for the analysis of 2,6-dichloro-*para*-phenylenediamine in rodent feed developed for the carcinogenesis study of the US National Toxicology Program (1982) involves extraction with methanol and gas chromatography with flame ionization detection; it was used for concentrations in the range of 1000-6000 ppm (mg/kg) in feed.

3. Biological Data Relevant to the Evaluation of Carcinogenic Risk to Humans

3.1 Carcinogenicity studies in animals

Oral administration

Mouse: Groups of 50 male and 50 female B6C3F$_1$ mice, six weeks of age, were fed diets containing 1000 or 3000 mg/kg [ppm] 2,6-dichloro-*para*-phenylenediamine (minimum purity, >98.2%; ammonium chloride, 1.6%) for 103 weeks. An equal number of untreated mice of each sex served as controls. All surviving animals were killed at 111 weeks. Survival at that time was: 39/50 control, 41/50 low-dose and 42/50 high-dose males and 40/50 control, 45/50 low-dose and 35/50 high-dose females. Increased incidences of hepatocellular adenomas and carcinomas combined were seen in animals of each sex: 16/50 control, 19/50 low-dose and 29/50 ($p = 0.008$) high-dose males and 6/50 control, 6/50 low-dose and 16/50 ($p = 0.014$) high-dose females. In males only, the incidence of adenomas was significantly increased when benign and malignant tumours were analysed separately (National Toxicology Program, 1982).

Rat: Groups of 50 male and 50 female Fischer 344/N rats, six weeks of age, were fed diets containing 1000 or 2000 mg/kg [ppm] (males) or 2000 or 6000 mg/kg [ppm] (females) 2,6-dichloro-*para*-phenylenediamine (minimum purity, >98.3%; ammonium chloride, 1.6%) for 103 weeks. An equal number of untreated rats of each sex served as controls. All surviving animals were killed at 111 weeks. Survival at that time was: 30/50 control, 30/50 low-dose and 21/50 high-dose males and 36/50 control, 32/50 low-dose and 38/50 high-dose females. No treatment-related neoplasm was observed. Moderate to severe decreases in body-weight gain were observed in high-dose animals of each sex (National Toxicology Program, 1982).

3.2 Other relevant biological data

(a) Experimental systems

Toxic effects

The oral LD_{50} of 2,6-dichloro-*para*-phenylenediamine in male rats is reported to be 700 mg/kg bw (National Toxicology Program, 1982).

In 13-week subchronic studies, mice and rats were fed diets containing 625-7500 and 1000-8000 mg/kg (ppm) 2,6-dichloro-*para*-phenylenediamine, respectively. In mice, depression of mean body-weight gain occurred at all doses, except in females receiving the lowest dose. In rats, weight-gain depression was dose-related among males and slight among females. In high-dose males, papillary necrosis of the kidney was found in 3/10, pyelonephritis in 4/10 and transitional-cell hyperplasia in 3/10 (National Toxicology Program, 1982).

In male and female rats given diets containing 1000-2000 and 1000-6000 mg/kg (ppm) 2,6-dichloro-*para*-phenylenediamine, respectively, for 103 weeks, an increased incidence of nephropathy was observed in animals of each sex. In treated rats, ectopic hepatocytes were associated with pancreatic islets (National Toxicology Program, 1982).

Effects on reproduction and prenatal toxicity

No data were available to the Working Group.

Absorption, distribution, excretion and metabolism

In rats administered a single dose of 1 g/kg bw 2,6-dichloro-*para*-phenylenediamine by gavage, the parent compound and a second compound, possibly its N^4-acetylated derivative, were found in the urine (Gallo *et al.*, 1976).

Mutagenicity and other short-term tests

2,6-Dichloro-*para*-phelynediamine (tested at 3.3-3333 μg/plate) was mutagenic to *Salmonella typhimurium* TA1537, TA98 and TA100, using the preincubation method in the presence of an Aroclor-induced rat or hamster metabolic system (S9); results with strain TA1535 were equivocal (Mortelmans *et al.*, 1986).

(*b*) *Humans*

No data were available to the Working Group.

3.3 Case reports and epidemiological studies of carcinogenicity to humans

No data were available to the Working Group.

4. Summary of Data Reported and Evaluation

4.1 Exposure data

2,6-Dichloro-*para*-phenylenediamine has been used to a limited extent as an intermediate in dye and resin manufacture. The main potential for exposure derives from its formation as a metabolite of the pesticide 2,6-dichloro-4-nitroaniline.

4.2 Experimental data

2,6-Dichloro-*para*-phenylenediamine was tested in mice and rats by oral administration in the diet. Increased numbers of liver-cell tumours were observed in mice; no treatment-related tumour was found in rats.

No data were available to evaluate the reproductive effects or prenatal toxicity of 2,6-dichloro-*para*-phenylenediamine to experimental animals.

2,6-Dichloro-*para*-phenylenediamine was mutagenic to *Salmonella typhimurium* in the presence and absence of an exogenous metabolic system.

4.3 Human data

No data were available to evaluate the reproductive effects or prenatal toxicity of 2,6-dichloro-*para*-phenylenediamine to humans.

No case report or epidemiological study was available to evaluate the carcinogenicity of 2,6-dichloro-*para*-phenylenediamine to humans.

4.4 Evaluation[1]

There is *limited evidence* for the carcinogenicity of 2,6-dichloro-*para*-phenylenediamine to experimental animals.

No data on humans were available.

In the absence of epidemiological data, no evaluation of the carcinogenicity of 2,6-dichloro-*para*-phenylenediamine to humans could be made.

---

[1]For definition of the italicized term, see Preamble, p. 18.

Overall assessment of data from short-term tests: 2,6-Dichloro-*para*-phenylene-diamine[a]

	Genetic activity			Cell transformation
	DNA damage	Mutation	Chromosomal effects	
Prokaryotes		+		
Fungi/Green plants				
Insects				
Mammalian cells (*in vitro*)				
Mammals (*in vivo*)				
Humans (*in vivo*)				
Degree of evidence in short-term tests for genetic activity: **Inadequate**				Cell transformation: no data

[a]The groups into which the table is divided and the symbol + are defined on pp. 19-20 of the Preamble; the degrees of evidence are defined on pp. 20-21.

5. References

Gallo, M.A., Bachmann, E. & Goldberg, L. (1976) Mitochondrial effects of 2,6-dichloro-4-nitroaniline and its metabolites. *Toxicol. appl. Pharmacol.*, *35*, 51-61

Hutzinger, O. (1969) Electron acceptor complexes for chromogenic detection and mass spectrometric identification of phenol and aniline derivatives, related fungicides, and metabolites. *Anal. Chem.*, *41*, 1662-1665

Jaglan, P.S. & Arnold, T.S. (1982) Metabolism of [^{14}C]dichloran (2,6-dichloro-4-nitroaniline) in the lactating goat. *J. agric. Food Chem.*, *30*, 1051-1056

Mortelmans, K., Haworth, S., Lawlor, T., Speck, W., Tainer, B. & Zeiger, E. (1986) *Salmonella* mutagenicity tests. II. Results from the testing of 270 chemicals. *Environ. Mutagenesis, 8* (Suppl. 7) (in press)

National Toxicology Program (1982) *Carcinogenesis Bioassay of 2,6-Dichloro-p-phenylene-diamine (CAS No. 609-20-1) in F344 Rats and B6C3F1 Mice (Feed Study)* (*Tech. Rep. Ser. No. 219*), Research Triangle Park, NC

NIH/EPA Chemical Information System (1983) *Carbon-13 NMR Spectral Search System, Mass Spectral Search System,* and *Infrared Spectral Search System*, Arlington, VA, Information Consultants

Sadtler Research Laboratories (1980) *The Sadtler Standard Spectra Collection, Cumulative Index*, Philadelphia, PA

Sax, N.I. (1984) *Dangerous Properties of Industrial Materials*, 6th ed., New York, Van Nostrand Reinhold, p. 883

von Stryk, F.G. (1967) Determination of 2,6-dichloro-4-nitroaniline (dichloran) and metabolites by thin-layer chromatography. *J. Chromatogr.*, *31*, 574-575

Toxicology Data Base (1985) *Toxicology Data Base*, Washington DC, National Library of Medicine

Van Alfen, N.K. & Kosuge, T. (1974) Microbial metabolism of the fungicide 2,6-dichloro-4-nitroaniline. *J. agric. Food Chem.*, *22*, 221-224

Van Alfen, N.K. & Kosuge, T. (1976) Metabolism of the fungicide 2,6-dichloro-4-nitroaniline in soil. *J. agric. Food Chem.*, *24*, 584-588

Weast, R.C., ed. (1984) *CRC Handbook of Chemistry and Physics*, 65th ed., Boca Raton, FL, CRC Press, p. C-445

MELAMINE

1. Chemical and Physical Data

1.1 Synonyms and trade names

Chem. Abstr. Services Reg. No.: 108-78-1

Chem. Abstr. Name: 1,3,5-Triazine-2,4,6-triamine

IUPAC Systematic Name: Melamine

Synonyms: Cyanuramide; cyanuric triamide; cyanurotriamide; cyanurotriamine; cyanurtriamide; isomelamine; NCI-C50715; triaminotriazine; 2,4,6-triaminotriazine; 2,4,6-triamino-s-triazine; 2,4,6-triamino-1,3,5-triazine; s-triazinetriamine; 1,3,5-triazine 2,4,6(1H,3H,5H)-triimine

Trade Names: Ammelide; Cymel; Hicophor PR; Teoharn; Theoharn; Virset 656-4

1.2 Structural and molecular formulae and molecular weight

$C_3H_6N_6$ Mol. wt: 126.13

1.3 Chemical and physical properties of the pure substance

(a) *Description*: Colourless-to-white monoclinic crystals or prisms (Sax, 1975; Hawley, 1981; Windholz, 1983; Weast, 1984)

(b) *Boiling-point*: Sublimes (Hawley, 1981; Weast, 1984)

(c)   *Melting-point*: 354°C (Hawley, 1981); 345°C (Weast, 1984)

(d)   *Density*: d_4^{18} 1.573 (Weast, 1984)

(e)   *Spectroscopy data*: Ultraviolet (Sadtler Research Laboratories, 1980 [1499[a]]), infrared (Sadtler Research Laboratories, 1980; prism [5460], grating [477]), nuclear magnetic resonance (Sadtler Research Laboratories, 1984 proton [39677]) and mass spectral data (NIH/EPA Chemical Information System, 1983) have been reported.

(f)   *Solubility*: Slightly soluble in water, ethanol (Grasselli & Ritchey, 1975), glycol, glycerol and pyridine; insoluble in diethyl ether, benzene and carbon tetrachloride (Hawley, 1981)

(g)   *Volatility*: Vapour pressure, 50 mm Hg at 315°C; relative vapour density (air = 1), 4.34 (Verschueren, 1983)

(h)   *Stability*: Sublimes when heated gently; emits highly toxic fumes of cyanides when heated to decomposition (Sax, 1975); noninflammable (Hawley, 1981)

(i)   *Conversion factor:* mg/m³ = 5.16 × ppm[b]

1.4 Technical products and impurities

Melamine is available commercially in crystal form; it is usually shipped as fine white crystalline powder in paper bags and in bulk quantities. It is a stable chemical when stored under normal warehouse conditions (Mannsville Chemical Products Corp., 1983) and can be kept for a year without any noticeable change in composition. Commercial melamine is available in 99.9% purity by a titration method, although chromatographic separation of samples used in animal carcinogenicity studies (National Toxicology Program, 1983) showed that several had impurities representing about 3% of the sample. Typical US analyses show: iron, <1 mg/kg; hardness as $CaCO_3$, <10 mg/kg; absorptivity at 292 nm, <0.01; water insolubles, <0.06 wt %; assay, melamine 99.8% min, moisture 0.1% max and ash 0.01% max (Melamine Chemicals, Inc., undated). 6-Amino-s-triazine-2,4-diol [ammelide], 4,6-diamino-s-triazine-2-ol [ammeline] and cyanuric acid have been reported to be common impurities in melamine (Hamprecht & Schwarzmann, 1968; CdF Chimie SA, 1984), although current commercial melamine reportedly contains less than 0.01% of these compounds (Melamine Chemicals, Inc., undated).

---

[a]Spectrum number in Sadtler compilation

[b]Calculated from: mg/m³ = (molecular weight/24.45) × ppm, assuming standard temperature (25°C) and pressure (760 mm Hg)

2. Production, Use, Occurrence and Analysis

2.1 Production and use

(a) Production

A commercial process for production of melamine was developed in 1939 using dicyanodiamide. Since 1963, urea has gradually replaced dicyanodiamide as a feed stock, and a high-pressure (80 atm) liquid-phase process was developed to convert urea to cyanuric acid (plus ammonia), which was then converted in the presence of ammonia to melamine. Since 1971, all melamine production in the USA and western Europe has been based on the urea process, which is cheaper than the dicyanodiamide process. In a modified urea process, a fertilizer-grade urea is melted and sprayed into a bed of aluminosilicate catalyst fluidized with ammonia at 7-8 atm and 330-450°C. Melamine vapours pass through the reactor to a cooling system where the melamine solidifies. The crude melamine product is then dissolved in the recycled mother liquor in a purification step. Coloured impurities are removed by treatment with charcoal, and pure melamine is recovered by vacuum crystallization. The product is air dried and stored for future use (Mannsville Chemical Products Corp., 1983).

In 1983, Japanese production of melamine by three major producers totalled 120 000 tonnes (Anon., 1984a). In the same year, US production by two major producers was 82 000 tonnes, decreased from 92 000 tonnes in 1978 (Anon., 1984b). About 25% of the melamine used in the USA is imported; exports are reported to be negligible (Mannsville Chemical Products Corp., 1983).

Among the major producers of melamine in Europe are (in hundred thousand tonnes): Federal Republic of Germany (62), The Netherlands (55), Austria (35), Poland (32), Italy (24), Spain (15), France (12), the USSR (10) and the German Democratic Republic (4). Taiwan and the Republic of Korea reported capacities of 10 000 and 5 000 tonnes, respectively. Saudi Arabia will have an estimated production capacity of 20 000 tonnes in 1988 (O'Sullivan, 1985).

(b) Use

The predominant use of melamine is in the manufacture of amino resins, made by condensation with aldehydes. Melamine-formaldehyde resins (see IARC, 1982) are extremely versatile and are available in various forms, formulations and grades, depending on the intended applications. Melamine is used in laminates (26%), surface coating resins (24%), plastic moulding compounds (18%), paper products (12%), textile resins (8%), bonding resins (6%) and miscellaneous applications (6%), e.g., gypsum-melamine resin mixture and orthopaedic casts (Logan & Perry, 1972; Fregert, 1981; Mannsville Chemical Products Corp., 1983).

Laminated resins

Most melamine-formaldehyde resins are used in laminated products. For this purpose, sheets of paper, glass cloth or other fillers are impregnated with solutions of the resin and dried under controlled conditions at 145-155°C for 15-20 min at 1000-1200 psi (70-80 atm). For table tops and related applications, the laminates are made of several plies of phenolic-resin impregnated kraft paper. The surface is made of a melamine resin barrier sheet on which the desired pattern is printed; this is covered by a clear melamine resin overlay (American Cyanamid Co., 1968; Mannsville Chemical Products Corp., 1983).

Surface coating resins

Melamine-formaldehyde resins that are soluble in organic solvents such as alcohols are used as clear finishes for paper, fabrics, wood and metals. These finishes are resistant to water and chemicals and are used for interior and exterior applications such as refrigerators, washing machines, automobiles, hospital equipment, toys and tin cans (American Cyanamid Co., 1968).

Plastic moulding compounds

Melamine-formaldehyde resins can be moulded into a variety of heat-resistant products that are odourless, tasteless and have good colour retention. They are used to make tableware, buttons, electrical panel boards (Melnick et al., 1984) and insulation. Inert fillers such as cellulose are used with melamine to make plastic dinnerware (Mannsville Chemical Products Corp., 1983).

Paper products

Melamine-formaldehyde resins are also used to improve the strength and stiffness of paper products, even when wet. The resins are added (0.5-3%) to the paper slush before it reaches the forming wire (American Cyanamid Co., 1968; Mannsville Chemical Products Corp., 1983).

Textile resins

Each year, millions of metres of rayon, cotton, nylon and other natural and synthetic fabrics are treated with melamine resins to make them wrinkle- and shrink-resistant and to increase their ability to retard fire and repel water (American Cyanamid Co., 1968; Mannsville Chemical Products Corp., 1983).

Bonding resins

Melamine resin adhesives can be used to bond a variety of surfaces. Melamine urea adhesives have been used extensively in plywood manufacture and as binders for glass fibres used at high temperatures (American Cyanamid Co., 1968).

Miscellaneous

Melamine and its derivatives are also used as rubber additives, chemotherapeutic agents, additives to animal and poultry feeds and stabilizers for aqueous formaldehyde solutions. Melamine-tanned leathers are resistant to heat and oxidation and do not darken with age and sunlight. Melamine-resins are also used in dyeing operations and as ion-exchange materials and sterilizing agents (American Cyanamid Co., 1968). Melamine may be used in silver tarnish cleaners, and melamine derivatives (perhydrates) may be used in neutralizer solutions for permanent wave preparations (Bann & Miller, 1958; Balsam & Sagarin, 1971).

(c)   *Regulatory status and guidelines*

No data on occupational exposure limits were available to the Working Group.

The US Food and Drug Administration (1984) permits use of melamine polymers as components of articles intended for use in contact with food in adhesives, resinous or polymeric coatings in epoxy resins as the basic polymer, resinous or polymeric coatings for polyolefin films as the basic polymer or modified with methanol, paper or paperboard in contact with dry food, and cellophane, as the basic polymer or in the modified form as a resin to anchor coatings to the substrate.

Melamine-formaldehyde resins may be used as surfaces in contact with food in moulded articles, providing the yield of chloroform-soluble extractives does not exceed 80 $\mu g/cm^2$ of food contact surface under specific solvent and temperature parameters (US Food and Drug Administration, 1984).

2.2 Occurrence

(a)   *Natural occurrence*

It is not known whether melamine occurs as a natural product.

It has been detected as an adulterant in potatoes processed for animal feeds to increase the apparent protein content; levels of 0-5.2% of the dry water-extractable protein have been found (Bisaz & Kummer, 1983).

In both rats and humans, melamine is a metabolite of the antineoplastic agent hexamethylmelamine (Worzalla *et al.*, 1974).

(b)   *Occupational exposure*

No data were available to the Working Group.

(c)   *Water*

Melamine has been detected in the waste-water from nitroguanidine production (a component of military propellants) at a level of 0.23 mg/l (Burrows *et al.*, 1984).

2.3 Analysis

Low-temperature reversed-phase high-performance liquid chromatography (HPLC) with gradient elution and ultraviolet detection (at 220 nm) has been used to determine melamine at levels as low as 0.3 nmol in water, in the presence of similar quantities of 16 other *s*-triazines (Beilstein *et al.*, 1981). For less complex waste waters (e.g., from nitroguanidine manufacture), a simpler isocratic ion-pair HPLC procedure with ultraviolet detection (at 235 nm) has been used to detect melamine at levels down to 28 ppb ($\mu g/l$; 0.044 nmol) (Burrows *et al.*, 1984).

Gas chromatography with flame ionization detection of the tris(trimethylsilyl) derivative of melamine and related s-triazines has been reported to have a lower quantifiable limit of approximately 0.02 nmol s-triazine (Stoks & Schwartz, 1979).

A method for the analysis of melamine in rodent feed developed for the carcinogenesis study of the US National Toxicology Program (1983) involves extraction with methanolic ammonium hydroxide, acidification with hydrochloric acid, filtration and direct spectro-photometric determination at 235 nm. The method was used for concentrations in the range 0.2-0.9% in feed.

A method has been reported for the analysis of melamine in urine and blood (Kechek & Kadzhoyan, 1975) using cyanuric acid and photocolorimetry and is reportedly sensitive to 0.01 mg/ml.

3. Biological Data Relevant to the Evaluation of Carcinogenic Risk to Humans

3.1 Carcinogenicity studies in animals[1]

(a) Oral administration

Mouse: Groups of 50 male and 50 female B6C3F$_1$ mice, six weeks of age, were fed a diet containing 2250 or 4500 mg/kg melamine (97% pure, with six unspecified impurities [possibly including ammeline (4,6-diamino-s-triazine-2-ol), ammelide (6-amino-s-triazine-2,4-diol) and cyanuric acid]) *ad libitum* for 103 weeks, followed by a basal diet for two weeks before sacrifice. Groups of 50 male and 50 female mice were maintained on basal diet and served as controls. No effect was observed on body-weight gain in either male or female mice. Survival at termination of the study was: 39/49 (80%) control, 36/50 (72%) low-dose and 28/50 (56%) high-dose males and 37/50 (74%) control, 43/50 (86%) low-dose and 41/50 (82%) high-dose females. The reduction in the survival of high-dose males was statistically significant ($p = 0.013$). No treatment-related increase in the incidence of tumours was observed. In male mice, treatment-related increases were observed in the incidence of urinary bladder stones (2/45 control, 40/47 low-dose and 41/44 high-dose animals), in the incidence of acute and chronic inflammation of the urinary bladder (0/45 controls, 25/47 low-dose and 24/44 high-dose animals) and in the incidence of epithelial hyperplasia of the bladder (1/45 controls, 11/47 low-dose and 13/44 high-dose mice). Urinary bladder stones were seen in 4/50 high-dose females (National Toxicology Program, 1983; Melnick *et al.*, 1984).

---

[1]The Working Group was aware of a completed but unpublished study in rats by oral administration (IARC, 1984).

Rat: Groups of 50 male and 50 female Fischer 344/N rats, six weeks of age, were fed diets containing 2250 or 4500 mg/kg (males) or 4500 or 9000 mg/kg (females) melamine (97% pure, see above), respectively, *ad libitum* for 103 weeks, followed by a basal diet for two weeks prior to sacrifice. Groups of 50 male and 50 female rats fed basal diet only served as controls. Survival was significantly reduced in high-dose males ($p = 0.03$) from 101 weeks on study. Survival rates at termination of the study were: 30/49 (61%) control, 30/50 (60%) low-dose and 19/50 (38%) high-dose males and 34/50 (68%) control, 30/50 (60%) in low-dose and 27/50 (54%) high-dose females. The incidence of transitional-cell carcinomas of the urinary bladder in males was: 0/45 controls, 0/50 low-dose and 8/49 high-dose (control *versus* high-dose animals, $p \leqslant 0.016$). There was also a dose-related incidence of bladder stones in male rats (0/45 controls, 1/50 low-dose and 10/49 high-dose). [In a separate study, X-ray microscopic analysis of two urinary bladder stones obtained from male Fischer 344/N rats fed diets containing 16 000 mg/kg and 19 000 mg/kg melamine indicated that the principal component of the stones was melamine (American Cyanamide Co., 1982).] Of 49 high-dose animals, seven had transitional-cell carcinomas and bladder stones, one had a carcinoma without stones and three had stones without carcinoma (one of these rats had a papilloma and one had epithelial hyperplasia). Female rats had no bladder stones, and one female in each of the low-dose and the high-dose group had a papilloma of the bladder (National Toxicology Program, 1983; Melnick *et al.*, 1984). [The Working Group considered that the presence of bladder stones in 7/8 rats with bladder tumours precluded a clear interpretation of the results; they agreed with the original author that there may have been a relationship.]

(*b*)   *Skin application*

Mouse: In an initiation-promotion study, a group of 20 female CD-1 mice, eight weeks old, received a single topical application of 1 μmol [6 mg/kg bw assuming a 20 g mouse] melamine [purity unspecified] in 0.2 ml acetone on shaven back skin, followed by twice-weekly applications of 10 nmol 12-*O*-tetradecanoylphorbol 13-acetate (TPA) in 0.2 ml acetone for 31 weeks, at which time they were killed. A control group of 20 female mice received a single application of acetone alone, followed by applications of TPA. No increase in the incidence of papillomas was observed in melamine-treated mice (19%) as compared to controls (14%) (Perrella & Boutwell, 1983). [The Working Group noted the low dose of melamine used.]

3.2   Other relevant biological data

(*a*)   *Experimental systems*

Toxic effects

Oral LD_{50} values for melamine given in corn oil by gavage have been reported to be 3.3 and 7.0 g/kg bw in male and female $B6C3F_1$ mice, respectively, and 3.2 and 3.8 g/kg bw in male and female Fischer 344/N rats, respectively (National Toxicology Program, 1983).

In male and female Fischer 344 rats and B6C3F$_1$ mice fed diets containing 5000-30 000 mg/kg melamine (purity, 97%) for 14 days, a hard crystalline solid was found in the urinary bladder in most male rats receiving 10 000 mg/kg or more and in all treated male mice. In females, this effect was noted at dose levels of 20 000 mg/kg or more in rats and in 2/5 mice given 30 000 mg/kg. In a subsequent study, diets containing 0, 6000, 9000, 12 000, 15 000 or 18 000 mg/kg melamine were fed to groups of 12 male and 12 female rats and to groups of 10 male and 10 female mice for 13 weeks. Stones were found in the urinary bladders of most male rats, in a dose-related incidence, and the bladders of some female rats receiving 15 000 mg/kg or more. Bladder stones were observed in both male and female mice receiving 12 000 mg/kg or more. Ulceration of the urinary bladder was also noted in treated mice of both sexes fed 12 000 mg/kg or more; 60% of the mice that had bladder ulcers also had stones. The distribution of bladder ulcers and stones was not considered to provide evidence for an association between ulceration and bladder stones in animals of either sex. In a second study of the same duration, diets containing 750, 1500, 3000, 6000 and 12 000 mg/kg melamine were fed to rats. Hyperplasia of the bladder epithelium was noted in male rats receiving 3000 mg/kg or more, but in none of the female rats. Urinary bladder stones were not observed in treated or control female rats, but among male rats the incidence increased in a dose-related manner from the lowest-dose group (2/10) to the 12 000 mg/kg level (9/9) (National Toxicology Program, 1983; Melnick et al., 1984).

X-ray and infrared analysis of two urinary bladder stones obtained from male F344/N rats indicated that the principal component of the bladder stones is melamine (see section 3.1) (American Cyanamid Co., 1982).

Effects on reproduction and prenatal toxicity

No toxic effect or gross malformation was found in foetuses of pregnant rats injected intraperitoneally with 70 mg/kg bw melamine on gestation days 5 and 6, 8 and 9, or 12 and 13 (Thiersch, 1957). [The Working Group noted that this study was inadequate for an evaluation of prenatal toxicity due to incomplete reporting of experimental methods and results of foetal examination.]

Absorption, distribution, excretion and metabolism

After administration of a single oral dose of 250 mg/kg bw melamine to rats, 50% of the dose was recovered from the urine within 6 h (Lipschitz & Stokey, 1945).

Recovery of a number of urinary metabolites, including melamine, following administration of hexamethylmelamine to rats indicated that the s-triazine ring is very stable and does not undergo cleavage in vivo (Worzalla et al., 1974).

After administration of a single oral dose of 0.38 mg ^{14}C-melamine to adult male Fischer 344/N rats, 90% of the administered dose was excreted in the urine within the first 24 h. Negligible radioactivity was detected in exhaled air and faeces; and radioactivity was concentrated in the kidney and bladder. Virtually no residual radioactivity was observed in tissue after 24 h or more. Chromatography of the radioactivity found in plasma or urine indicated that melamine is not metabolized in rats (Mast et al., 1983).

Mutagenicity and other short-term tests

Melamine (tested at up to 5550 μg/plate) was not mutagenic to *Salmonella typhimurium* TA1535, TA1537, TA98 or TA100 in the presence or absence of a metabolic system (S9) from the liver of Aroclor-induced rats or hamsters, when tested in the liquid preincubation assay (Haworth *et al.*, 1983; National Toxicology Program, 1983). In an abstract, Mast *et al.* (1982a) reported negative results (at levels of up to 5000 μg/plate) in a plate incorporation assay with these strains, in the presence and absence of liver S9. In the absence of an exogenous metabolic system, melamine was not mutagenic to *S. typhimurium his*G46, TA1530, TA1531, TA1532 or TA1534 [details not given] (Seiler, 1973).

It was reported in an abstract that melamine (600-1000 μg/ml) did not induce HGPRT forward mutations in Chinese hamster ovary cells and did not induce sister chromatid exchange in the presence or absence of liver S9 (Mast *et al.*, 1982a). In another abstract, it was reported that the compound did not induce unscheduled DNA synthesis in cultured rat hepatocytes (Mirsalis *et al.*, 1983).

Sex-linked recessive lethal mutations were not induced in *Drosophila melanogaster* given melamine in the diet (Röhrborn, 1962).

It was reported in an abstract that melamine did not induce micronuclei in mouse bone marrow (Mast *et al.*, 1982b). Negative results were obtained at two sampling times with a single oral dose (1000 mg/kg bw) or with two oral doses separated by 24 h.

(b) *Humans*

Toxic effects

Dermatitis has been reported in persons exposed to melamine-formaldehyde resins (Logan & Perry, 1972; Soubrier & Burlet, 1972; Fregert, 1981).

Effects on reproduction and prenatal toxicity

No data were available to the Working Group.

Absorption, distribution, excretion and metabolism

Recovery of urinary metabolites following administration of hexamethylmelamine to two patients indicated that the *s*-triazine ring is very stable and does not undergo cleavage *in vivo* (Worzalla *et al.*, 1974).

Mutagenicity and chromosomal effects

No data were available to the Working Group.

3.3 Case reports and epidemiological studies of carcinogenicity to humans

No data were available to the Working Group.

4. Summary of Data Reported and Evaluation

4.1 Exposure data

Melamine has been available commercially since the late 1930s. Occupational exposure to this compound may occur during its production and use in the manufacture of laminates, surface coatings, moulding compounds and textiles. No measurement of such exposure was available to the Working Group.

4.2 Experimental data

Melamine was tested for carcinogenicity by oral administration in the diet in one study in mice and in one study in rats, and for initiating activity by skin application in one study in mice. No neoplasm related to treatment was observed after oral administration to mice. Male rats fed diets containing melamine developed transitional-cell tumours of the urinary bladder; with one exception, all tumour-bearing animals had bladder stones probably consisting of melamine. This finding precluded a clear interpretation of the results. In a two-stage mouse-skin assay in which melamine was tested at one dose level, it did not show initiating activity.

The available data were inadequate to evaluate the reproductive effects or prenatal toxicity of melamine to experimental animals.

Melamine was not mutagenic to *Salmonella typhimurium* in the presence or absence of an exogenous metabolic system nor was it mutagenic to *Drosophila melanogaster*.

4.3 Human data

No data were available to evaluate the reproductive effects or prenatal toxicity of melamine to humans.

No case report or epidemiological study was available to evaluate the carcinogenicity of melamine to humans.

4.4. Evaluation[1]

There is *inadequate evidence* for the carcinogenicity of melamine to experimental animals.

No data on humans were available.

In the absence of epidemiological data, no evaluation of the carcinogenicity of melamine to humans could be made.

---

[1]For definition of the italicized term, see Preamble, p. 18.

Overall assessment of data from short-term tests: Melamine[a]

	Genetic activity			Cell transformation
	DNA damage	Mutation	Chromosomal effects	
Prokaryotes		−		
Fungi/Green plants				
Insects		−		
Mammalian cells (*in vitro*)				
Mammals (*in vivo*)				
Humans (*in vivo*)				
Degree of evidence in short-term tests for genetic activity: **Inadequate**				Cell transformation: no data

[a]The groups into which the table is divided and the symbol − are defined on pp. 19-20 of the Preamble; the degrees of evidence are defined on pp. 20-21.

5. References

American Cyanamid Co. (1968) *Aero (R) Melamine, an Intermediate for the Process Industries*, Wayne, NJ

American Cyanamid Co. (1982) *Evaluation of Urolithiasis Induction by Melamine (CAS No. 108-78-1) in Male Weanling Fischer 344 Rats*, Wayne, NJ

Anon. (1984a) Plastic material production in 1983. Japan: Thermosetting resins output. *Jpn. chem. Week*, April 19, 2

Anon. (1984b) Facts and figures for the chemical industry. *Chem. Eng. News*, *62*, 32-74

Balsam, M.S. & Sagarin, E., eds (1971) *Cosmetics. Science and Technology*, 2nd ed., Vol. 2, New York, John Wiley & Sons, p. 229

Bann, B. & Miller, S.A. (1958) Melamine and derivatives of melamine *Chem. Rev.*, *58*, 131-172

Beilstein, P., Cook, A.M. & Hutter, R. (1981) Determination of seventeen *s*-triazine herbicides and derivatives by high-pressure liquid chromatography. *J. agric. Food Chem.*, *29*, 1132-1135

Bisaz, K. & Kummer, A. (1983) Determination of 2,4,6-triamino-1,3,5-triazine (melamine) in potato proteins (Ger.). *Mitt. Geb. Lebensmittelunters. Hyg.*, *74*, 74-79

Burrows, E.P., Brueggeman, E.E. & Hoke, S.H. (1984) Chromatographic trace analysis of guanidine, substituted guanidines and *s*-triazines in water. *J. Chromatogr.*, *294*, 494-498

CdF Chimie SA (1984) *Melamine*, Paris

Fregert, S. (1981) Formaldehyde dermatitis from a gypsum-melamine resin mixture. *Contact Dermatol.*, *7*, 56

Grasselli, J.G. & Ritchey, W.M., eds (1975) *CRC Atlas of Spectral Data and Physical Constants for Organic Compounds*, Vol. 3, Cleveland, OH, CRC Press, p. 581

Hamprecht, G. & Schwarzmann, M. (1968) Synthesis of melamine from urea by pressureless single-stage process (Ger.). *Chem. Ing. Tech.*, *40*, 462-464

Hawley, G.G., ed. (1981) *The Condensed Chemical Dictionary*, 10th ed., New York, Van Nostrand Reinhold, p. 649

Haworth, S., Lawlor, T., Mortelmans, K., Speck, W. & Zeiger, E. (1983) *Salmonella* mutagenicity test results for 250 chemicals. *Environ. Mutagenesis, Suppl. 1*, 3-142

IARC (1982) *IARC Monographs on the Evaluation of the Carcinogenic Risk of Chemicals to Humans*, Vol. 29, *Some Industrial Chemicals and Dyestuffs*, Lyon, pp. 345-389

IARC (1984) *Information Bulletin on the Survey of Chemicals Being Tested for Carcinogenicity, No. 11*, Lyon, p. 287

Kechek, Y.A. & Kadzhoyan, D.N. (1975) Method of determining the content of melamine in urine and blood (Russ.). *Gig. Tr. prof. Zabol.*, *6*, 55-57

Lipschitz, W.L. & Stokey, E. (1945) The mode of action of three new diuretics: Melamine, adenine and formoguanamine. *J. Pharmacol. exp. Ther.*, *83*, 235-249

Logan, W.S. & Perry, H.O. (1972) Cast dermatitis due to formaldehyde sensitivity. *Arch. Dermatol.*, *106*, 717-721

Mannsville Chemical Products Corp. (1983) *Melamine (Chemical Products Synopsis)*, Cortland, NY

Mast, R.W., Friedman, M.A. & Finch, R.A. (1982a) Mutagenicity testing of melamine (Abstract No. 602). *Toxicologist*, *2*, 172

Mast, R.W., Naismith, R.W. & Friedman, M.A. (1982b) Mouse micronucleus assay of melamine (Abstract No. Bi-8). *Environ. Mutagenesis*, *4*, 340-341

Mast, R.W., Jeffcoat, A.R., Sadler, B.M., Kraska, R.C. & Friedman, M.A. (1983) Metabolism, disposition and excretion of [^{14}C]melamine in male Fischer 344 rats. *Food chem. Toxicol.*, *21*, 807-810

Melamine Chemicals, Inc. (undated) *Melamine Crystal (Technical Data Sheet)*, Donaldsonville, CA

Melnick, R.L., Boorman, G.A., Haseman, J.K., Montali, R.J. & Huff, J. (1984) Urolithiasis and bladder carcinogenicity of melamine in rodents. *Toxicol. appl. Pharmacol.*, *72*, 292-303

Mirsalis, J., Tyson, K., Beck, J., Loh, F., Steinmetz, K., Contreras, C., Austere, L., Martin, S. & Spalding, J. (1983) Induction of unscheduled DNA synthesis (UDS) in hepatocytes following in vitro and in vivo treatment (Abstract No. Ef-5). *Environ. Mutagenesis, 5*, 482

National Toxicology Program (1983) *Carcinogenesis Bioassay of Melamine (CAS No. 108-78-1) in F344/N Rats and B6C3F1 Mice (Feed Study) (Technical Report No. 245)*, Research Triangle Park, NC

NIH/EPA Chemical Information System (1983) *Carbon-13 NMR Spectral Search System, Mass Spectral Search System,* and *Infrared Spectral Search System*, Arlington, VA, Information Consultants, Inc.

O'Sullivan, D.A. (1985) Saudi chemicals buildup worries West European firms. *Chem. Eng. News, 63*, 16-18

Perrella, F.W. & Boutwell, R.K. (1983) Triethylenemelamine: An initiator of two-stage carcinogenesis in mouse skin which lacks the potential of a complete carcinogen. *Cancer Lett., 21*, 37-41

Röhrborn, G. (1962) Chemical constitution and mutagenic activity. II. Triazine derivatives (Ger.). *Z. Verbungslehre, 93*, 1-6

Sadtler Research Laboratories (1980) *The Sadtler Standard Spectra Collection, Cumulative Index*, Philadelphia, PA

Sadtler Research Laboratories (1984) *The Sadtler Standard Spectra Collection, 1981-1984 Supplementary Index*, Philadelphia, PA

Sax, N.I. (1975) *Dangerous Properties of Industrial Materials*, 4th ed., New York, Van Nostrand Reinhold, p. 891

Seiler, J.P. (1973) A survey on the mutagenicity of various pesticides. *Experientia, 29*, 622-623

Soubrier, R. & Burlet, P. (1972) Dermatoses induced by melamine (Fr.). *Arch. Mal. prof. Trav. Séc. soc., 33*, 202-204

Stoks, P.G. & Schwartz, A.W. (1979) Determination of s-triazine derivatives at the nanogram level by gas-liquid chromatography. *J. Chromatogr., 168*, 455-460

Thiersch, J.B. (1957) Effect of 2,4,6-triamino-'S'-triazine (TR), 2,4,6-'tris' (ethyleneimino)-'S'-triazine (TEM) and N,N',N''-triethylenephosphoramide (TEPA) on rat litter *in utero. Proc. Soc. exp. biol. Med., 94*, 36-40

US Food and Drug Administration (1984) Food and drugs. *US Code Fed. Regul., Title 21*, Parts 175.105, 175.300, 175.320, 176.180, 177.1200, 177.1460, pp. 130, 145, 157, 188, 209, 232

Verschueren, K. (1983) *Handbook of Environmental Data on Organic Chemicals*, 2nd ed., New York, Van Nostrand Reinhold, p. 808

Weast, R.C., ed. (1984) *CRC Handbook of Chemistry and Physics*, 65th ed., Boca Raton, FL, CRC Press, p. C-368

Windholz, M., ed. (1983) *The Merck Index*, 10th ed., Rahway, NJ, Merck & Co., p. 827

Worzalla, J., Kaiman, B.D., Johnson, B.M., Ramirez, G. & Bryan, G.T. (1974) Metabolism of hexamethylmelamine-ring-^{14}C in rats. *Cancer Res.*, *34*, 2669-2674

4,4′-METHYLENEDIANILINE AND ITS DIHYDROCHLORIDE

4,4′-Methylenedianiline was considered by a previous Working Group, in June 1973 (IARC, 1974a). Since that time, new data have become available, and these have been incorporated into the monograph and taken into consideration in the present evaluation.

1. Chemical and Physical Data

4,4′-Methylenedianiline

1.1 Synonyms and trade names

Chem. Abstr. Services Reg. No.: 101-77-9

Chem. Abstr. Name: Benzenamine, 4,4′-methylenebis-

IUPAC Systematic Name: 4,4′-Methylenedianiline

Synonyms: 4-(4-Aminobenzyl)aniline; bis(aminophenyl)methane; bis(4-aminophenyl)-methane; bis(*para*-aminophenyl)methane; dadpm; DAPM; DDM; diaminodiphenyl-methane; 4,4′-diaminodiphenylmethane; *para,para*′-diaminodiphenylmethane; di(4-aminophenyl)methane; dianilinemethane; dianilinomethane; 4,4′-diphenylmethane-diamine; MDA; methylenebis(aniline); 4,4′-methylenebis(aniline); 4,4′-methylenebis-benzenamine; 4,4′-methylenebis(benzeneamine); methylenedianiline; methylene-dianiline (VAN); *para,para*-methylenedianiline; *para,para*′-methylenedianiline; 4,4′-methylenedibenzenamine

Trade Names: Ancamine TL; Araldite Hardener 972; Epicure DDM; Epikure DDM; HT972; Jeffamine AP-20; Sumicure M; Tonox

1.2 Structural and molecular formulae and molecular weight

$$H_2N - \bigcirc - CH_2 - \bigcirc - NH_2$$

$C_{13}H_{14}N_2$ Mol. wt: 198.26

1.3 Chemical and physical properties of the pure substance

(a) *Description*: Crystalline solid (Hawley, 1981); pearly leaflets (Buckingham, 1982); colourless to pale-yellow flakes (BASF Wyandotte Corp., 1983); tan flakes or lumps, faint amine-like odour (Sax, 1984)

(b) *Boiling-point*: 398-399°C at 768 mm Hg (Windholz, 1983)

(c) *Melting-point*: 91.5-92°C (Windholz, 1983); 93°C (Buckingham, 1982; Verschueren, 1983)

(d) *Density*: Specific gravity, 1.1 (National Fire Protection Association, 1984); d^{100}_4 1.056 (Moore, 1978)

(e) *Spectroscopy data*: Ultraviolet (Sadtler Research Laboratories, 1980 [18517^a]), infrared (Sadtler Research Laboratories, 1980; prism [7846], grating [24038]), nuclear magnetic resonance (Sadtler Research Laboratories, 1980; proton [11592], C-13 [6819]) and mass spectral data (NIH/EPA Chemical Information System, 1983) have been reported.

(f) *Solubility*: Very slightly soluble in water (0.1 g/100 g at 25°C) (Moore, 1978); very soluble in ethanol, benzene, diethyl ether (Hawley, 1981; Windholz, 1983) and acetone (273 g/100 g) (Moore, 1978)

(g) *Volatility*: Vapour pressure, 1 mm Hg at 197°C; relative vapour density (air = 1), 6.8 (Upjohn Co., 1984)

(h) *Stability*: Flash-point, 220°C (National Fire Protection Association, 1984); stable for about six months when protected from heat, light and oxygen (BASF Wyandotte Corp., 1983)

(i) *Reactivity*: Reactions involve substitution of amine or aromatic hydrogens; diazo groups are formed by treatment with nitrous acid; reaction with epoxides replaces all amine hydrogens; reaction with phosgene yields the 4,4'-methylenediphenyl diisocyanate (see IARC, 1979) (Moore, 1978); heat causes decomposition to aniline (see IARC, 1974b, 1982a), and oxygen and light cause formation of polymeric amines (BASF Wyandotte Corp., 1983).

(j) *Conversion factor:* mg/m³ = 8.11 × ppm^b

---

^{a}Spectrum number in Sadtler compilation

^{b}Calculated from: mg/m³ = (molecular weight/24.45) × ppm, assuming standard temperature (25°C) and pressure (760 mm Hg)

4,4-Methylenedianiline dihydrochloride

1.1 Synonyms and trade names

Chem. Abstr. Services Reg. No.: 13552-44-8
Chem. Abstr. Name: Benzenamine, 4,4'-methylenebis-, dihydrochloride
Chem. Abstr. Services Reg. No.: 13552-44-8
Chem. Abstr. Name: Benzenamine, 4,4'-methylenebis-, dihydrochloride
IUPAC Systematic Name: 4,4'-Methylenedianiline dihydrochloride
Synonym: para,para'-Methylenedianiline dihydrochloride

1.2 Structural and molecular formulae and molecular weight

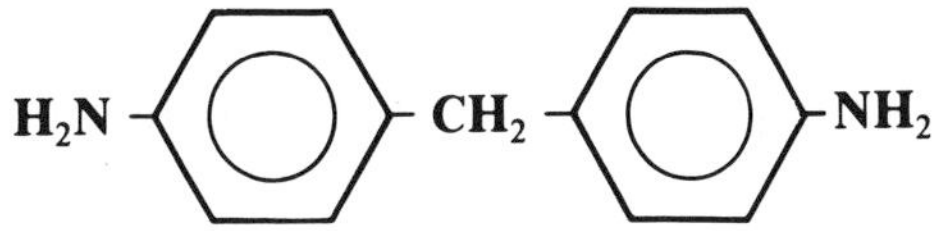

$$H_2N \langle\bigcirc\rangle - CH_2 - \langle\bigcirc\rangle - NH_2$$

(2 HCl)

$C_{13}H_{14}N_2 \cdot 2HCl$ Mol. wt: 271.21

1.3 Chemical and physical properties of the pure substance

(a) *Spectroscopy data*: Ultraviolet (Sadtler Research Laboratories, 1980 [19954[a]]), infrared (Sadtler Research Laboratories, 1980; prism [42877], grating [23877]) and nuclear magnetic resonance (Sadtler Research Laboratories, 1980; C-13 [14566]) spectral data have been reported.

(b) *Melting-point*: 288°C (National Toxicology Program, 1983)

(c) *Conversion factor*: mg/m^3 = 11.09 × ppm[b]

1.4 Technical products and impurities

4,4'-Methylenedianiline is available commercially as the free amine in bulk quantities. An assay of a commercial sample indicated a minium content of 99% aromatic amine; this would contain approximately 3% isomeric amines and traces of aniline (see IARC, 1974b, 1982a) (BASF Wyandoote Corp., 1983).

---

[a]Spectrum number in Sadtler compilation

[b]Calculated from: mg/m^3 = (molecular weight/24.45) × ppm, assuming standard temperature (25°C) and pressure (760 mm Hg)

2. Production, Use, Occurrence and Analysis

2.1 Production and use

(a) Production

4,4'-Methylenedianiline has been produced commercially since the early 1920s (US Tariff Commission, 1922). It is produced by the acid-catalysed condensation of formaldehyde (see IARC, 1982b) and aniline (see IARC, 1974b, 1982a). This reaction proceeds through a series of intermediates, resulting in N-(4-aminobenzyl)aniline. This product cleaves into aniline and a short-lived intermediate, which subsequently alkylates the aniline to form the final diamine product. All of these steps can be carried out in one reaction vessel (Moore, 1978). Unreacted aniline is removed from the 4,4'-methylenedianiline by a distillation process, and the purified product is either isolated for shipment or is used on-site (Anon., 1984a).

Seven manufacturers (National Institute for Occupational Safety and Health, 1978) currently produce approximately 90 000-180 000 tonnes of 4,4'-methylenedianiline in the USA (Anon., 1984a). One firm markets a crude aromatic diamine mixture containing 4,4'-methylenedianiline plus other related aromatic and polymeric amines (Uniroyal Chemical Co., 1983). Polymethylene polyphenylamine, a polyamine with approximately 70% 4,4'-methylenedianiline by weight, is available from one US company (Upjohn Co., 1984). Two firms in the USA have recently ceased production of 4,4'-methylenedianiline (Anon., 1984b). The majority of the 4,4'-methylenedianiline produced in the USA is for internal ('captive') use by the company (Moore, 1978).

Five companies are listed as producers/distributors of 4,4'-methylenedianiline in Europe: one each in Belgium, the Federal Republic of Germany and The Netherlands, and two in the UK (Baker et al., 1980). In Japan, there are three major producers (Chemical Daily Co., 1980).

(b) Use

Over 90% of the 4,4'-methylenedianiline produced in the USA is used as a closed-system intermediate in the production of 4,4'-methylenediphenyl diisocyanate (see IARC, 1979) (Anon., 1984a). 4,4'-Methylenediphenyl diisocyanate, a 4,4'-methylenedianiline mixture containing 30% or more polymeric isocyanate (Moore, 1978), is used primarily in rigid urethane foams for insulation material. The isocyanates developed from 4,4'-methylenedianiline are also incorporated into semiflexible polyurethane foams for automobile safety cushioning (National Institute for Occupational Safety and Health, 1978). 4,4'-Methylenediphenyl diisocyanate produced from the highly purified 4,4'-methylene dianiline isomer is used for the manufacture of elastomers such as spandex fibres (Moore, 1978).

4,4'-Methylenedianiline is used extensively as a curing agent for epoxy resins, acting as a cross-linking agent for the polyhydric phenolpolyepoxide polymer (Moore, 1978).

Isolated 4,4'-methylenedianiline can undergo catalytic hydrogenation to yield 4,4'-methylenebis(cyclohexaneamine). The hydrogenated amine can be polymerized with dodecanedioic acid to yield a polyamide which is the raw material for Qiana® nylon. This yarn was introduced in 1968 for clothing manufacture as a silk substitute (Moore, 1978).

4,4'-Methylenedianiline can be reacted to form a polyamide-imide or a polyester imide, which is used as a wire coating (Moore, 1978).

This compound has also been used in the preparation of azo dyes, as a reagent for the determination of tungsten and sulphates, as a corrosion inhibitor for iron under acidic conditions, as a curative for neoprene rubber, in a heat-sensitive hair-setting cream, and in the formulation of polyurethanes for encapsulating instruments for measuring water flow (Clement Associates, Inc., 1978; Moore, 1978; Lewis, 1980; Windholz, 1983).

(c) *Regulatory status and guidelines*

The American Conference of Governmental Industrial Hygienists (1984) and the UK Health and Safety Executive (1985) recommend that employee exposure to 4,4'-methylenedianiline not exceed a threshold limit value of 0.8 mg/m^3 time-weighted average for any 8-h shift of a 40-h working week and a short-term exposure limit of 4 mg/m^3.

4,4'-Methylenedianiline has been approved by the US Food and Drug Administration (1984) as a catalyst and cross-linking agent for epoxy resins, for use only in coatings for containers with a capacity of 1000 gallons (3785 l) or more, when the containers are intended for repeated use in contact with alcoholic beverages containing up to 8% of alcohol by volume.

2.2 Occurrence

(a) *Natural occurrence*

It is not known whether 4,4'-methylenedianiline occurs as a natural product.

(b) *Occupational exposure*

4,4'-Methylenedianiline is formed as a hydrolysis product of 4,4'-methylenediphenyl diisocyanate.

4,4'-Methylenedianiline has been detected in the air of working areas during: (1) its production, at levels of 0.2-31 mg/m^3 (American Conference of Government Industrial Hygienists, 1980); (2) its use in the manufacture of insulation materials, at levels of 0.8 mg/m^3 (McGill & Moto, 1974); (3) its use as part of a polyurethane mixture in the encapsulation of instruments, at a level of 10 μg/m^3 (Lewis, 1980); and (4) during core-making in iron and steel foundries (where polymers are used as binders in moulding), at levels up to 1.6 mg/m^3 (Toeniskoetter, 1981).

Boeniger (1984a,b,c) has recently reported exposure levels to 4,4'-methylenedianiline in two industries (Table 1).

Table 1. Occupational exposure to 4,4'-methylenedianiline

Industry	Type of sample	Concentration range (μg/m^3)	Reference
4,4'-Methylenedianiline production	personal	5-74	Boeniger (1984a)
	area	13-651	Boeniger (1984a)
	surface wipe	0.04-4.9[a]	Boeniger (1984a)
	dermal pad	4.2-54[a]	Boeniger (1984a)
Reinforced plastics production	area	<0.3-5.7	Boeniger (1984b)
	surface wipe	0.03-0.015[a]	Boeniger (1984b)
	area	2-99	Boeniger (1984c)
	personal	1-690	Boeniger (1984c)

[a] μg/cm^2

The percentage of urine samples found to contain 4,4'-methylenedianiline from a group of 27 workers producing the compound was 14.9% (levels, >200 μg/l) in 1970 and 0.09% (levels, >20 μg/l) in 1980 (Vaudaine et al., 1982).

2.3 Analysis

Skarping et al. (1983a) reported that 4,4'-methylenedianiline can be determined in trace quantities (detection limit, 10-20 pg) by formation of the bis(perfluoropropionamide) or bis(perfluorobutyramide) derivative and analysis by capillary gas chromatography with a thermionic nitrogen-selective detector. Electron capture detection offers greater sensitivity (about pg) but less selectivity (Skarping et al., 1983b).

Residual 4,4'-methylenedianiline has been determined in polyurethane films by aqueous extraction, conversion to the N,N'-dibenzamide derivative, and analysis by high-performance liquid chromatography (HPLC) with dual-wavelength ultraviolet detection. The minimum detectable concentration in the aqueous extract was 5 ng/ml (Ernes & Hanshumaker, 1983).

A method has also been developed for the detection of 4,4'-methylenedianiline contamination on metal, painted and concrete surfaces. The surface is contacted with solvent-moistened filter paper, and the filter paper is treated with a visualization reagent. The limit of detection, using fluorescamine with ultraviolet light (at 366 nm) as the visualization system, was 3 ng/cm^2 (Weeks et al., 1976).

4,4'-Methylenedianiline has been measured in urine following alkaline hydrolysis and extraction by gas chromatography/electron capture detection, with a detection limit of 10 μg/l (Vaudaine et al., 1982).

4,4'-Methylenedianiline has been determined by extraction with dimethyl sulphoxide/-acetonitrile and HPLC with ultraviolet detection after collection from air in glass-fibre filter/silica gel sampling tubes or from surfaces by wiping. Limits of detection ranged from 0.1 to 1.6 μg/sample, depending on the sampling technique (Boeniger, 1984a).

3. Biological Data Relevant to the Evaluation of Carcinogenic Risk to Humans

3.1 Carcinogenicity studies in animals[1]

(a) Oral administration

Mouse: Groups of 50 male and 50 female B6C3F1 mice, 12 weeks of age, were given 0.015% (150 ppm, mg/l) or 0.03% (300 ppm, mg/l) 4,4'-methylenedianiline dihydrochloride (98.6% pure) in the drinking-water for 103 weeks, followed by one week without treatment prior to terminal sacrifice. Groups of 50 male and 50 female mice receiving drinking-water adjusted with 0.1 N HCl to pH 3.7 (equivalent to the pH of the 0.03% 4,4'-methylenedianiline dihydrochloride solution) served as controls. Survival at termination of the study was 40/50 (80%) control, 39/50 (78%) low-dose and 32/50 (64%) high-dose males and 40/50 (80%) control, 38/50 (76%) low-dose and 37/50 (74%) high-dose females. An increased incidence of follicular-cell adenomas of the thyroid was observed in high-dose animals: 0/47 control, 3/49 (6%) low-dose and 16/49 (33%) high-dose males ($p < 0.001$) and 0/50 control, 1/47 (2%) low-dose and 13/50 (26%) high-dose females ($p < 0.001$). In addition, a dose-related incidence of thyroid-gland follicular-cell hyperplasia was observed in both males and females, and 2/50 high-dose females developed thyroid follicular-cell carcinomas. An increased incidence of hepatocellular adenomas occurred in females: 3/50 (6%) controls, 9/50 (18%) low-dose and 12/50 (24%) high-dose animals ($p = 0.01$, Fisher exact and Cochran-Armitage trend tests), but not in males. Increased incidences of hepatocellular carcinomas were observed in treated males [10/49 (20%) controls, 33/50 (66%; $p < 0.001$) low-dose and 29/50 (58%; $p < 0.001$) high-dose animals] and in treated females [1/50 (2%) controls, 6/50 (12%) low-dose and 11/50 (22%; $p = 0.002$, Fisher exact and Cochran-Armitage trend tests) high-dose animals] (National Toxicology Program, 1983; Weisburger *et al.*, 1984).

Rat: A group of 20 female Sprague-Dawley rats, 40 days old, received 30 mg (maximum tolerated dose) 4,4'-methylenedianiline dihydrochloride [purity unspecified] in 1 ml sesame oil by gastric intubation every three days for 30 days (total dose, 300 mg/rat) and were observed for a further nine months. A group of 140 female rats receiving sesame oil alone served as negative controls and a group of 40 females receiving single doses of 18 mg 7,12-dimethylbenz[*a*]anthracene (DMBA) served as positive controls. Survival after nine months was 14/20 in the 4,4'-methylenedianiline dihydrochloride-treated group, 127/140 in the negative-control group and 19/40 in the DMBA-treated group. Mammary lesions were found in 5/132 negative controls (three carcinomas, one fibroadenoma, five hyperplasias), 29/29 DMBA-treated (75 carcinomas, ten fibroadenomas, 47 hyperplasias) and 1/14 4,4'-methylenedianiline dihydrochloride-treated (one hyperplasia) animals (Griswold

---

[1]The Working Group was aware of a study on 4,4'-methylenedianiline in progress in mice by skin application and of a completed study, not yet published, on subcutaneous administration of 4,4'-methylenedianiline to rats (IARC, 1984).

et al., 1968). [The Working Group noted the limited duration of the study, the small number of test animals, which were of one sex only, and the fact that this study was aimed principally at examining use of the mammary gland in female Sprague-Dawley rats as a tool for identifying chemical carcinogens.]

Groups of eight male and eight female rats [strain and age unspecified] received four or five doses of 20 mg/rat 4,4'-methylenedianiline [purity not stated] by gastric intubation over a period of less than eight months and were observed until death. One hepatoma and a haemangioma-like tumour of the kidney were found in a male rat after 18 months. An adenocarcinoma of the uterus was found in one female after 24 months. Most animals had varying degrees of liver fibrosis and inflammation (Schoental, 1968). [The Working Group noted that this experiment was reported as a pilot study — hence, the small number of animals involved and the paucity of experimental detail.]

Groups of 50 male and 50 female Fischer 344/N rats, six weeks old, were given 0.015% (150 ppm, mg/l) or 0.03% (300 ppm, mg/l) 4,4'-methylenedianiline dihydrochloride (98.6% pure) in the drinking-water for 103 weeks, followed by one week without treatment, after which time the animals were sacrificed. Groups of 50 males and 50 females receiving drinking-water adjusted with 0.1 N HCl to the pH 3.7 (equivalent to the pH of the 0.03% 4,4'-methylenedianiline dihydrochloride solution) served as controls. There was no significant effect on survival in males or females. The incidences of thyroid follicular-cell carcinomas in high-dose animals were significantly increased over those in controls: 0/49 control, 0/47 low-dose and 7/48 high-dose males ($p < 0.012$, life-table test) and 0/47 control, 2/47 low-dose and 17/48 high-dose females ($p < 0.001$). A significant increase in the incidence of liver neoplastic nodules was also observed in male rats: 1/50 controls, 12/50 low-dose ($p = 0.002$) and 25/50 high-dose ($p < 0.001$) animals, and a statistically nonsignificant increase in these lesions was seen in treated females: 4/50 controls, 8/50 low-dose and 8/50 high-dose (National Toxicology Program, 1983; Weisburger, 1984).

Dog: A group of five female pure-bred beagle dogs, five to six months of age, received oral administrations of 70 mg 4,4'-methylenedianiline ('highly purified', dissolved in corn oil and placed in gelatinous capsules) thrice weekly. A further four female beagles received capsules containing 'crude' 4,4'-methylenedianiline (50% 4,4'-methylenedianiline; 50% higher molecular weight analogues). Total doses were 5.0-6.26 g/kg bw 'pure' 4,4'-methylenedianiline over periods of four-and-a-half to seven years, at which time there was one survivor, and 4.0-6.25 g/kg bw 'crude' 4,4'-methylenedianiline over periods of four to seven years, at which time there were two survivors. No tumour of the urinary bladder or liver was found (Deichmann, 1978). [The Working Group noted the small number of animals and the limited duration of the study.]

(b) Subcutaneous administration

Rat: Groups of 25 male and 25 female Wistar rats [age unspecified] received subcutaneous injections of 30-50 mg/kg bw 4,4'-methylenedianiline in physiological saline at one- to three-week intervals over a period of 705 days (total dose, 1.4 g/kg bw). Mean survival times were 970 days for treated males and 1060 days for treated females, compared to 1007 days in controls. A total of 29 benign tumours [types unspecified] and 33 malignant tumours [types unspecified] were found in treated rats compared with 15 benign and 16 malignant tumours in controls. Four hepatomas were reported (Steinhoff & Grundmann, 1970). [The Working Group noted the limited reporting of this study.]

(c) *Administration with known carcinogens and other chemicals*

A series of studies was undertaken to investigate the possible protective effect of 4,4'-methylenedianiline against the induction of tumours in various organs by known carcinogens, including 1,2-dimethylhydrazine (see IARC, 1974c), quinoline, *N*-ethyl-*N*-hydroxyethylnitrosamine, *N*-butyl-*N*-(4-hydroxybutyl)nitrosamine and *N*-nitrosomorpholine (see IARC, 1978). In some cases, a reduction in the incidence of tumours was seen; in others, no protective effect was observed nor was there evidence for carcinogenicity of 4,4'-methylenedianiline when given alone (Fukushima *et al.*, 1977; Shinohara *et al.*, 1977; Fukushima *et al.*, 1981; Ito *et al.*, 1984). [The Working Group noted the limited nature and short duration of some of these studies.]

Rat: In a study to investigate the possible promoting activity of 4,4'-methylenedianiline on the development of thyroid tumours in rats treated with *N*-bis(2-hydroxypropyl)-nitrosamine (DHPN), a group of 21 male inbred W rats, seven weeks old, received a single intraperitoneal injection of 2800 mg/kg bw DHPN [purity unspecified] and were maintained on a diet containing 1000 mg/kg 4,4'-methylenedianiline [purity unspecified] for 19 weeks. A second group of 21 males were fed a diet containing 1000 mg/kg of diet 4,4'-methylenedianiline. Groups of 21 rats each received a single intraperitoneal injection of either 2800 mg bw DHPN (positive controls) or 0.5 ml saline/100 g bw (negative controls), followed by basal diet for 19 weeks. All animals were still alive at the termination of the experiment. There was a significant ($p < 0.05$) increase in the incidence of thyroid tumours (polymorphofollicular, microfollicular and papillary adenomas, and follicular carcinomas) in the rats treated with DHPN plus 4,4'-methylenedianiline (19/21) over that in the group treated with DHPN alone (6/21) (Hiasa *et al.*, 1984). [The Working Group noted the small number of animals used, of one sex only, and the short duration of the experiment.]

3.2 Other relevant biological data

(a) *Experimental sytems*

Toxic effects

The oral LD_{50} value for 4,4'-methylenedianiline was 830 mg/kg bw in Wistar rats (Pludro *et al.*, 1969). Dose-related reductions in body weight were observed in male Fischer 344/N rats receiving 1600 or 3200 mg/l 4,4'-methylenedianiline dihydrochloride in the drinking-water for 14 days (National Toxicology Program, 1983).

Increased weights of adrenal gland, uterus and thyroid gland were observed in ovariectomized female Sprague-Dawley rats given 14 daily doses of 150 mg/kg bw 4,4'-methylenedianiline dihydrochloride by gavage. Thyroid weights nearly doubled during the dosing period (Tullner, 1960).

4,4'-Methylenedianiline produced toxic effects in the liver (enlargement) and bile duct when administered to rats by gavage. Hepatotoxic effects seen in rats administered 4,4'-methylenedianiline by gavage daily for ten days included necrotizing cholangitis with 8-600 mg/kg bw and periportal necrosis and glycogen loss with 200 mg/kg bw or more; marked mitotic activity was observed in hepatocytes and bile duct epithelium (Gohlke & Schmidt, 1974). Atrophy of liver parenchyma was observed in Wistar rats given 83 mg/kg bw per day for 12 weeks (Pludro et al., 1969). Cirrhosis occurred in all of 21 male rats administered an average dose of 38 mg/kg bw 4,4'-methylenedianiline by gavage on five days per week for 17 weeks (Munn, 1967). Administration to rats of 1000 mg/kg 4,4'-methylenedianiline in the diet for 12 weeks caused severe bile-duct proliferation with concurrent oval-cell and inflammatory cell infiltration, fibrosis and dilatation of smooth endoplasmic reticulum (Miyamoto et al., 1977). Bile-duct hyperplasia was found in all male and female rats that received 800 mg/l 4,4'-methylenedianiline dihydrochloride in the drinking-water for 13 weeks and in approximately one-third of those receiving 400 mg/l under similar conditions (National Toxicology Program, 1983). Bile-duct proliferation occurred in male rats fed a diet containing 1000 mg/kg 4,4'-methylenedianiline for 40 weeks. The hepatic parenchyma was replaced by proliferating bile ducts, and eventually portal cirrhosis developed. These alterations were reversed when treatment was discontinued (Fukushima et al., 1979). Bile-duct proliferation was also observed in rats receiving an oral dose of 20 mg/kg bw 4,4'-methylenedianiline per day for 16 weeks (Gohlke, 1978).

Necrosis of the proximal convoluted tubules has been associated with 4,4'-methylene-dianiline treatment (Calder et al., 1973) and liver haemangiomas were found in 1/10 albino rats receiving 20 mg/kg bw and in 1/10 rats given 8 mg/kg bw per day by gavage for 16 weeks (Gohlke, 1978). Mineralization of the kidney was observed in rats and mice administered 4,4'-methylenedianiline in the drinking-water for two years (National Toxicology Program, 1983) (see section 3.1).

Increased relative spleen weights associated with hyperplasia of the lymphatic system were observed in Wistar rats given 83 mg/kg bw 4,4'-methylenedianiline per day for 12 weeks (Pludro et al., 1969).

Effects on reproduction and prenatal toxicity

Injection of 0.05 ml of a 10% solution of 4,4'-methylenedianiline in ethanol into the yolk of fertilized chicken eggs before incubation reduced hatching to 30% and induced malformations in over 90% of the surviving chicks. The same volume of ethanol alone resulted in hatching of 95% of eggs, but 0.1 and 0.3 ml ethanol resulted in hatching of 60% and 0%, respectively (McLaughlin et al., 1963). [The Working Group considered that the observed effect of 4,4'-methylenedianiline may be attributable in part to synergistic interaction with a toxic vehicle.]

Absorption, distribution, excretion and metabolism

No data were available to the Working Group.

Mutagenicity and other short-term tests

4,4'-Methylenedianiline was mutagenic to *Salmonella typhimurium* TA98 and TA100 in the presence of an exogenous metabolic system from the livers of Aroclor- or phenobarbital-induced rats or phenobarbital-induced mice (Darby *et al.*, 1978; Lavoie *et al.*, 1979; Andersen *et al.*, 1980; Gałkiewicz *et al.*, 1980; Parodi *et al.*, 1981; McCarthy *et al.*, 1982; Rao *et al.*, 1982; Shimizu *et al.*, 1982).

It was reported in an abstract that 4,4'-methylenedianiline induced mutation in yeast, in the presence or absence of an exogenous metabolic system. In the same abstract, it was reported that 4,4'-methylenedianiline failed to induce sex-linked recessive lethal mutations in *Drosophila melanogaster* (Ho *et al.*, 1979).

Alkaline-elution analysis revealed that 4,4'-methylenedianiline (1-3 mM) induced DNA damage in cultured Chinese hamster V79 cells in the presence of rat-liver S9 (Swenberg, 1981).

It was reported in an abstract that 4,4'-methylenedianiline failed to induce chromosomal aberrations or sister chromatid exchange in cultured human peripheral lymphocytes either in the presence or absence of rat-liver microsomal enzymes (Ho *et al.*, 1978, 1979).

Intraperitoneal injection of 0.37 mmol/kg bw (74 mg/kg bw) 4,4'-methylenedianiline into male Sprague-Dawley rats induced DNA damage (detected by alkaline elution analysis) in the liver 4 and 24 h after injection (Parodi *et al.*, 1981).

Male Swiss mice received 9 or 18 mg/kg bw 4,4'-methylenedianiline by intraperitoneal injection; the incidence of sister chromatid exchange in femoral bone-marrow cells was determined 24 h after treatment in the presence of a BUdR tablet. Both dose levels induced statistically significant increases (1.35- and 1.39-fold for the low and high dose, respectively) (Parodi *et al.*, 1983). A statistically significant dose-related increase in sister chromatid exchange was observed in bone-marrow cells recovered from BALB/c mice treated with 1-35 mg/kg bw 4,4'-methylenedianiline, a doubling in frequency being seen with 35 mg/kg (Górecka-Turska *et al.*, 1983).

(b)   Humans

Toxic effects

Exposure to 4,4'-methylenedianiline can cause dermatitis (Melli *et al.*, 1983; Emmett, 1976; LeVine, 1983).

The inadvertent contamination of flour with 4,4'-methylenedianiline and the subsequent ingestion of bread made with that flour led to an outbreak of 84 cases of jaundice in Epping, UK (Kopelman *et al.*, 1966a). Biopsies from seven of the patients showed portal inflammation, eosinophil infiltration, cholangitis, cholestasis and different degrees of hepatocellular damage. All patients made a good clinical recovery (Kopelman *et al.*, 1966b). Occupational exposure to 4,4'-methylenedianiline caused toxic hepatitis in 12 workers, all of whom recovered within seven weeks; follow-up more than five years later showed no biochemical or clinical evidence of chronic hepatic disease. A skin rash was seen in five of the cases. Another case of hepatitis developed in a worker in another factory who had used the compound (McGill & Motto, 1974).

A case of acute myocardiopathy attributed to 4,4′-methylenedianiline has been reported (Brooks *et al.*, 1979).

Effects on reproduction and prenatal toxicity
No data were available to the Working Group.

Absorption, distribution, excretion and metabolism
Among a group of 27 workers producing 4,4′-methylenedianiline, the percentage of urine samples found to contain 4,4′-methylenedianiline was 14.9% (levels, >200 μg/l) in 1970 and 0.09% (levels, >20 μg/l) in 1980 (Vaudaine *et al.*, 1982).

Mutagenicity and chromosomal effects
No data were available to the Working Group.

3.3 Case reports and epidemiological studies of carcinogenicity to humans

No data were available to the Working Group.

4. Summary of Data Reported and Evaluation

4.1 Exposure data

4,4′-Methylenedianiline has been available commercially since the 1920s. It is used mainly as an intermediate in 4,4′-methylenediphenyl diisocyanate production and as a curing agent for epoxy resins. Exposure occurs during the production of 4,4′-methylenedianiline and the use of 4,4′-methylenediphenyl diisocyanate resins.

4.2 Experimental data

4,4′-Methylenedianiline and its dihydrochloride were tested for carcinogenicity by oral administration in mice, rats and dogs. Treatment-related increases in the incidences of thyroid follicular-cell adenomas and hepatocellular neoplasms were observed in both male and female mice. In rats, treatment-related increases in the incidences of thyroid follicular-cell carcinomas and hepatic nodules were observed in males, and thyroid follicular-cell adenomas occurred in females. In a study in rats in which 4,4′-methylenedianiline was administered orally in conjunction with a known carcinogen, the incidence of thyroid tumours was greater than that produced by the carcinogen alone.

The available data were inadequate to evaluate the reproductive effects or prenatal toxicity of 4,4′-methylenedianiline to experimental animals.

4,4′-Methylenedianiline was mutagenic to *Salmonella typhimurium* in the presence of an exogenous metabolic system. It induced DNA damage in Chinese hamster V79 cells in the presence of an exogenous metabolic system, and induced DNA damage in the liver of rats and sister chromatid exchanges in the bone marrow of mice treated *in vivo*.

Overall assessment of data from short-term tests: 4,4′-Methylenedianiline [a]

	Genetic activity			Cell transformation
	DNA damage	Mutation	Chromosomal effects	
Prokaryotes		+		
Fungi/Green plants				
Insects				
Mammalian cells (*in vitro*)	+			
Mammals (*in vivo*)	+		+	
Humans (*in vivo*)				
Degree of evidence in short-term tests for genetic activity: **Sufficient**				Cell transformation: no data

[a]The groups into which the table is divided and the symbol + are defined on pp. 19-20 of the Preamble; the degrees of evidence are defined on pp. 20-21.

4.3 Human data

4,4′-Methylenedianiline is hepatotoxic. No data were available to evaluate the reproductive effects or prenatal toxicity of 4,4′-methylenedianiline to humans.

No case report or epidemiological study was available to evaluate the carcinogenicity of 4,4′-methylenedianiline to humans.

4.4 Evaluation[1]

There is *sufficient evidence*[2] for the carcinogenicity of 4,4′-methylenedianiline and its dihydrochloride to experimental animals.

No data on humans were available.

---

[1]For definition of the italicized term, see Preamble, p. 18.

[2]In the absence of adequate data in humans, it is reasonable, for practical purposes, to regard chemicals for which there is sufficient evidence of carcinogenicity in animals as if they represented a carcinogenic risk to humans.

5. References

American Conference of Government Industrial Hygienists (1980) *Documentation of the Threshold Limit Values*, 4th ed, Cincinnati, OH, p. 278

American Conference of Governmental Industrial Hygienists (1984) *Threshold Limit Values for Chemical Substances and Physical Agents in the Work Environment and Biological Exposure Indices with Intended Changes for 1984-85*, Cincinnati, OH, pp. 24, 36, 42

Andersen, M., Binderup, M.-L., Kiel, P., Larsen, H. & Maxild, J. (1980) Mutagenic action of isocyanates used in the production of polyurethanes. *Scand. J. Work Environ. Health*, 6, 221-226

Anon. (1984a) More tests ahead for MDA in workers. *Chem. Week*, 134, 42

Anon. (1984b) Chemical profile: MDI. *Chem. Mark. Rep.*, 26 November, 54

Baker, M.J., Gandenberger, C.L., Gandenberger, R. & Merz, J.B. (1980) *Chemical Sources Europe*, 6th ed., Mountain Lakes, NJ, Chemical Sources Europe, p. 335

BASF Wyandotte Corp. (1983) *Methylene Dianiline (Technical Bulletin No. D423)*, Parsippany, NJ

Boeniger, M. (1984a) *Industrial Hygiene Survey Report of Olin Corporation, Moundsville, West Virginia. Dates of Survey 30-31 August, 1983*, Cincinnati, OH, National Institute for Occupational Safety and Health, Centers for Disease Control, Industrial Hygiene Section, Industrywide Studies Branch, Division of Surveillance, Hazard Evaluations and Field Studies

Boeniger, M. (1984b) *Industrial Hygiene Walk-Through Survey Report of Hercules Aerospace Division, Hercules, Inc., Clearfield, Utah. Dates of Survey 20-21 March 1984*, Cincinnati, OH, National Institute for Occupational Safety and Health, Centers for Disease Control, Industrial Hygiene Section, Industrywide Studies Branch, Division of Surveillance, Hazard Evaluations and Field Studies

Boeniger, M. (1984c) *Industrial Hygiene Survey Report of A.O. Smith Inland Incorporated, Little Rock, Arkansas, Dates of Survey 28-29 July 1983*, Cincinnati, OH, National Institute for Occupational Safety and Health, Centers for Disease Control, Industrial Hygiene Section, Industrywide Studies Branch, Division of Surveillance, Hazard Evaluations and Field Studies

Brooks, L.J., Neale, J.M. & Pieroni, D.R. (1979) Acute myocardiopathy following tripathway exposure to methylenedianiline. *J. Am. med. Assoc.*, 242, 1527-1528

Buckingham, J., ed. (1982) *Dictionary of Organic Compounds*, 5th ed., Vol. 2, New York, Chapman and Hall, p. 1554 [D-00854]

Calder, I.C., Williams, P.J., Funder, C.C., Green, C.R., Ham, K.N. & Tange, J.D, (1973) Nephrotoxicity and hepatoxicity from substituted anilines. *Nephron*, 10, 361

Chemical Daily Co. (1980) *JCW (Japan Chemical Week) Chemical Guide*, Tokyo, p. 125

Clement Associates, Inc. (1978) *Dossier on 4,4'-Methylenedianiline*, Washington DC

Darby, T.D., Johnson, H.J. & Northup, S.J. (1978) An evaluation of a polyurethane for use as a medical grade plastic. *Toxicol. appl. Pharmacol.*, *46*, 449-453

Deichmann, W.B., MacDonald, W.E., Coplan, M., Woods, F. & Blum, E. (1978) Di-(4-aminophenyl)-methane (MDA): 4-7 year dog feeding study. *Toxicology*, *11*, 185-188

Emmett, E.A. (1976) Allergic contact dermatitis in polyurethane plastic moulders. *J. occup. Med.*, *18*, 802-804

Ernes, D.A. & Hanshumaker, D.T. (1983) Determination of extractable methylenebis(aniline) in polyurethane films by liquid chromatography. *Anal. Chem.*, *55*, 408-409

Fukushima, S., Hibino, T., Shibata, M., Murasaki, G., Ogiso, T. & Ito, N. (1977) Effect of hepatotoxic or nephrotoxic agents on the induction of colon cancers in rats by 1,2-dimethylhydrazine. *Toxicol. appl. Pharmacol.*, *40*, 561-570

Fukushima, S., Shibata, M., Hibino, T., Yoshimura, T., Hirose, M. & Ito, N. (1979) Intrahepatic bile duct proliferation induced by 4,4'-diaminodiphenylmethane in rats. *Toxicol. appl. Pharmacol.*, *48*, 145-155

Fukushima, S., Hirose, M., Hagiwara, A., Hasegawa, R. & Ito, N. (1981) Inhibitory effect of 4,4'-diaminodiphenylmethane on liver, kidney and bladder carcinogenesis in rats ingesting *N*-ethyl-*N*-hydroxyethylnitrosamine or *N*-butyl-*N*-(4-hydroxybutyl)-nitrosamine. *Carcinogenesis*, *2*, 1033-1037

Gałkiewicz, E., Sikora, M., Chomiczewski, J. & Gorski, T. (1980) Effect of some chemical compounds on induction of the reversion of histidine mutants of *Salmonella typhimurium* (Pol.). *Med. Dośw. Mikrobiol.*, *32*, 243-251

Gohlke, R. (1978) 4,4-Diaminodiphenylmethane in a chronic experiment (Ger.). *Z. Ges. Hyg.*, *24*, 159-162

Gohlke, R. & Schmidt, P. (1974) 4,4'-Diaminodiphenylmethane: Histological, enzyme-histochemical and autoradiographic investigations in acute and subacute experiments in rats with and without additional heat stress (Ger.). *Int. Arch. Arbeitsmed.*, *32*, 217-231

Górecka-Turska, D., Mekler, U. & Górski, T. (1983) Sister chromatid exchanges in BALB/c mice bone-marrow induced by carcinogenic and non-carcinogenic products and intermediate products from the dyestuff industry (Pol.). *Bromat. Chem. Toksykol.*, *16*, 37-42

Griswold, D.P., Jr, Casey, A.E., Weisburger, E.K. & Weisburger, J.H. (1968) The carcinogenicity of multiple intragastric doses of aromatic and heterocyclic nitro or amino derivatives in young female Sprague-Dawley rats. *Cancer Res.*, *28*, 924-933

Hawley, G.G., ed. (1981) *The Condensed Chemical Dictionary*, 10th ed., New York, Van Nostrand Reinhold, p. 319

Health and Safety Executive (1985) *Occupational Exposure Limits* (*Guidance Note EH 40/85*), London, Her Majesty's Stationery Office, p. 16

Hiasa, Y., Kitahori, Y., Enoki, N., Konishi, N. & Shimoyama, T. (1984) 4,4'-Diaminodiphenyl-methane: Promoting effect on the development of thyroid tumors in rats treated with N-bis(2-hydroxypropyl)nitrosamine. *J. natl Cancer Inst.*, *72*, 471-476

Ho, T., Tipton, S.C. & Epler, J.L. (1978) Cytogenetic effects of m-phenylene diamine (MDPA) and methylene dianiline (MDA) on human leukocytes *in vitro* (Abstract No. 65). *In Vitro*, *14*, 350

Ho, T., Hardigree, A.A., Larimer, F.W., Nix, C.E., Rao, T.K., Tipton, S.C. & Epler, J.L. (1979) Comparative mutagenicity study of potentially carcinogenic industrial compounds (Abstract No. Ea-10). *Environ. Mutagenesis*, *1*, 167-168

IARC (1974a) *IARC Monographs on the Evaluation of Carcinogenic Risk of Chemicals to Man*, Vol. 4, *Some Aromatic Amines, Hydrazine and Related Substances, N-Nitroso Compounds and Miscellaneous Alkylating Agents*, Lyon, pp. 79-85

IARC (1974b) *IARC Monographs on the Evaluation of Carcinogenic Risk of Chemicals to Man*, Vol. 4, *Some Aromatic Amines, Hydrazine and Related Substances, N-Nitroso Compounds and Miscellaneous Alkylating Agents*, Lyon, pp. 27-39

IARC (1974c) *IARC Monographs on the Evaluation of Carcinogenic Risk of Chemicals to Man*, Vol. 4, *Some Aromatic Amines, Hydrazine and Related Substances, N-Nitroso Compounds and Miscellaneous Alkylating Agents*, Lyon, pp. 145-152

IARC (1978) *IARC Monographs on the Evaluation of the Carcinogenic Risk of Chemicals to Humans*, Vol. 17, *Some N-Nitroso Compounds*, Lyon, pp. 263-280

IARC (1979) *IARC Monographs on the Evaluation of the Carcinogenic Risk of Chemicals to Humans*, Vol. 19, *Some Monomers, Plastics and Synthetic Elastomers, and Acrolein*, Lyon, pp. 303-340

IARC (1982a) *IARC Monographs on the Evaluation of the Carcinogenic Risk of Chemicals to Humans*, Vol. 27, *Some Aromatic Amines, Anthraquinones and Nitroso Compounds, and Inorganic Fluorides used in Drinking-water and Dental Preparations*, Lyon, pp. 39-61

IARC (1982b) *IARC Monographs on the Evaluation of the Carcinogenic Risk of Chemicals to Humans*, Vol. 29, *Some Industrial Chemicals and Dyestuffs*, Lyon, pp. 345-389

IARC (1984) *Information Bulletin on the Survey of Chemicals Being Tested for Carcinogenicity*, No. 11, pp. 34, 193

Ito, N., Moore, M.A. & Bannasch, P. (1984) Modification of the development of N-nitrosomorpholine-induced hepatic lesions by 2-acetylaminofluorene, phenobarbital and 4,4'-diaminodiphenylmethane: A sequential histological and histochemical analysis. *Carcinogenesis*, *5*, 335-342

Kopelman, H., Robertson, M.H., Sanders, P.G. & Ash, I. (1966a) The Epping jaundice. *Br. med. J.*, *i*, 514-516

Kopelman, H., Scheuer, P.J. & Williams, R. (1966b) The liver lesion of the Epping jaundice. *Q. J. Med.*, *35*, 553-564

Lavoie, E., Tulley, L., Fow, E. & Hoffmann, D. (1979) Mutagenicity of aminophenyl and nitrophenyl ethers, sulfides and disulfides. *Mutat. Res.*, *67*, 123-131

LeVine, M.J. (1983) Occupational photosensitivity to diaminodiphenylmethane. *Contact Dermatol.*, *9*, 488-490

Lewis, F.A. (1980) *Health Hazard Evaluation Determination Report No. HHE-79-141-711 (US NTIS PB81-167918)*, Cincinnati, OH, National Institute for Occupational Safety and Health, US Department of Health and Human Services, Public Health Service, Center for Disease Control

McCarthy, D.J., Struck, R.F., Shih, T.-W., Suling, W.J., Hill, D.L. & Enke, S.E. (1982) Disposition and metabolism of the carcinogen reduced Michler's ketone in rats. *Cancer Res.*, *42*, 3475-3479

McGill, D.B. & Motto, J.D. (1974) An industrial outbreak of toxic hepatitis due to methylenedianiline. *New Engl. J. Med.*, *291*, 278-282

McLaughlin, J., Jr, Marliac, J.-P., Verrett, M.J., Mutchler, M.K., Fitzhugh, O.G. (1963) The injection of chemicals into the yolk sac of fertile eggs prior to incubation as a toxicity test. *Toxicol. appl. Pharmacol.*, *5*, 760-771

Melli, M.C., Giorgini, S. & Sertoli, A. (1983) Occupational dermatitis in a bee-keeper. *Contact Dermatol.*, *9*, 427-428

Miyamoto, J., Okuno, Y., Kadota, T. & Mihara, K. (1977) Experimental hepatic lesions and drug metabolizing enzymes in rats. *J. Pest. Sci.*, *2*, 257-269

Moore, W.M. (1978) *Methylenedianiline*. In: Mark, H.F., Othmer, D.F., Overberger, C.G. & Seaborg, G.T., eds, *Kirk-Othmer Encyclopedia of Chemical Technology*, 3rd ed., Vol. 2, New York, John Wiley & Sons, pp. 338-348

Munn, A. (1967) *Occupational bladder tumors and carcinogens: Recent developments in Britain*. In: Deichmann, W. & Lampe, K., eds, *Bladder Cancer. A Symposium*, Birmingham, AL, Aesculapius, pp. 187-193

National Fire Protection Association (1984) *Fire Protection Guide on Hazardous Materials*, 8th ed., Quincy, MA, p. 325M-68

National Institute for Occupational Safety and Health (1978) *Current Intelligence Bulletin Reprints — Bulletins 1 Through 18 (1975-1977) (DHEW (NIOSH) Pub. No. 78-127)*, Cincinnati, OH, pp. 59-64

National Toxicology Program (1983) *Carcinogenesis Studies of 4,4'-Methylenedianiline Dihydrochloride (CAS No. 13552-44-8) in F344/N Rats and B6C3F$_1$ Mice (Drinking Water Studies) (Technical Report No. 248)*, Research Triangle Park, NC

NIH/EPA Chemical Information System (1983) *Carbon-13 NMR Spectral Search System, Mass Spectral Search System,* and *Infrared Spectral Search System*, Arlington, VA, Information Consultants, Inc.

Parodi, S., Taningher, M., Russo, P., Pala, M., Tamaro, M. & Monti-Bragadin, C. (1981) DNA-damaging activity *in vivo* and bacterial mutagenicity of sixteen aromatic amines and azo-derivatives, as related quantitatively to their carcinogenicity. *Carcinogenesis*, *2*, 1317-1326

Parodi, S., Zunino, A., Ottaggio, L., De Ferrari, M. & Santi, L. (1983) Lack of correlation between the capability of inducing sister-chromatid exchanges *in vivo* and carcinogenic potency, for 16 aromatic amines and azo derivatives. *Mutat. Res.*, *108*, 225-238

Pludro, G., Karłowski, K., Mańkowska, M., Woggon, H. & Uhde, W.-J. (1969) Toxicological and chemical studies of some epoxy resins and hardeners. I. Determination of acute and subacute toxicity of phthalic acid anhydride, 4,4'-diaminodiphenylmethane and of the epoxy resin: Epilox EG-34. *Acta pol. pharmacol.*, *26*, 352-357

Rao, T.K., Dorsey, G.F., Allen, B.E. & Epler, J.L. (1982) Mutagenicity of 4,4'-methylenedianiline derivatives in the *Salmonella* histidine reversion assay. *Arch. Toxicol.*, *49*, 185-190

Sadtler Research Laboratories (1980) *The Sadtler Standard Spectra Collection, Cumulative Index*, Philadelphia, PA

Sax, N.I. (1984) *Dangerous Properties of Industrial Materials*, 6th ed., New York, Van Nostrand Reinhold, p. 1845

Schoental, R. (1968) Carcinogenic and chronic effects of 4,4'-diaminodiphenylmethane, an epoxyresin hardener. *Nature*, *219*, 1162-1163

Shimizu, H., Suzuki, Y., Suzuki, T., Akiyama, I., Sakitani, T. & Takemura, N. (1982) Mutagenicity of epoxy resin hardners (Jpn.). *Jpn. J. ind. Health*, *24*, 498-503

Shinohara, T., Ogiso, T., Hananouchi, M., Nakanishi, K., Yoshimura, T. & Ito, N. (1977) Effect of various factors on the induction of liver tumors in animals by quinoline. *Gann*, *68*, 785-796

Skarping, G., Renman, L. & Dalene, M. (1983a) Trace analysis of amines and isocyanates using glass capillary gas chromatography and selective detection. II. Determination of aromatic amines as perfluorofatty acid amides using nitrogen-selective detection. *J. Chromatogr.*, *270*, 207-218

Skarping, G., Renman, L. & Smith, B.E.F. (1983b) Trace analysis of amines and isocyanates using glass capillary gas chromatography and selective detection. I. Determination of aromatic amines as perfluoro fatty acid amides using electron-capture detection. *J. Chromatogr.*, *267*, 315-327

Steinhoff, D. & Grundmann, E. (1970) Carcinogenic action of 4,4'-diaminodiphenylmethane and 2,4'-diaminodiphenylmethane (Ger.). *Naturwissenschafften*, *57*, 247-248

Swenberg, J.A. (1981) *Utilization of the alkaline elution assay as a short-tem test for chemical carcinogens.* In: Stich, H.F. & San, R.H.C., eds, *Short-Term Tests for Chemical Carcinogens*, New York, Springer-Verlag, pp. 48-58

Toeniskoetter, R.H. (1981) *Urethane foundry binders — An industrial hygiene appraisal.* In: *Proceedings of the Symposium on Occupational Health Hazard Control Technology in Foundry and Secondary Non-Ferrous Smelting Industries* (*NIOSH Publ. No. 81-114*), Cincinnati, OH, National Institute for Occupational Safety and Health, pp. 142-152

Tullner, W.W. (1960) Endocrine effects of methylenedianiline in the rat, rabbit and dog. *Endocrinology*, *66*, 470-474

Uniroyal Chemical Co. (1983) *Tonox 22, Material Safety Data Sheet*, Middlebury CT

Upjohn Co. (1984) *Material Safety Data Sheet: Polymethylene Polyphenylamine*, Kalamazoo, MI

US Food and Drug Administration (1984) Food and drugs. *US Code Fed. Regul.*, *Title 21*, Part 175.300, pp. 143-144

US Tariff Commission (1922) *Census of Dyes and Other Synthetic Chemicals 1921* (*Tariff Information Series No. 26*), Washington DC, US Government Printing Office, p. 23

Vaudaine, M., Lery, N., Diter, J.N., Droin, M. & Chamaillard, C. (1982) Diaminodiphenyl-methane: An example of toxicological surveillance in production workshops at Rhone-Poulenc (Fr.). *J. Toxicol. Méd.*, *2*, 207-212

Verschueren, K. (1983) *Handbook of Environmental Data on Organic Chemicals*, 2nd ed., New York, Van Nostrand Reinhold, p. 454

Weeks, R.W., Jr, Dean, B.J. & Yasuda, S.K. (1976) Detection limits of chemical spot tests toward certain carcinogens on metal, painted, and concrete surfaces. *Anal. Chem.*, *48*, 2227-2233

Weisburger, E.K., Murthy, A.S.K., Lilja, H.S. & Lamb, J.C., IV (1984) Neoplastic response of F344 rats and B6C3F$_1$ mice to the polymer and dyestuff intermediates, 4,4'-methylenebis(*N,N*-dimethyl)benzenamine, 4,4'-oxydianiline, and 4,4'-methylenedianiline. *J. natl Cancer Inst.*, *72*, 1457-1463

Windholz, M., ed. (1983) *The Merck Index*, 10th ed., Rahway, NJ, Merck & Co., pp. 430-431

RELATED COMPOUND

DICHLOROACETYLENE

1. Chemical and Physical Data

1.1 Synonyms and trade names

Chem. Abstr. Services Reg. No.: 7572-29-4

Chem. Abstr. Name: Ethyne, dichloro-

IUPAC Systematic Name: Dichloroacetylene

1.2 Structural and molecular formulae and molecular weight

$$ClC \equiv CCl$$

C_2Cl_2 Mol. wt: 94.93

1.3 Chemical and physical properties of the pure substance

(a) *Description*: Volatile liquid (Buckingham, 1982)

(b) *Boiling-point*: 33°C (Buckingham, 1982)

(c) *Melting-point*: -66°C (Weast, 1984)

(d) *Spectroscopy data*: Mass spectral data have been reported (NIH/EPA Chemical Information System, 1983).

(e) *Solubility*: Soluble in ethanol, diethyl ether and acetone (Weast, 1984)

(f)   *Stability*: Explodes on heating strongly, ignites on contact with air (Buckingham, 1982); severe explosion hazard when shocked or exposed to heat or air, can react vigorously with oxidizing materials (Sax, 1984). In air, unstabilized dichloroacetylene decomposes to phosgene, chloroform (see IARC, 1979a, 1982a), carbon tetrachloride (see IARC, 1979b, 1982b), trichloroacetyl chloride, tetrachloroethylene (see IARC, 1979c, 1982c), trichloroacryloyl chloride and hexachlorobutadiene (see IARC, 1979d) (Reichert *et al.*, 1980). Acetylene is used as a stabilizer (Reichert *et al.*, 1979); the stability of dichloroacetylene is considerably increased in the presence of trichloroethylene (Reichert *et al.*, 1980).

(g)   *Conversion factor:* $mg/m^3 = 3.88 \times ppm$[a]

1.4 Technical products and impurities

Dichloroacetylene is not produced commercially.

2. Production, Use, Occurrence and Analysis

2.1 Production and use

(a)   *Production*

Dichloroacetylene is not available in commercial quantitites. It is reported to be a by-product in the synthesis of vinylidene chloride (see p. 195 of this volume) (Reichert *et al.*, 1980). Patents have been awarded for processes to isolate chloroacetylenes found as impurities in hydrogen chloride gas.

A synthetic route for chloroacetylenes involves dehydrochlorination of trichloroethylene by strong alkalis. Dichloroacetylene can be prepared from trichloroethylene in the presence of epoxides and ionic halides (McNeill, 1979). The compound may also be produced from the pyrolysis of various chlorohydrocarbons.

(b)   *Use*

Dichloroacetylene is not known to be used commercially.

---

[a]Calculated from: mg/m^3 = (molecular weight/24.45) $\times$ ppm, assuming standard temperature (25°C) and pressure (760 mm Hg)

(c)   Regulatory status and guidelines

Occupational exposure limits to dichloroacetylene have been set by six countries by regulation or recommended guideline (Table 1). Dichloroacetylene is recognized as an animal carcinogen in the Federal Republic of Germany; as a consequence, a previously existing maximal occupational level (MAK value) has been suspended (Deutsche Forschungsgemeinschaft, 1984).

Table 1. National occupational exposure limits for dichloroacetylene[a]

Country	Year	Concentration (mg/m³)	Interpretation[b]
Australia	1978	0.4	Ceiling
Belgium	1978	0.4	Ceiling
Finland	1981	0.4	Ceiling
		1.2 (15 min)	STEL
Netherlands	1978	0.4	Ceiling
Switzerland	1978	0.4	Ceiling
UK	1985	0.4	Ceiling
USA (ACGIH)	1984	0.4	Ceiling

[a]From International Labour Office (1980); Työsuojeluhallitus (1981); American Conference of Governmental Industrial Hygienists (ACGIH) (1984); Health and Safety Executive (1985)

[b]STEL, short-term exposure limit

2.2 Occurrence

(a)   Natural occurrence

It is not known whether dichloroacetylene occurs as a natural product.

(b)   Occupational exposure

Dichloroacetylene has been identified several times in special occupational situations. In one incident, it was identified in air samples from a fully enclosed and contained environmental life support system being evaluated for the US space programme. Dichloroacetylene was also identified in the atmosphere of a nuclear submarine. In both cases, the source of dichloroacetylene was attributed to the presence and degradation of trichloroethylene (Saunders, 1967). When trichloroethylene is used for closed circuit anaesthesia, dichloroacetylene may be produced in the heat and moisture generated from soda-lime carbon dioxide absorbers (Sittig, 1981).

Airborne dichloroacetylene may have been formed when trichloroethylene was used for removing a wax coating from a concrete-lined stone floor. Incubation of commercial samples of trichloroethylene with alkaline mortar and tile filling materials resulted in the formation of dichloroacetylene (Greim *et al.*, 1984).

2.3 Analysis

Dichloroacetylene in air has been measured quantitatively over the range 0.4-40 mg/m^3 by gas chromatography with electrolytic conductivity detection (Reichert *et al.*, 1979).

3. Biological Data Relevant to the Evaluation of Carcinogenic Risk to Humans

3.1 Carcinogenicity studies in animals

Inhalation exposure

Mouse: Groups of 30 male and 30 female NMRI mice, six to seven weeks old, were exposed by inhalation to a mixture of 20 ppm (21.2 mg/m^3) acetylene (as stabilizer) and either 9 ppm (36 mg/m^3) dichloroacetylene (freshly synthesized from trichloroethylene; no other chlorinated hydrocarbon detected in the mixture) in air for 6 h per day on one day per week for 12 months (group I), 2 ppm (8 mg/m^3) dichloroacetylene in air for 6 h per day on one day per week for 18 months (group II) or 2 ppm dichloroacetylene in air for 6 h per day on two days per week for 18 months (group III). Three groups of 30 males and 30 females exposed to air and acetylene served as controls. The mice were observed for lifetime. An exposure-dependent reduction in body-weight gain and mean survival time was observed in all treated male mice and in females in groups I and III. Treatment-related increases in the incidence of adenocarcinomas of the kidney were observed in male mice: controls, 0/30 (all groups); group I, 4/30 ($p = 0.0006$); group II, 12/30 ($p = 0.0001$); and group III, 3/30 ($p = 0.0038$). The incidence of kidney cystadenomas and adenocarcinomas combined in males was: group I, 8/30 controls *versus* 27/30 treated; group II, 4/30 controls *versus* 27/30 treated; and group III, 4/30 controls *versus* 19/30 treated. The incidence of kidney cystadenomas in females was: group I, 0/30 controls *versus* 15/30 treated; group II, 0/30 controls *versus* 7/30 treated; and group III, 4/30 controls *versus* 6/30 treated (Reichert *et al.*, 1984). [The Working Group noted that *p* values were apparently calculated using methods which accounted for survival differences between control and treated groups.]

Rat: Groups of 30 male and 30 female Wistar rats, six to seven weeks old, were exposed by inhalation to a mixture of 14 ppm (56 mg/m^3) dichloroacetylene (freshly prepared from trichloroethylene; no other chlorinated hydrocarbon detected in the mixture) and 20 ppm (21.2 mg/m^3) acetylene (as stabilizer) in air for 6 h per day on two days per week for 18 months. Control groups of 30 males and 30 females exposed to air plus acetylene were available. The rats were observed for lifetime. A reduction in body-weight gain and mean survival time was observed in treated animals. Increased incidences of cystadenomas of the kidney were observed in treated animals: males, 0/30 controls *versus* 7/30 treated (p < 0.0001); females, 0/30 controls *versus* 3/30 treated ($p = 0.0012$). One adenocarcinoma of the kidney was observed in a treated male. Increased incidences of cholangiomas of the liver were observed in treated animals: males, $0/30$ controls *versus* $6/30$ treated ($p = 0.0001$); females, $4/30$ controls *versus* $11/30$ treated ($p < 0.0001$). Malignant lymphomas occurred in $4/30$ control *versus* $11/30$ treated females ($p = 0.0081$) (Reichert *et al.*, 1984). [The Working Group was aware of the controversy concerning the neoplastic nature of cholangiomas in the rat, and that p values were apparently calculated using methods which accounted for survival differences between control and treated groups.]

3.2 Other relevant biological data

(*a*) *Experimental systems*

Toxic effects

The LC_{50} of dichloroacetylene (with trichloroethylene as stabilizer) in female NMRI mice was 480 mg/m³ (124 ppm) for a 1-h inhalation exposure and 74 mg/m³ (19 ppm) for 6 h of exposure (Reichert *et al.*, 1975). Values in male rats exposed for 4 h were 213 mg/m³ (55 ppm) (1:7 parts by volume with trichloroethylene as stabilizer) and 850 mg/m³ (219 ppm) (1:9 parts by volume with diethyl ether as stabilizer). In guinea-pigs, the LC_{50} for a 4-h exposure was 58 mg/m³ (15 ppm) (1:10 parts by volume with trichloroethylene) or 200 mg/m³ (52 ppm) (1:9 parts by volume with diethyl ether) (Siegel *et al.*, 1971). Death was due to acute renal failure caused by necrosis of the kidney tubules in the corticomedullary area (Jackson *et al.*, 1971).

Neuropathological changes induced by dichloroacetylene are highly characteristic. After a single exposure of male rabbits to 490, 780 or 1200 mg/m³ (126, 202 or 307 ppm) dichloroacetylene for 1 h, or to 66 mg/m³ (17 ppm) for 6 h, the sensory trigeminal nucleus was severely affected. Histological findings included chromatolysis, disintegration of the Nissl bodies and cell shrinkage (Reichert *et al.*, 1976). Nephrotoxic and hepatotoxic effects in these rabbits included extensive tubular and focal necrosis in the collecting tubules of the kidney and increased mitotic activity in the renal epithelium. In the liver, fatty degeneration of the parenchyma was observed (Reichert *et al.*, 1978).

Continuous exposure of rats to 20 or 130 mg/m³ (4.8 or 33 ppm) dichloroacetylene for 28 days or repeated exposures to 60 mg/m³ (15.5 ppm) for six weeks (6 h/day on five days/week) resulted in renal changes similar to those observed after acute exposure (Jackson *et al.*, 1971; Siegel *et al.*, 1971).

Effects on reproduction and prenatal toxicity

No data were available to the Working Group.

Absorption, distribution, excretion and metabolism

No data were available on the biotransformation of dichloroacetylene. However, the spontaneous decomposition into reactive, toxic products that occurs when unstabilized dichloroacetylene comes into contact with air has been well established (see section 1.3).

Mutagenicity and other short-term tests

Under aerobic conditions, dichloroacetylene (at 20 000 mg/m^3 [5000 ppm] for up to 9 h) was mutagenic to *Salmonella typhimurium* TA100 but not to TA98. Mixtures of dichloroacetylene with acetylene (used as a stabilizer in the experiments described in section 3.1) were not mutagenic to *S. typhimurium* in the presence or absence of a metabolic system from the liver of Aroclor-induced rats (Reichert *et al.*, 1983).

Mutagenicity of decomposition products

Trichloroacryloyl chloride was mutagenic to *S. typhimurium* TA100 in the presence and absence of S9, whereas *trichloroacetyl chloride* was not. *Hexachlorobutadiene* (see IARC, 1979d) was toxic and could not be tested (Reichert *et al.*, 1983). Tardiff *et al.* (1976) reported that *hexachlorobutadiene* was mutagenic to *S. typhimurium* TA100 in a spot test [details not given].

(b)   Humans

Toxic effects

Toxic effects have been reported after accidental exposure to dichloroacetylene in various settings: its generation during use of trichloroethylene as an anaesthetic (Humphrey & McClelland, 1944; Defalque, 1961), after use of a solvent mixture containing trichloroethylene as a cleaning agent either domestically (Greim *et al.*, 1984) or in enclosed work spaces (Saunders, 1967), and during the cleaning of tank cars containing vinylidene chloride copolymers where dichloroacetylene was present (Henschler *et al.*, 1970). The signs and symptoms observed in each of these reports included headache, dizziness, nausea, vomiting, irritation of the mucous membranes of the mouth and throat as well as eye irritation, facial and oral herpes and neurological disorders. The latter were manifested in paresis and neuralgia in several cranial and cervical nerves. In some cases, the signs and symptoms of cranial-nerve involvement persisted for periods ranging from several days to years. These effects were closely related to findings in dichloroacetylene-exposed animals (Reichert *et al.*, 1976).

Extreme nausea was reported by persons exposed to concentrations as low as 2-4 mg/m^3 (0.5-1 ppm) dichloroacetylene (Marhold, 1983).

Effects on reproduction and prenatal toxicity

No data were available to the Working Group.

Absorption, distribution, excretion and metabolism

No data were available to the Working Group.

Mutagenicity and chromosomal effects

No data were available to the Working Group.

3.3 Case reports and epidemiological studies of carcinogenicity to humans

No data were available to the Working Group.

4. Summary of Data Reported and Evaluation

4.1 Exposure data

Dichloroacetylene is not available commercially. It can be formed from the decomposition of trichloroethylene.

4.2 Experimental data

Dichloroacetylene was tested for carcinogenicity in mice and rats by inhalation. Treatment-related increases were observed in the incidence of adenocarcinomas of the kidney in male mice. In rats, the occurrence of benign tumours of the liver and kidney and an increased incidence of lymphomas were reported.

No data were available to evaluate the reproductive effects or prenatal toxicity of dichloroacetylene to experimental animals.

Dichloroacetylene and one of its decomposition products, trichloroacryloyl chloride, were mutagenic to *Salmonella typhimurium* in the presence or absence of an exogenous metabolic system. Under the same conditions a mixture of dichloroacetylene and acetylene was not mutagenic.

Overall assessment of data from short-term tests: Dichloroacetylene[a]

	Genetic activity			Cell transformation
	DNA damage	Mutation	Chromosomal effects	
Prokaryotes		+		
Fungi/Green plants				
Insects				
Mammalian cells (*in vitro*)				
Mammals (*in vivo*)				
Humans (*in vivo*)				
Degree of evidence in short-term tests for genetic activity: **Inadequate**				Cell transformation: no data

[a]The groups into which the table is divided and the symbol + are defined on pp. 19-20 of the Preamble; the degrees of evidence are defined on pp. 20-21.

4.3 Human data

Dichloroacetylene is a neurotoxin, with a special affinity for the cranial nerves. No data were available to evaluate the reproductive effects or prenatal toxicity of dichloroacetylene to humans.

No case report or epidemiological study was available to evaluate the carcinogenicity of dichloroacetylene to humans.

4.4 Evaluation[1]

There is *limited evidence* for the carcinogenicity of dichloroacetylene to experimental animals.

No data on humans were available.

In the absence of epidemiological data, no evaluation of the carcinogenicity of dichloroacetylene to humans could be made.

5. References

American Conference of Governmental Industrial Hygienists (1984) *Threshold Limit Values for Chemical Substances and Physical Agents in the Work Environment and Biological Exposure Indices with Intended Changes for 1984-85*, Cincinnati, OH, p. 16

Buckingham, J., ed. (1982) *Dictionary of Organic Compounds*, 5th ed., Vol. 2, New York, Chapman and Hall, pp. 1698-1699 [D-02297]

Defalque, R.J. (1961) Pharmacology and toxicology of trichloroethylene: A critical review of the world literature. *Clin. Pharmacol. Ther.*, *2*, 665-688

Deutsche Forschungsgemeinschaft (1984) *Maximal Concentrations in the Workplace and Biological Occupational Limit Value* (Ger.), Part XX, Weinheim, Verlag Chemie GmbH, pp. 27, 58

Greim, H., Wolff, T., Höfler, M. & Lahaniatis, E. (1984) Formation of dichloroacetylene from trichloroethylene in the presence of alkaline material — Possible cause of intoxication after abundant use of chloroethylene-containing solvents. *Arch. Toxicol.*, 256, 74-77

Health and Safety Executive (1985) *Occupational Exposure Limits 1985* (*Guidance Note EH 40/85*), London, Her Majesty's Stationery Office, p. 11

---

[1]For definition of the italicized term, see Preamble, p. 18.

Henschler, D., Broser, F. & Hopf, H.C. (1970) 'Polyneuritis cranialis' following poisoning with chlorinated acetylenes while handling vinylidene chloride copolymers (Ger.). *Arch. Toxicol.*, *26*, 62-75

Humphrey, J.A. & McClelland, M. (1944) Cranial-nerve palsies with herpes following general anaesthesia. A report from the central Middlesex County hospital. *Br. med. J.*, *i*, 315-318

IARC (1979a) *IARC Monographs on the Evaluation of the Carcinogenic Risk of Chemicals to Humans*, Vol. 20, *Some Halogenated Hydrocarbons*, Lyon, pp. 401-427

IARC (1979b) *IARC Monographs on the Evaluation of the Carcinogenic Risk of Chemicals to Humans*, Vol. 20, *Some Halogenated Hydrocarbons*, Lyon, pp. 371-379

IARC (1979c) *IARC Monographs on the Evaluation of the Carcinogenic Risk of Chemicals to Humans*, Vol. 20, *Some Halogenated Hydrocarbons*, Lyon, pp. 491-514

IARC (1979d) *IARC Monographs on the Evaluation of the Carcinogenic Risk of Chemicals to Humans*, Vol. 20, *Some Halogenated Hydrocarbons*, Lyon, pp. 179-193

IARC (1982a) *IARC Monographs on the Evaluation of the Carcinogenic Risk of Chemicals to Humans*, Suppl. 4, *Chemicals, Industrial Processes and Industries Associated with Cancer in Humans, IARC Monographs Volumes 1 to 29*, Lyon, pp. 87-88

IARC (1982b) *IARC Monographs on the Evaluation of the Carcinogenic Risk of Chemicals to Humans*, Suppl. 4, *Chemicals, Industrial Processes and Industries Associated with Cancer in Humans, IARC Monographs Volume 1 to 29*, Lyon, pp. 74-75

IARC (1982c) *IARC Monographs on the Evaluation of the Carcinogenic Risk of Chemicals to Humans*, Suppl. 4, *Chemicals, Industrial Processes and Industries Associated with Cancer in Humans, IARC Monographs Volume 1 to 29*, pp. 243-245

International Labour Office (1980) *Occupational Exposure Limits for Airborne Toxic Substances, A Tabular Compilation of Values from Selection Countries*, 2nd (rev.) ed. (*Occupational Safety and Health Series No. 37*), Geneva, pp. 88-89

Jackson, M.A., Lyon, J.P. & Siegel, J. (1971) Morphologic changes in kidneys of rats exposed to dichloroacetylene-ether. *Toxicol. appl. Pharmacol.*, *18*, 175-184

Marhold, J.V. (1983) *Hydrocarbons, halogenated aliphatic.* In: Parmeggiani, L., ed., *Encyclopedia of Occupational Health and Safety*, 3rd rev. ed., Vol. 1, Geneva, International Labour Office, pp. 1080-1084

McNeill, W.C., Jr (1979) *Trichloroethylene.* In: Mark, H.F., Othmer, D.F., Overberger, C.G. & Seaborg, G.T., eds, *Kirk-Othmer Encyclopedia of Chemical Technology*, 3rd ed., Vol. 5, New York, John Wiley & Sons, pp. 745-753

NIH/EPA Chemical Information System (1983) *Carbon-13 NMR Spectral Search System, Mass Spectral Search System*, and *Infrared Spectral Search System*, Arlington, VA, Information Consultants, Inc.

Reichert, D., Ewald, D. & Henschler, D. (1975) Generation and inhalation toxicity of dichloroacetylene. *Food Cosmet. Toxicol.*, *13*, 511-515

Reichert, D., Liebaldt, G. & Henschler, D. (1976) Neurotoxic effects of dichloroacetylene. *Arch. Toxicol.*, *37*, 23-38

Reichert, D., Henschler, D. & Bannasch, P. (1978) Nephrotoxic and hepatotoxic effects of dichloroacetylene. *Food Cosmet. Toxicol.*, *16*, 227-235

Reichert, D., Spengler, U. & Henschler, D. (1979) Selective detection of dichloroacetylene and its decomposition product phosgene with the electrolytic conductivity detector combined with a special gas-sampling system. *J. Chromatogr.*, *179*, 181-183

Reichert, D., Metzler, M. & Henschler, D. (1980) Decomposition of the neuro- and nephrotoxic compound dichloroacetylene in the presence of oxygen: Separation and identification of novel products. *J. environ. Pathol. Toxicol.*, *4*, 525-532

Reichert, D., Neudecker, T., Spengler, U. & Henschler, D. (1983) Mutagenicity of dichloroacetylene and its degradation products, trichloroacetyl chloride, trichloroacryloyl chloride and hexachlorobutadiene. *Mutat. Res.*, *117*, 21-29

Reichert, D., Spengler, U., Romen, W. & Henschler, D. (1984) Carcinogenicity of dichloroacetylene: An inhalation study. *Carcinogenesis*, *5*, 1411-1420

Saunders, R.A. (1967) A new hazard in closed environment atmospheres. *Arch. environ. Health*, *14*, 380-384

Sax, N.I. (1984) *Dangerous Properties of Industrial Materials*, 6th ed., New York, Van Nostrand Reinhold Co., p. 931

Siegel, J., Jones, R.A., Coon, R.A. & Lyon, J.P. (1971) Effects on experimental animals of acute, repeated and continuous inhalation exposures to dichloroacetylene mixtures. *Toxicol. appl. Pharmacol.*, *18*, 168-174

Sittig, M. (1981) *Handbook of Toxic and Hazardous Chemicals*, Park Ridge, NJ, Noyes Publications, pp. 226-227

Tardiff, R.G., Carlson, G.P. & Simmon, V. (1976) *Halogenated organics in tap water: A toxicological evaluation.* In: Jolley, R.L., ed., *The Environmental Impact of Water Chlorination*, Springfield, VA, National Technical Information Service, pp. 213-227

Työsuojeluhallitus (National Finnish Board of Occupational Safety and Health) (1981) *Airborne Contaminants in the Workplace (Safety Bull. 3)*, (Finn.), Tampere, p. 10

Weast, R.C., ed. (1984) *CRC Handbook of Chemistry and Physics*, 65th ed., Boca Raton, FL, CRC Press, Inc., p. C-79

CUMULATIVE INDEX TO IARC MONOGRAPHS
ON THE EVALUATION OF THE CARCINOGENIC RISK
OF CHEMICALS TO HUMANS

Numbers in italics indicate volume, and other numbers indicate page. References to corrigenda are given in parentheses. Compounds marked with an asterisk(*) were considered by the working groups in the year indicated, but monographs were not prepared because adequate data on carcinogenicity were not available.

A

Acetaldehyde	*36*, 101
Acetaldehyde formylmethylhydrazone	*31*, 163
Acetamide	*7*, 197
Acetylsalicylic acid (1976)*	
Acridine orange	*16*, 145
Acriflavinium chloride	*13*, 31
Acrolein	*19*, 479
	36, 133
Acrylamide	*39*, 41
Acrylic acid	*19*, 47
Acrylic fibres	*19*, 86
Acrylonitrile	*19*, 73
	Suppl. 4, 25
Acrylonitrile-butadiene-styrene copolymers	*19*, 9
Actinomycins	*10*, 29 (corr. *29*, 399; *34*, 197)
Adipic acid (1978)*	
Adriamycin	*10*, 43
	Suppl. 4, 29
AF-2	*31*, 47
Aflatoxins	*1*, 145 (corr. *7*, 319; *8*, 349)
	10, 51
	Suppl. 4, 31
Agaritine	*31*, 63
Aldrin	*5*, 25
	Suppl. 4, 35
Allyl chloride	*36*, 39
Allyl isothiocyanate	*36*, 55
Allyl isovalerate	*36*, 69
Aluminium production	*34*, 37
Amaranth	*8*, 41

IARC MONOGRAPHS ON THE EVALUATION OF THE CARCINOGENIC RISK OF CHEMICALS TO HUMANS
(English editions only)

(Available from WHO Sales Agents)

Volume 1
Some inorganic substances, chlorinated hydrocarbons, aromatic amines, N-nitroso compounds, and natural products (1972)
184 pp.; out of print

Volume 2
Some inorganic and organometallic compounds (1973)
181 pp.; out of print

Volume 3
Certain polycyclic aromatic hydrocarbons and heterocyclic compounds (1973)
271 pp.; out of print

Volume 4
Some aromatic amines, hydrazine and related substances, N-nitroso compounds and miscellaneous alkylating agents (1974)
286 pp.

Volume 5
Some organochlorine pesticides (1974)
241 pp.; out of print

Volume 6
Sex hormones (1974)
243 pp.; US$7.20; Sw.fr. 18.-

Volume 7
Some anti-thyroid and related substances, nitrofurans and industrial chemicals (1974)
326 pp.

Volume 8
Some aromatic azo compounds (1975)
357 pp.

Volume 9
Some aziridines, N-, S- and O-mustards and selenium (1975)
268 pp.

Volume 10
Some naturally occurring substances (1976)
353 pp.

Volume 11
Cadmium, nickel, some epoxides, miscellaneous industrial chemicals and general considerations on volatile anaesthetics (1976)
306 pp.

Volume 12
Some carbamates, thiocarbamates and carbazides (1976)
282 pp.

Volume 13
Some miscellaneous pharmaceutical substances (1977)
255 pp.

Volume 14
Asbestos (1977)
106 pp.

Volume 15
Some fumigants, the herbicides 2,4-D and 2,4,5-T, chlorinated dibenzodioxins and miscellaneous industrial chemicals (1977)
354 pp.

Volume 16
Some aromatic amines and related nitro compounds - hair dyes, colouring agents and miscellaneous industrial chemicals (1978)
400 pp.

Volume 17
Some N-nitroso compounds (1978)
365 pp.

Volume 18
Polychlorinated biphenyls and poly brominated biphenyls (1978)
140 pp.

Volume 19
Some monomers, plastics and synthetic elastomers, and acrolein (1979)
513 pp.

Volume 20
Some halogenated hydrocarbons (1979)
609 pp.

Volume 21
Sex hormones (II) (1979)
583 pp.

Volume 22
Some non-nutritive sweetening agents (1980)
208 pp.

IARC MONOGRAPHS SERIES

INFORMATION BULLETINS ON THE
SURVEY OF CHEMICALS BEING
TESTED FOR CARCINOGENICITY

(Available from IARC)

No. 8 (1979)
Edited by M.-J. Ghess, H. Bartsch
& L. Tomatis
604 pp.

No. 9 (1981)
Edited by M.-J. Ghess, J.D. Wilbourn,
H. Bartsch & L. Tomatis
294 pp.

No. 10 (1982)
Edited by M.-J. Ghess, J.D. Wilbourn
H. Bartsch
326 pp.

No. 11 (1984)
Edited by M.-J. Ghess, J.D. Wilbourn,
H. Vainio & H. Bartsch
336 pp.

PUBLICATIONS OF THE INTERNATIONAL AGENCY FOR RESEARCH ON CANCER

SCIENTIFIC PUBLICATIONS SERIES

(Available from Oxford University Press)

No. 19 ENVIRONMENTAL ASPECTS
OF *N*-NITROSO COMPOUNDS (1978)
Edited by E.A. Walker, M. Castegnaro,
L. Griciute & R.E. Lyle
566 pages

No. 20 NASOPHARYNGEAL
CARCINOMA: ETIOLOGY AND
CONTROL (1978)
Edited by G. de-Thé & Y. Ito,
610 pages

No. 21 CANCER REGISTRATION
AND ITS TECHNIQUES (1978)
Edited by R. MacLennan, C.S. Muir,
R. Steinitz & A. Winkler
235 pages

No. 22 ENVIRONMENTAL CARCINO-
GENS - SELECTED METHODS OF
ANALYSIS
Editor-in-Chief H. Egan
Vol. 2 - METHODS FOR THE MEASURE-
MENT OF VINYL CHLORIDE IN
POLY(VINYL CHLORIDE), AIR, WATER
AND FOODSTUFFS (1978)
Edited by D.C.M. Squirrell & W. Thain,
142 pages

No. 23 PATHOLOGY OF TUMOURS IN
LABORATORY ANIMALS. VOLUME II.
TUMOURS OF THE MOUSE (1979)
Editor-in-Chief V.S. Turusov
669 pages

No. 24 ONCOGENESIS AND HERPES-
VIRUSES III (1978)
Edited by G. de-Thé, W. Henle & F. Rapp
Part 1, 580 pages
Part 2, 522 pages

No. 25 CARCINOGENIC RISKS -
STRATEGIES FOR INTERVENTION
(1979)
Edited by W. Davis & C. Rosenfeld,
283 pages

No. 26 DIRECTORY OF ON-GOING
RESEARCH IN CANCER EPI-
DEMIOLOGY 1978 (1978)
Edited by C.S. Muir & G. Wagner,
550 pages; out of print

No. 27 MOLECULAR AND CELLULAR
ASPECTS OF CARCINOGEN
SCREENING TESTS (1980)
Edited by R. Montesano, H. Bartsch &
L. Tomatis
371 pages

No. 28 DIRECTORY OF ON-GOING
RESEARCH IN CANCER EPI-
DEMIOLOGY 1979 (1979)
Edited by C.S. Muir & G. Wagner,
672 pages; out of print

No. 29 ENVIRONMENTAL CARCINO-
GENS - SELECTED METHODS OF
ANALYSIS
Editor-in-Chief H. Egan
Vol. 3 - ANALYSIS OF POLYCYCLIC
AROMATIC HYDROCARBONS IN
ENVIRONMENTAL SAMPLES (1979)
Edited by M. Castegnaro, P. Bogovski,
H. Kunte & E.A. Walker
240 pages

No. 30 BIOLOGICAL EFFECTS OF
MINERAL FIBRES (1980)
Editor-in-Chief J.C. Wagner
Volume 1, 494 pages
Volume 2, 513 pages

No. 31 *N*-NITROSO COMPOUNDS:
ANALYSIS, FORMATION AND
OCCURRENCE (1980)
Edited by E.A. Walker, M. Castegnaro,
L. Griciute & M. Börzsönyi
841 pages

No. 32 STATISTICAL METHODS IN
CANCER RESEARCH
Vol. 1. THE ANALYSIS OF CASE-
CONTROL STUDIES (1980)
By N.E. Breslow & N.E. Day
338 pages

No. 33 HANDLING CHEMICAL
CARCINOGENS IN THE LABORATORY
- PROBLEMS OF SAFETY (1979)
Edited by R. Montesano, H. Bartsch,
E. Boyland, G. Della Porta, L. Fishbein,
R.A. Griesemer, A.B. Swan & L. Tomatis,
32 pages

No. 34 PATHOLOGY OF TUMOURS
IN LABORATORY ANIMALS. VOLUME
III. TUMOURS OF THE HAMSTER
(1982)
Editor-in-Chief V.S. Turusov,
461 pages

No. 35 DIRECTORY OF ON-GOING
RESEARCH IN CANCER EPI-
DEMIOLOGY 1980 (1980)
Edited by C.S. Muir & G. Wagner,
660 pages; out of print

SCIENTIFIC PUBLICATIONS SERIES

SCIENTIFIC PUBLICATIONS SERIES

No. 68 ENVIRONMENTAL
CARCINOGENS — SELECTED
METHODS OF ANALYSIS.
VOL. 7: SOME VOLATILE HALOGENATED
ALKANES AND
ALKENES (1985)
Edited by L. Fishbein & I.K. O'Neill
479 pages

No. 69 DIRECTORY OF ON-GOING
RESEARCH IN CANCER
EPIDEMIOLOGY 1985 (1985)
Edited by C.S. Muir & G. Wagner
756 pages

No. 70 THE ROLE OF CYCLIC NUCLEIC
ACID ADDUCTS IN CARCINOGENESIS AND
MUTAGENESIS (1986)
Edited by B. Singer & H. Bartsch
467 pages

No. 71 ENVIRONMENTAL CARCINOGENS.
SELECTED METHODS OF ANALYSIS
VOL. 8:. SOME METALS: As, Be, Cd,
Cr, Ni, Pb, Se, Zn (1986)
Edited by I.K. O'Neill, P. Schuller
& L. Fishbein (in press)

No. 72 ATLAS OF CANCER IN
SCOTLAND 1975-1980: INCIDENCE AND
EPIDEMIOLOGICAL PERSPECTIVE (1985)
Edited by I. Kemp, P. Boyle, M. Smans
& C. Muir
282 pages

No. 73 LABORATORY DECONTAMI-
NATION AND DESTRUCTION OF
CARCINOGENS IN LABORATORY
WASTES: SOME ANTINEOPLASTIC
AGENTS (1985)
Edited by M. Castegnaro, J. Adams,
M. Armour, J. Barek, J. Benvenuto,
C. Confalonieri, U. Goff, S. Ludeman,
D. Reed, E.B. Sansone & G. Telling
163 pages

No. 74 TOBACCO: A MAJOR INTER-
NATIONAL HEALTH HAZARD (1986)
Edited by D. Zaridze and R. Peto
(in press)

No. 75 CANCER OCCURRENCE IN
DEVELOPING COUNTRIES (1986)
Edited by D.M. Parkin
(in press)

No. 76 SCREENING FOR CANCER OF THE
UTERINE CERVIX (1986)
Edited by M. Hakama, A.B. Miller &
N.E. Day
311 pages

No. 77 HEXACHLOROBENZENE.
PROCEEDINGS OF AN INTERNATIONAL
SYMPOSIUM (1986)
Edited by C.R. Morris & J.R.P. Cabral
(in press)

No. 78 CARCINOGENICITY OF CYTOSTATIC
DRUGS (1986)
Edited by D. Schmähl & J. Kaldor
(in press)

No. 79 STATISTICAL METHODS IN CANCER
RESEARCH, VOL. 3, THE DESIGN AND
ANALYSIS OF LONG-TERM ANIMAL
EXPERIMENTS (1986)
By J.J. Gart, D. Krewski, P.N. Lee,
R.E. Tarone & J. Wahrendorf
(in press)

No. 80 DIRECTORY OF ON-GOING
RESEARCH IN CANCER EPIDEMIOLOGY
1986 (1986)
Edited by G. Wagner & C. Muir
(in press)

No. 81 ENVIRONMENTAL CARCINOGENS.
SELECTED METHODS OF ANALYSIS, VOL. 9,
PASSIVE SMOKING (1986)
Edited by I.K. O'Neill, K.D. Brunnemann,
B. Dodet & D. Hoffmann
(in press)

NON SERIAL PUBLICATIONS

(Available from IARC)

ALCOOL ET CANCER (1978)
By A.J. Tuyns (in French only)
42 pages

CANCER MORBIDITY AND CAUSES OF
DEATH AMONG DANISH BREWERY
WORKERS (1980)
By O.M. Jensen
145 pages

Imprimé en Suisse